APOPTOSIS IN CARDIAC BIOLOGY

BASIC SCIENCE FOR THE CARDIOLOGIST

1. B. Levy, A. Tedgui (eds.): *Biology of the Arterial Wall.* 1999
   ISBN 0-7923-8458-X
2. M.R. Sanders, J.B. Kostis (eds): *Molecular Cardiology in Clinical Practice.* 1999.
   ISBN 0-7923-8602-7
3. B. Swynghedauw (ed.): *Molecular Cardiology for the Cardiologist.* Second Edition. 1998.
   ISBN: 0-7923-8323-0
4. B. Ostadal, F. Kolar (eds.): *Cardiac Ischemia: From Injury to Protection.* 1999.
   ISBN: 0-7923-8642-6
5. H. Schunkert, G.A.J. Riegger (eds.): *Apoptosis in Cardiac Biology*
   ISBN: 0-7923-8648-5

KLUWER ACADEMIC PUBLISHERS - DORDRECHT/BOSTON/LONDON

APOPTOSIS IN CARDIAC BIOLOGY

Edited by:

Heribert Schunkert
G.A.J. Riegger
Klinik und Poliklinik fur Innere
Germany

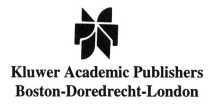

Kluwer Academic Publishers
Boston-Doredrecht-London

Distributors for North, Central and South America:
Kluwer Academic Publishers
101 Philip Drive
Assinippi Park
Norwell, Massachusetts 02061 USA
Telephone (781) 871-6600
Fax (781) 681-9045
E-Mail <kluwer@wkap.com>

Distributors for all other countries:
Kluwer Academic Publishers Group
Distribution Centre
Post Office Box 322
3300 AH Dordrecht, THE NETHERLANDS
Telephone 31 78 6392 392
Fax 31 78 6546 474
E-Mail <services@wkap.nl>

 Electronic Services <http://www.wkap.nl>

Library of Congress Cataloging-in-Publication Data

A C.I.P. Catalogue record for this book is available
from the Library of Congress.

Printed on acid-free paper.

Printed in the United States of America

Contents

List of Contributors

Privatdozent Dr. med. Hermann Aebert
Klinik und Poliklinik für Herz-, Thorax-
und herznahe Gefäßchirurgie
University of Regensburg
Franz-Josef-Strauß-Allee 11
D-93053 Regensburg
Germany

Laura Agnoletti, M.D.
Cardiovascular Research Center
„Salvatore Maugeri" Foundation
Via Pinidolo, 23
I-25064 Gussago (Brescia)
Italy

Dr. med. Harald Bär
Department of Internal Medicine
University of Heidelberg
Bergheimer Straße 58
D-69115 Heidelberg
Germany

**Prof. Dr. med. Gerhard Bauriedel,
FACC, FESC**
Associate Professor, Department of Internal
Medicine II/Cardiology
University of Bonn
Sigmund-Freud-Straße 25
D-53105 Bonn
Germany

Alan Chesley, Ph.D.
Laboratory of Cardiovascular Sciences
Gerontology Research Center
National Institute on Aging, National Institutes
of Health
5600 Nathan Shock Drive
Baltimore, MD 21224
USA

Laura Comini, M.D.
Cardiovascular Research Center
„Salvatore Maugeri" Foundation
Via Pinidolo, 23
I-25064 Gussago (Brescia)
Italy

Michael T. Crow, Ph.D.
Laboratory of Cardiovascular Sciences
Gerontology Research Center
National Institute on Aging, National Institutes
of Health
5600 Nathan Shock Drive
Baltimore, MD 21224
USA

Salvatore Curello, M.D.
Chair of Cardiology
Spedali Civili
P.le Spedali Civili
I-25123 Brescia
Italy

Dr. rer. nat. Dorothea Darmer
Martin-Luther Universität Halle-Wittenberg
Institut für Pathophysiologie
Magdeburger Straße 18
D-06097 Halle
Germany

Denis deBlois, Ph.D.
CHUM Research Center
3840 St-Urbain
Montreal, Quebec
H2W IT8
Canada

Mahboubeh Eghbali-Webb, Ph.D.
Department of Anesthesiology
Yale School of Medicine
333 Cedar Street
New Haven, CT 065/0
USA

Dr. rer. nat. Dirk Eick
Institut für Klinische Molekularbiologie
und Tumorgenetik
GSF-Forschungszentrum für Umwelt und
Gesundheit
Marchioninistraße 25
D-81377 München
Germany

Roberto Ferrari, M.D.
Chair of Cardiology
University of Ferrara
„Salvatore Maugeri" Foundation
Via Pinidolo, 23
I-25064 Gussago (Brescia)
Italy

Giora Z. Feuerstein, M.D.
Senior Director, Cardiovascular Sciences
DuPont Pharmaceuticals Corporation
E400/3255
Route 141 & Henry Clay Road
Wilmington, DE 19880-0400
USA

Guiseppina Gaia, M.D.
Cardiovascular Research Center
„Salvatore Maugeri" Foundation
Via Pinidolo, 23
I-25064 Gussago (Brescia)
Italy

Dr. med. Daniela Grimm
Institute of Clinical Pharmacology and
Toxicology
Benjamin Franklin Medical Center
FU-Berlin
Garystraße 5
D-14195 Berlin
Germany

Privatdozent Dr. med. Christian Grohé
Rheinische Friedrich-Wilhelms-Universität
Medizinische Univ.-Poliklinik
Wilhelmstraße 35–37
D-53111 Bonn
Germany

Dr. med. Markus Haass
Department of Cardiology
University of Heidelberg
Bergheimer Straße 58
D-69115 Heidelberg
Germany

Pavel Hamet, M.D., Ph.D.
Professor of Internal Medicine
CHUM Research Center
3840 St-Urbain
Montreal, Quebec
H2W IT8
Canada

David J. Harrison, M.D.
Professor of Pathology
Department of Pathology
The University of Edinburgh
Medical School
Teviot Place
Edinburgh EH8 9AG.
United Kingdom

Dr. med. Rüdiger von Harsdorf
Franz-Volhard-Klinik
Humboldt-Universität
Universitätsklinikum Charité
Wiltbergstraße 50
D-13125 Berllin
Germany

Dr. med. Armin Haunstetter
Department of Cardiology
University of Heidelberg
Bergheimer Straße 58
D-69115 Heidelberg
Germany

LIST OF CONTRIBUTORS

Prof. Dr. med. Jürgen Holtz
Professor of Physiology
Martin-Luther Universität Halle-Wittenberg
Institut für Pathophysiologie
Magdeburger Straße 18
D-06097 Halle
Germany

Dr. med. Randolph Hutter
Department of Internal Medicine II/Cardiology
University of Bonn
Sigmund-Freud-Straße 25
D-53105 Bonn
Germany

Seigo Izumo, M.D.
Cardiovascular Division
Beth Israel Deaconess Medical Center
Harvard Medical School
330 Brookline Ave.
Boston, MA 02215
USA

Privatdozent Dr. med. Lothar Jahn
Department of Internal Medicine
University of Heidelberg
Bergheimer Straße 58
D-69115 Heidelberg
Germany

Lee Baines Jordan, B.Sc.(Hons), M.B., Ch.B.
Department of Pathology
The University of Edinburgh
Medical School
Teviot Place
Edinburgh EH8 9AG.
United Kingdom

Dr. rer. nat. Franz Kohlhuber
Institut für Klinische Molekularbiologie
und Tumorgenetik
GSF-Forschungszentrum für Umwelt und
Gesundheit
Marchioninistraße 25
D-81377 München
Germany

Edward G. Lakatta, M.D., Ph.D.
Laboratory of Cardiovascular Sciences
Gerontology Research Center
National Institute on Aging, National Institutes
of Health
5600 Nathan Shock Drive
Baltimore, MD 21224
USA

Xilin Long, M.D.
Laboratory of Cardiovascular Sciences
Gerontology Research Center
National Institute on Aging, National Institutes
of Health
5600 Nathan Shock Drive
Baltimore, MD 21224
USA

Prof. Dr. med. Berndt Lüderitz, FACC, FESC
Professor of Internal Medicine
Department of Internal Medicine II/Cardiology
University of Bonn
Sigmund-Freud-Sraße 25
D-53105 Bonn
Germany

Ziad Mallat, M.D.
U141-INSERM-Hospital Lariboisière
41 Bd de la Chapelle
F-75475 Paris Cedex
France

Privatdozent Dr. rer. nat. Rainer Meyer
Rheinische Friedrich-Wilhelms-Universität
Physiologisches Institut
Wilhelmstraße 31
D-53111 Bonn
Germany

Sergei Orlov, Ph.D.
CHUM Research Center
3840 St-Urbain
Montreal, Quebec
H2W IT8
Canada

Prof. Dr. med. Martin Paul
Professor of Pharmacology and Toxicology
Institute of Clinical Pharmacology and
Toxicology
Benjamin Franklin Medical Center
FU-Berlin
Garystraße 5
D-14195 Berlin
Germany

Dr. med. Gilbert Schönfelder
Institute of Clinical Pharmacology and
Toxicology
Benjamin Franklin Medical Center
FU-Berlin
Garystraße 5
D-14195 Berlin
Germany

Prof. Dr. med. Günter A.J. Riegger
Professor of Internal Medicine
University of Regensburg
Franz-Josef-Strauß-Allee 11
D-93053 Regensburg
Germany

Prof. Dr. med. Heribert Schunkert
Professor of Clinical and Molecular Cardiology
University of Regensburg
Franz-Josef-Strauß-Allee 11
D-93053 Regensburg
Germany

Dr. rer. nat. Thomas Rudel
Max-Planck-Institute for Infection Biology
Department of Molecular Biology
Monbijoustraße 2
D-10117 Berlin
Germany

Dr. rer. nat. Herbert Schwarz
Department of Pathology
University of Regensburg
Franz-Josef-Strauß-Allee 11
D-93053 Regensburg
Germany

Dr. med. Klaus Schlottmann
Department of Internal Medicine
University of Regensburg
Franz-Josef-Strauß-Allee 11
D-93053 Regensburg
Germany

Dr. med. Andreas V. Sigel
Department of Internal Medicine
University of Regensburg
Franz-Josef-Strauß-Allee 11
D-93053 Regensburg
Germany

Dr. med. Joachim P. Schmitt
Klinik und Poliklinik für Herz-, Thorax-
und herznahe Gefäßchirurgie
University of Regensburg
Franz-Josef-Strauß-Allee 11
D-93053 Regensburg
Germany

Ioakim Spyridopoulos, M.D.
Department of Cardiology and Cardiovascular
Research
Medizinische Klinik Tübingen
Otfried-Müller-Straße 10
D-72076 Tübingen
Germany

Prof. Dr. med. Jürgen Schölmerich
Professor of Internal Medicine
University of Regensburg
Franz-Josef-Strauß-Allee 11
D-93053 Regensburg
Germany

Bernard Swynghedauw, M.D.
Professor of Physiology
U127-INSERM-Hospital Lariboisière
41 Bd de la Chapelle
F-75475 Paris Cedex
France

Prof. Dr. med. Hans Vetter
Rheinische Friedrich-Wilhelms-Universität
Medizinische Univ.-Poliklinik
Wilhelmstraße 35–37
D-53111 Bonn
Germany

Dr. med. Ulrich Welsch
Department of Anatomy III
University of Munich
Pettenkoferstraße 11
D-80336 München
Germany

Dr. med. Kai C. Wollert
Department of Cardiology and Angiology
Medizinische Hochschule Hannover
Carl-Neuberg-Straße 1
D-30625 Hannover
Germany

Introduction

Cardiac myocytes are, for the most part, terminally differentiated and non-renewing cells. Thus, the functional and structural integrity of cardiac myocytes needs to be maintained during the entire lifespan. In this context, it appears almost contra-intuitively that cardiac myocytes accommodate a complex machinery for self destruction. Obviously, this machinery has to be kept under tight control such that coordinated self elimination does not occur accidentally. Rather, apoptosis must be reserved for rather desperate conditions in which necrosis with inflammatory responses may be the only alternative fate for a malfunctioning cell.

The question arises if excessive or unintentional activation of apoptosis is involved in the precipitation or progression of cardiovascular diseases, i.e. the leading causes for morbidity and mortality in industrialized countries. Moreover, what are the factors that push cardiac cells involuntarily into death and what are the precise mechanisms that are activated along this path. Comprehensive answers to these questions are certainly a major challenge for nowadays cardiovascular research.

Deepening our knowledge on apoptosis in cardiac biology emerges to be a timely goal in this context, both for clinical practice as well as basic research in cardiology. In particular, the appropriate integration of the functional consequences related to apoptosis appear to be essential for a complete understanding of the pathophysiology of cardiac diseases. Likewise, the potential benefits achieved by the abrogation of apoptosis need to be defined by future research. Subsequently, new treatment modalities focused on apoptotic cell death will require careful evaluation in experimental models and ultimately in patients with heart failure or myocardial infarction.

Fortunately, the forefront of apoptosis research is in a phase of rapid expansion and creative molecular biological techniques are being increasingly introduced for the exploration of cardiac cell death. This book reflects these advances and starts with a series of chapters on basic mechanisms of apoptosis. The complex system required to keep apoptosis in custody, for the most part, as well as the components of the death machinery itself will be distinctly presented. Next, the cellular targets of apoptosis in the heart and the cardiovascular system will be lined up and discussed with respect to their susceptibility to programmed cell death. The current conception of the role of apoptosis in the course of myocardial infarction, heart failure, and hypertension is next being presented. Finally, pharmacological interventions that are directed to the genuine mechanisms as well as the initiating factors of programmed cell death are being described.

Thus, *Apoptosis in Cardiac Biology,* written by a team of internationally renowned researchers, gives a timely synopsis of programmed cell death in the heart. We hope that the book will provide candid guidance into the emerging fields of apoptosis for the cardiologist with interest in basic mechanisms of heart disease as well as the basic scientist with interest in a comprehensive overview on the subject.

Our appreciation goes to Professor Bernard Swynghedauw who encouraged us and our fellow contributors to edit this volume. The Working Group on Heart Failure of the European Society of Cardiology as well as the Arbeitsgruppe für Molekularbiologie und Gentechnologie of the German Society of Cardiology provided further in valuable support. Finally, our special thanks go to Frau Irene Brandl, University of Regensburg, and Ms Elaine Bello, Kluwer Academic Publishers, who have to be acknowledged for their outstanding expertise and patience during the realization of this book.

Regensburg   H. Schunkert and G. Riegger

PART ONE:
Basic mechanisms of apoptosis

I.1
The initiation of apoptosis

I.1.1
Death receptors and their ligands

Jürgen Holtz, M.D., Dorothea Darmer, Ph.D.
Martin-Luther-Universität Halle-Wittenberg, Halle/Saale, Germany

INTRODUCTION

The identification and description of an intrinsic program of regulated cellular suicide or apoptosis was originally obtained from morphological analyses in developmental biology (76, 77). This program exists in all multicellular organisms, and genetic analyses in the nematode *Caenorhabditis elegans* identified three ced-genes (for *C. elegans* death) as basal, highly conserved components of this program, see (39, 57). In mammals, several structural and functional homologs of these ced-encoded proteins are involved in the apoptosis regulating complex formation at the outer mitochondrial membrane (Fig. 1), the apoptosome (56, 124), such as Apaf-1 (for "apoptosis protease activating factor") or proteins of the Bcl-2 family (see chapter I.2.2). Another important discovery from *C. elegans* genetics was the identification of interleukin-1ß-converting enzyme (ICE or caspase-1) as a functional homolog of the ced-3 gene product. This discovery triggered the

Abbreviations: **ASK-1:** apoptosis signal regulating kinase 1, **A-SMase:** acidic sphingomyelinase, **CAF:** caspase-activated factor, **CARD:** caspase recruitment domain, **CAPK:** ceramide activated protein kinase, **CASH:** caspase homology, **Casper:** caspase eight related protein, **CLARP:** caspase-like apoptosis regulatory protein, **CIF:** cytochrome c efflux-inducing factor, **cIAP:** cellular inhibitor of apoptosis protein, **Daxx:** Fas death domain associated protein xx (xx for later nomenclature refinements), **DcR:** decoy receptor, **DD:** death domain, **DED:** death effector domain, **DISC:** death-inducing signaling complex, **DR:** death receptor, **ERK:** extracellular signal-regulated kinase, **FADD:** Fas-associating protein with death domain, **FAF-1:** Fas associated factor, **FAN:** factor associated with neutral sphingomyelinase activation, **FAP-1:** Fas associated phosphatase-1, **FLAME-1:** FADD-like antiapoptotic molecule, **FLICE:** FADD-like ICE, **FLIP:** FLICE-inhibitory protein, **JNK:** Jun N-terminal kinase, **LARD:** lymphocyte associated receptor of death, **LIT:** Lymphocyte inhibitor of TRAIL, **I-FLICE:** inhibitor of FLICE, **MEKK1:** MAPK/ERK kinase kinase, **MORT1:** mediator of receptor-induced toxicity, identification of a whole cascade of caspases (for "cysteine-containing aspartic acid proteases", see chapter I.3.1). This cascade is involved in the execution phase of apoptosis (164), and one source for activating the cascade is the mitochondrial apoptosome (Fig. 1).

The other important source for apoptosis induction via caspase activation in mammalian cells, illustrated in Fig.1, could not be identified from genetic analyses in *C. elegans*. In 1989, two groups independently identified cell-killing antibodies raised against virus-transformed B-cells (166) or against FS-7-fibroblasts (183). These antibodies recognized and activated cell surface proteins, which were called Apo-1 or Fas, respectively, and their cDNA cloning (68, 116) revealed their identity. At the same time, the two receptors of TNF, the 55 kDa type 1 receptor TNF-R1 (or CD120a) and the 75 kDa type 2 receptor TNF-R2 (or CD120b) were identified and cloned (41, 61, 134, 148, 163). The TNF-R1 mediates the cytolytic activity of TNF (162). Mutational analyses of Fas and TNF-R1 identified a cytoplasmic domain of about 80 amino acids, highly conserved between the two receptors, which was necessary and sufficient for the transduction of the apoptotic signal elicited by ligand-induced receptor activation, and therefore this domain has been called "death domain" (67, 161). In their extracellular domain, Fas and TNF-R1 have several imperfect repeats of "cysteine rich repeats" (6 cysteine residues within 40 amino acids), which is the hallmark of a larger superfamily of type I transmembrane proteins, the NGF/TNF receptor family (112). These cysteine rich repeats are required for binding of the cognate ligand to the receptor (119). Table I shows those human receptors from this family, which have cytosolic death domains and which can induce apoptosis upon activation by their cognate ligands. This induction of apoptosis and caspase activation depends on the complexation of several cytosolic signaling peptides with the intracellular death domains of these "death receptors", forming DISCs or "death-inducing signal complexes" (79).

(**Abbreviations continued**) **NDPF:** NF-κB-dependent cell death protective factor, **NGF:** nerve growth factor, **NIK:** NF-κB-inducing kinase, **NSD:** neutral sphingomyelinase activating domain, **N-SMase:** neutral sphingomyelinase, **OCIF:** osteoclastogenesis-inhibitory factor, **ODF:** osteoclast differentiation factor, **OPG:** osteoprotegerin, **RAIDD:** RIP-associated ICH-1/CED-3 homologous protein with death domain, **RANK(L):** receptor activator of NF-κB (ligand), **RICK:** RIP-like interacting CLARP kinase, **RIP:** receptor interacting protein, **TACE:** TNF α converting enzyme, **TNF:** tumor necrosis factor, **TRADD:** TNF-R1-associated death domain protein, **TRAF:** TNFR-associated factor, **TRAIL:** TNF-related apoptosis-inducing ligand, **TRAMP:** TNF receptor-related apoptosis mediating protein, **TRANCE:** TNF-related activation-induced cytokine, **TRICK2:** TRAIL receptor inducer of cell killing 2, **TRID:** TRAIL receptor without an intracellular domain, **TRIP:** TRAF-interacting protein, **TRUNDD:** TRAIL receptor with a truncated death domain,

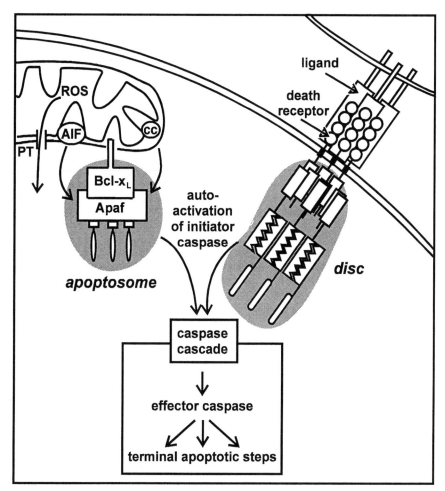

Figure 1 Apoptosis is mediated by a cascade of caspases, which can be started by autoactivation of initiator caspases. This autoactivation is induced by aggregation of death receptors, induced by trimeric, cell-bound ligands. Cytosolic domains of aggregated death receptors act as core for further association of other adapters, forming a "death-inducing signaling complex" (disc). The autoactivation of initiator caspases in a similar complex at the mitochondria, the apoptosome, is activated by release of proapoptotic signals from the mitochondrial intermembrane space, such as cytochrome c (cc) or apoptosis inducing factor (AIF) during permeability transition (PT), i.e.: the collapse of mitochondrial membrane potential and mitochondrial compartmentation of reactive oxygen species (ROS) formation.

Table I Death receptor systems

Ligands [Synonyms]	Receptors [Synonyms]	Activated signal cascades and death domain complex adapters	Competitive antagonists [Synonyms]
FasL [Apo-1L, CD95L] (153, 159)	Fas (68, 183) [Apo-1, CD95] (116, 166)	Apoptosis via - FADD → caspase-8 Daxx → JNK - RIP → RAIDD → caspase-2 NF-κB activation via - RIP → TRAF-2 → NIK - FADD/TRADD/TRAF-2→NIK (6, 127, 139, 172)	5 sFas isoforms (21, 93, 125) splice variants of the Fas gene encode secreted FasL-binding Fas-isoforms without a transmembrane domain DcR3 (128) Secreted FasL-binding protein, not encoded by the Fas gene
TNFα LTα (138)	p55 TNF-R1 [TNFR60] (41, 61, 134, 148, 168)	NF-κB-activation[a] via - TRADD → TRAF-2 → NIK - TRADD/RIP/TRAF-2 → NIK Apoptosis via - TRADD → FADD →caspase-8 - TRADD/RIP/RAIDD → casp.-2 AP-1 activation via - TRADD/TRAF-2→MEKK1/JNK N-SMase activation via FAN(4670) (6, 139, 172)	Soluble TNF-Rs cleaved from membrane-inserted TNF-Rs by metallo-proteinases (32, 110) sTNF-Rs attenuate TNF-mediated signaling (41, 47), but prolong halflife of circulating TNF by acting as a "slow-release reservoir" (3, 12, 33, 106)
	p75 TNF-R2[b] (61) [TNFR80][b]	Lowering of NDPF via unknown mechanism (61)	
Apo-3L (99) [TWEAK] (27)	DR3 (28)[c], [Apo-3(98), WSL-1(80), LARD (142), TRAMP (15)][c]	NF-κB activation and apoptosis as induced by TNF-R1 (6, 139, 172)	LARD-9 (142) Truncated splice variant without the transmembrane domain encodes secreted Apo3L-binding protein[d]

Table I (continued)

TRAIL (177) [Apo2L] (129)	DR4 (123)[e] [TRAIL-R1] (123)[e]	Apoptosis via FADD[f] and NF-κB activation (23, 136)	DcR1 (37, 96, 143)[g] [TRAIL-R3 (135), TRID (121), LIT (107)][g] no cytoplasmic domain, membrane-anchored via glyco-phosphoinositol
	DR 5 (23, 96)[h] [TRAIL-R2 (96, 135, 171), KILLER (179), TRICK2 (141)][h]	Apoptosis via FADD[f] and NF-κB activation (23, 136)	DcR2 (36)[g, i] [TRUNDD] (100, 122[g, i]) truncated cytoplasmic death domain OPG (108, 147, 180), [OCIF] (167, 182) Secreted TRAIL-binding protein
Unknown	DR6 (120)	Apoptosis via TRADD-mediated caspase activation (120) NF-κB and JNK activation(120)	Unknown

[a] In most cells, TRAF-2-mediated NF-κB activation attenuates the TNF-induced apoptosis (11, 95, 170, 173)

[b] The p75 TNF-R2/TNFR80 is not a death domain-containing receptor, but enhances p55 TNF-R1/TNFR60-mediated apoptosis, partially by silencing the apoptosis attenuating TRAF-2/NF-κB signaling of TNF-R1 (175), partially by "ligand passing" to TNF-R1 (13, 160)

[c] An extended DR3 splice isoform encodes a full-length transmembrane DR3β with a 28 amino acid extracellular extension (174)

[d] 9 other truncated LARD splice-isoforms are not yet functionally defined (142).

[e] 2 truncated DR4 splice isoforms are not yet functionally defined (121)

[f] Data concerning the role of FADD-coupling in DR4- or DR5-mediated apoptosis are controversial (48)

[g] DcR1 and DcR2 compete with DR4 and DR5 for binding of TRAIL, but cannot induce apoptosis

[h] DR5 and TRAIL-R2 may be splice variants from the same receptor gene, with TRAIL-R2 lacking the "TAPE repeat" (for threonine-, alanine-, proline- and glutamine-rich repeat)

[i] DcR2/TRUNDD antagonizes TRAIL-induced apoptosis by acting as TRAIL-binding decoy receptor and, concomitantly, as signal-transducing receptor activating NF-κB (36)

9

In addition to the TNF-related receptors with cysteine-rich repeats in table I, a receptor with a cytoplasmic death domain appears to be the low affinity p75 receptor of NGF, although its functional homology to the death domains of other death receptors is debatable (92, 103). Activation of this low affinity p75 NGF receptor by endogenous NGF contributes to death of neurons under certain conditions (24, 43), and the receptor also contributes to cell death under NGF withdrawal *in vitro* (8). However, the apoptotic signaling from this receptor is not well understood and the receptor is not included into the group of death receptors by all authors (113, 139).

Other transmembrane proteins from the TNF/NGF receptor superfamily or receptors for other interleukins do not contain cytoplasmic death domains and are not considered as death receptors, although many functional data indicate a substantial involvement in apoptotic regulation. This involvement includes phosphorylations of DISC- and apoptosome-associated proteins and apoptotic effector proteins via kinase signal cascades, alterations in gene expression of apoptosis regulating proteins and, finally, the physical connection of DISCs and interleukin receptor signal-complexes by adapter proteins (Fig. 2). An example of such a connecting adapter molecule with modular organization is the "myeloid differentiation protein" MyD88, which contains a N-terminal death domain with the capability to interact with the respective domains in DISC proteins and a C-terminal "Toll" domain mediating interactions with various interleukin-1-like receptors (20, 54, 111). Furthermore, this versatile adapter MyD88 can associate with the actin-containing microfilament network of the cytoskeleton and the nucleus during early or advanced stages of apoptosis, suggesting an involvement in apoptotic body formation and nucleocytoplasmic trafficking during apoptosis (70).

Recently, an involvement of integrins (a family of membrane proteins involved in cell adhesion) in apoptosis has been detected, which classifies these molecules as a further group of death-regulating receptors under certain conditions (131). Most integrins recognize the tripeptide-motif arginine-glycine-aspartate (RGD in the single letter code of amino acids) as binding site in extracellular matrix molecules, in coagulation factors or in other cellular membrane proteins (130). Synthetic peptides with this RGD motif act as inhibitors of integrin-ligand interactions, thereby inhibiting cell attachment and inducing apoptosis in cell models of inflammation and metastasis (18, 105). This apoptosis due to loss of intercellular contacts by RGD-blockade (or by enzymatic isolation of cells) has been called "anoikis" (greek for "homelessness") (25, 44). In this anoikis, RGD-containing peptides can enter the cells and induce activation of procaspase-3 by auto-processing, resulting in apoptosis by the active effector caspase-3 (19). Procaspase-3 contains an RGD-binding motif, aspartate-aspartate-methionine, called DDX-motif (126) and it was suggested inactive procaspase-3 is kept in an inactive configuration in resting cells by DDX-mediated binding to the cytoplasmic part of integrins, actively involved in cell attachment (131). RGD peptides entering the cell appear to outcompete this DDX-mediated binding of procaspase-3 to the integrins, allowing conformational change and autoactivation of this procaspase to an important effector caspase of the caspase cascade (19). It can be speculated that during enzymatic cleavage of integrin/integrin-ligand-mediated cellular

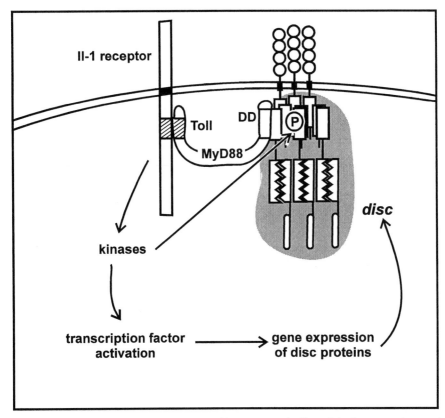

Figure 2 Disc formation and autoactivation of initiator caspases in discs of death receptors is strongly modified by activated interleukin receptors via binding by adapter proteins with modular organization, binding at death domains (DD) in discs and, simultaneously, at Toll domains of activated interleukin receptors. Furthermore, activated interleukin receptors modify disc formation by phosphorylating disc proteins and by altering gene expression of disc proteins.

attachments, soluble RGD-containing peptide fragments are formed, which enter the cells and trigger the release of DDX-bound procaspase-3 (131).

By analogy, therefore, integrines could also be considered as "death receptors", which keep procaspases complexed in an inactive form at their cytoplasmic binding domains. Presently, however, the term "death receptors" is used only for the death domain-containing transmembrane proteins of the TNF receptor family, the nomenclature of which is still full of synonyms (Table I). This text will follow this informal convention with the tacit understanding that many more membrane peptides can more or less directly contribute to caspase activation. (It should be mentioned for sake of completeness, that the term "death domain" is also discussed for the BH3 domains of Bcl-2-family proteins (75), which mediate important protein-protein interactions within the mitochondrial apoptosomes, see chapter I.2.2).

DEATH RECEPTOR LIGANDS AND ANTAGONISTS

The ligands of the death receptors (TNFα, LTα, FasL, Apo3L and TRAIL, see table 1) belong to the larger family of TNF-ligands (50) and are type II transmembrane proteins with the exception of LTα, which is a secreted protein with structural homologies to the transmembrane ligands of the family (138). The ligands of this family must form homotrimers to effectively activate their cognate receptors by inducing aggregation of these receptors (see below), and they are most effective activators in their transmembrane configuration. Fas and TNF occur also as shedded soluble ligands due to proteolytic cleavage near the transmembrane domain (159), mediated by the TNFα converting enzyme TACE (14, 109), but these shed forms are less effective agonists and may even act as competitive blockers for the signal transduction by their transmembrane forms (47, 158). Other competitive antagonists of this ligand family, competing for the ligand instead of the receptor, are circulating soluble receptor isoforms and socalled "decoy receptors" (table 1). Soluble receptor isoforms are synthesized by alternative splicing of the receptor mRNA, as is documented for Fas (21, 26, 93), DR3/LARD (142) and DR4 (121), and can prevent ligand-induced apoptosis (21). Decoy receptors have at first been detected as modulators of TRAIL-induced signaling: as membrane-associated receptors without a cytoplasmic signal domain (DcR1) or as transmembrane receptor with a truncated death domain (DcR2), they cannot induce apoptosis upon ligand binding, but they compete for TRAIL and thereby can protect cells with TRAIL receptors DR4 and DR5 from TRAIL-induced apoptosis (48, 100). Finally, the term "decoy receptor" is also used for certain secreted circulating proteins, which can bind ligands of the TNF family, but which are never inserted as membrane proteins (40, 128, 147). Therefore, the term "receptor" is somewhat misleading, but is derived from the structural homologies of these circulating proteins to TNFR family proteins. The DcR3 is a FasL binding molecule formed by some tumors which are resistant to FasL-induced apoptosis (128), and OPG (osteoprotegerin) is a TRAIL-binding protein under some (not all) experimental conditions (40). Furthermore, osteoprotegerin also binds (and inactivates) the osteoclast differentiation factor ODF (or TRANCE or RANK-L, 5, 88, 178). Thus, osteoprotegerin acts protective against osteoporosis and is also called OCIF (osteoclastogenesis inhibitory factor, 180). It is not known, whether TRAIL interferes with this antiosteoporotic function by binding of OPG.

Thus, the ligand-death receptor interaction is modulated at the extracellular level by soluble, receptor-blocking ligands, by soluble, ligand-binding receptor isoforms or shed receptors, by membrane-inserted decoy receptors competing for ligands, and, finally by secreted, ligand-binding decoy "receptors". This attenuation of ligand efficacy by a number of circulating proteins explains why it is so difficult to understand the activity of these ligand systems from analyzing only the ligand plasma concentrations. However, the death receptor ligand efficacy is not only modulated at the extracellular level.

CYTOPLASMIC DISCS AT RECEPTOR DEATH DOMAINS

As mentioned above, ligands of the death receptors do act as homotrimers and activate the receptors by associating the bound receptors to trimeric complexes, and the self-association of the cytoplasmic death domains of these receptors further supports this receptor aggregation, which is the decisive step in activating the ligand-induced signal cascade (6, 172). Intracellular signal transduction from these receptor aggregates is mediated by association of cytosolic death domain containing adapter molecules, and these complexes have been called "death inducing signaling complexes" or DISCs (79, 104). However, these signaling complexes do not only transduce the deadly apoptotic signal, but also a number of control mechanisms with antiapoptotic effects as well as other signal cascades involved in the control of growth and differentiation. Therefore, they are signaling complexes with "death" only as one of several signal messages. They have functional homologies in the signaling "apoptosomes" at the outer mitochondrial membrane (Fig. 1) and in similar complexes at the membranes of the endoplasmatic reticulum, which appear to contribute to apoptotic regulation, but will not be considered here.

Initiator caspase activation

Three types of protein-protein interaction domains cooperate in the DISC formation and activation of the caspase cascade (Fig. 1): the death domains (DDs), which contribute to the receptor trimerization and associate the adapter proteins FADD, TRADD and others to the activated receptor trimers; the death effector domains (DEDs), which associate the primary adapters (FADD, TRADD) to various signal cascades; and the caspase recruitment domains (CARDs), which associate several caspases to DISCs and apoptosomes (for review see, 60, 114). Although the sequence data indicate that these three domains belong to different domain families, the threedimensional structures show certain spatial homologies between these three domains (30, 91).

The cytosolic, death domain-containing proteins FADD/MORT-1 and TRADD are the primary adapter molecules involved in DISC formation at most death receptors (Table 1). There is still some debate on the exact functional role of these adapters in death signaling: analyses with gene knockout of an adapter or with transgenic introduction of a dominant negative version of the adapter can only identify the role of this adapter, if no other redundant transduction pathway exists. This appears to be the case for the role of FADD in Fas-mediated apoptosis, but in principle, this approach must severely underestimate the real role of the molecule under study. On the other hand, overexpression of complex forming molecules in a cell might generate a transduction pathway, which does not exist in a nontransfected cell. Therefore, it is not clear whether further primary adapters besides FADD and TRADD may contribute to DD signaling, for instance for the TRAIL receptors DR4 and DR5 (table 1). Furthermore, FADD appears to bind to still unknown receptors: bacterial lipopolysaccharide (LPS) causes apoptosis in mammalian endothelial cells in a FADD-dependent manner (29), which suggests that FADD directly or indirectly associates with the still unknown mammalian endothelial LPS receptor.

The main effect of the binding of the adapters FADD/TRADD to the activated death receptors is the binding to the large prodomain of initiator caspases, such as FLICE or caspase-8 (see chapter I.3.1). This association allows autoactivation of the initiator caspase by prodomain and subdomain cleavage, complexation to the active caspase and proteolytic activation of further caspases in the cascade (see I.3.1). At the DED of FADD or TRADD, the formation of intracellular filaments has been demonstrated (146), these "death effector filaments" appear to contribute to the recruitment of caspases to the DISCs of activated death receptors. Furthermore, RICK, a serine-threonine kinase with a C-terminal caspase recruitment domain can interact with the DISC of FAS via the adapter protein CLARP, and this CLARP-mediated binding of the protein kinase RICK potentiates Fas-stimulated apoptosis (64).

Besides the FADD/TRADD-mediated activation of initiator caspase-8 per complexation to the death domain of Fas or TNFR1, respectively, there are further apoptotic pathways activated by other adapter proteins associating with the DDs of activated death receptors: a further death receptor-stimulated pathway to caspase activation is mediated by the adapter protein RAIDD, which associates to the TRADD/RIP or FADD/RIP complex of receptor trimers (38). RAIDD is an adapter protein similar to FADD with a C-terminal death domain and a N-terminal caspase recruitment domain (CARD), which recruits and activates the initiator caspase-2 to the activated DISC of TNF-R1 (38). CARD/CARD interactions mediate also the association and activation of caspase-9 to Apaf-1 in the mitochondrial apoptosomes (30), see chapter I.2.2. The role of this redundant RAIDD pathway for death receptor-mediated caspase activation is not yet clear.

Similarly, the adapter protein Daxx can associate to the death domains of activated Fas trimers, resulting in the activation of the Jun N-terminal kinase (JNK) pathway and in an enhancement of Fas-mediated apoptosis. This JNK activation by Daxx is started by association of an apoptosis signal-regulating kinase 1 (22). This pathway appears to be implicated in the deletion of autoreactive lymphocytes (78). The apoptosis resulting from FADD-mediated activation of the caspase cascade is further potentiated by another protein associating with activated Fas: the FAF1 (31). FAF1-binding to Fas occurs membrane-proximally to the death domain at a site, which binds the ubiquitin-conjugating enzyme UBC9 in the yeast two-hybrid assay, and FAF1 contains sequences similar to ubiquitin (10). Therefore, it was speculated that the ubiquination pathway may modify the apoptotic Fas signaling via FAF1 binding (10).

Silencers of death domains (SODD)

Death receptor trimerization with DISC formation is not only induced by ligand binding, but is also possible without ligand interaction, for instance under irradiation, which oligomerizes death receptors also in absence of any activating ligands (139). Self-association of intracellular receptor death domains by protein-protein interaction does occur (149) and this is assumed to be the reason, why it is so difficult to generate stable cell lines with substantial overexpression of death receptors: constitutive death domain-mediated receptor aggregation and caspase activation appears to kill those transfected cells. However, several death receptors are naturally expressed at a remarkably high level in several tissues and yet maintain an inactive state, suggesting the existence of physiological cellular mechanisms against ligand-independent signaling by self-associating death receptors. During the search for such a mechanism, a cDNA was cloned encoding a 457-amino acid protein, which associates with the intracellular part of TNF-R1 and DR3 in the yeast two-hybrid assay (71). This protein interacts with the death domains of TNF-R1 (and DR3) under normal conditions in nonstimulated cells and prevents the apoptotic signal transducing molecule TRADD (see above) from interacting with the death domains of nonstimulated TNF-R1. After treatment of cells with trimeric TNF, this protein is rapidly released from TNF-R1 and TRADD association to the aggregated receptors occurs (71). Therefore, this protein was called "silencer of death domains" (SODD) under the assumption that SODD acts as a negative regulatory protein, normally associated to the death domain of nonstimulated TNF-R1 (or DR3), preventing death domain self association and maintaining the receptor in an inactive, monomeric state. Ligand-induced receptor trimerization results in a release of SODD from the receptor, enabling TRADD association and DISC formation at the death domains with subsequent caspase activation. In agreement with this model, cells with SODD overexpression were resistant against TNF-induced apoptosis and other TNF-typical cell responses, while reductions of SODD expression induced by antisense RNA rendered cells more susceptible to TNF-mediated apoptosis (71). Although SODD does not associate to the death domains of Fas, DR4 or DR5, this regulation by death domain silencing appears to be a general principle for death receptors, since cDNA clones encoding other proteins with predicted structure homologies to SODD can be found in gene databases (71). It remains to be established, whether SODD has signal functions of its own, when it is released from death domains upon receptor activation.

Apoptosis inhibiting ligands in DISCs

At the death domains of activated death receptors or at their primary adapters there is multiple interaction with cytosolic ligands, which mediate antiapoptotic signaling and which appear to act as a system of checks and balances in the decision to cellular suicide. These cellular control systems have been compared with the safeguard procedures in the capital punishment verdicts of the *Sanhedrin*, the supreme Jewish court in ancient Isreal (172). Many of these antiapoptotic ligands in the apoptic cellular signal pathway exist also as viral proteins, which help the viruses to keep infected cells alive against the attack of the immune system (169).

A mammalian homolog to some of these viral inhibitors is the FLICE inhibitory protein (FLIP), which exists in a long (FLIP$_L$) and a short isoform (FLIP$_S$), contains two DEDs and inhibits apoptosis induced by all death receptors,when it is overexpressed (66). This cellular apoptosis inhibitor has been independently detected and described by several groups under various acronyms: CASH (45), Casper (144), CLARP (65), FLAME-1 (150), I-FLICE (63) or MRIT (51). Its inhibitory effect is not quite clear and appears to interfere with the association and/or autoactivation of the initiator procaspase at the receptor DISC (63, 66).

However, in some cells, the induction of FLIP expression is sufficient to induce caspase activation and apoptosis (45, 144), which is somewhat reminiscent to the function of a membrane receptor blocker with some intrinsic agonist activity.

Another group of antiapoptotic signal adapters is activated by association with the DISCs of Fas, TNF-R1, DR3 and probably DRs -4, -5 and -6 via the adapter molecule TRAF-2 (table 1). At least three types of apoptosis-inhibiting proteins bind to the docking protein TRAF-2, when it is incorporated into the DISCs: the "zinc-finger" protein A20, which inhibits receptor-mediated apoptosis in an unknown way (69, 118); the "cellular inhibitor of apoptosis proteins" $cIAP_1$ and $cIAP_2$, (145, 168), which act as inhibitors of caspases, and the protein kinase NIK (151), which is the starter of a cascade resulting in the activation of the transcription factor NF-κB (see below).

A further protein associating with the death domains of Fas or TNF-R1 is sentrin, which inhibits death receptor-mediated apoptosis, when it is overexpressed (117). This protective protein has sequence homologies with ubiquitin and a *S. cerevisiae* gene, Smt3 (117). Ubiquitin-like sentrins (two mammalian proteins of the family are identified) occur in a monomeric form in the cytosol, and in multimeric forms in the nucleus together with sentrin-bound proteins (74). The ubiquitin-conjugating enzyme Ubc9 is probably the enzyme conjugating sentrins during protein "sentrinization" (46). The RING-finger protein PML, which has tumor suppressor activity, is normally sentrinizated, while this sentrinization of PML-fusion proteins cannot take place in acute promyelocytic leukemia, suggesting defective apoptotic regulation (73). Presently, no model is available explaining the antiapoptotic efficacy of sentrin and the context of this protective function with its association to the death receptors or its conjugation to nuclear proteins.

Finally, FAP-1 is a protein tyrosine phosphatase, which interacts with the C-terminal 15 amino acids of the cytoplasmic part of Fas, but not within the death domain of Fas (132, 181). Cytoplasmic microinjection of small peptides blocking this Fas/FAP-1 association substantially potentiated Fas-mediated apoptosis in cells, which express Fas and FAP-1 (181). This suggests that binding of this tyrosine phosphatase to activated Fas has an attenuating function on Fas-mediated apoptosis via an unknown mechanism, which may antagonize the effecs of some non-identified protein tyrosine kinase (132).

These examples of apoptosis-inhibiting signals arising from the binding of docking proteins into the DISCs of death receptors indicate the janus-faced nature of these signal complexes. The net effect in the "signal outcome" is open to multiple regulatory influences, which can be mediated by altered expression of adapter proteins for the DISCs via NF-κB activation (see below), via tumor suppressor p53 activation (see chapter I.2.2) or via signaling from interleukin receptors (Fig.2), by altered phosphorylations of DISC proteins via signal cascades from receptors for growth factors, interleukins and/or survival signals, and finally, by selective alterations of ubiquitin-dependent degradation of DISC elements. The "Sanhedrin" procedures of apoptosis control at the DISC level are far from being unraveled, and they are just a part of a broader set of control mechanisms at the apoptosomes and within the terminal effector pathway of apoptosis.

DEATH RECEPTOR-ACTIVATED NONAPOPTOTIC SIGNAL CASCADES

A strong argument for death receptor actions apart from the induction of apoptosis came from experiments with cells with eliminations of FADD, which were unresponsive to the cytocidal effects of Fas or TNF (as could be expected), but demonstrated also attenuated proliferation, implying an involvement of death domain signaling in growth control (115, 185). While the mechanism of such a putative growth control by death receptors remains to be unraveled, several possibilities can be outlined.

During activation of TNF-R1 or Fas , the second messenger ceramide is formed (81). In the case of TNF-R1-activation, the production of ceramide from membrane sphingomyelin is stimulated via two pathways: a membrane bound neutral sphingomyelinase (N-SMase) is activated via the adapter protein Fan (2), which binds to a small cytoplasmic domain of the TNF-R1 adjacent to its death domain and which is designated N-SMase activating domain (1); furthermore, a C-terminal domain (probably the death domain itself) of activated TNF-R1 appears to initiate the activation of an acidic SMase (176). The second messenger ceramide (which is also formed under stimuli of physical cell damage, such as ionizing radiation, ultraviolet light, heat and oxidative stress) appears to modify several stages of the apoptotic program in a cell type- and stimulus-specific way. This modification is mediated via the ceramide-activated protein kinase (CAPK), the ERK signal cascade and the MEKK1 or stress-activated protein kinase (SAPK) cascade (81), cascades involved also in growth reactions. However, the apoptosis-modulating role of ceramide formation cannot be considered as a general phenomenon, but appears to be rather restricted to certain tissues or cells under specific conditions.

A well known nonapoptotic or antiapoptotic signal system activated by death receptors is the activation of the transcription factor NF-κB (Table 1), which occurs by the signal kinase NIK and/or by the mitogen-activated kinases (97). NF-κB is the prototype member of an important transcription factor family, orchestrating gene expression during inflammation, cellular proliferation and apoptosis, which exists inactive in the cytoplasm of resting cells, bound to an inhibitory subunit, and is translocated to the nucleus upon activation and release from the inhibitor (7, 137). NF-κB induced gene transcription and protein synthesis during death receptor-stimulated apoptosis results in an attenuation or even complete inhibiton of the apoptotic program (11, 170, 173), which explains the better apoptotic efficacy of TNF-R1 activation under blockade of protein synthesis. Simultaneously with the death receptor-mediated activation of NF-κB, there is also an inhibition of NF-κB activation by TRIP, which complexes also with the adapter protein TRAF-2 (90). The NF-κB activation during death receptor stimulation appears an attractive candidate as mediator of nonapoptotic, trophic actions of this stimulation.

MITOCHONDRIA AND DEATH RECEPTOR-INDUCED APOPTOSIS

As indicated in Figure 2, the caspase cascade can be activated by DISCs at the death receptors and by apoptosomes at the outer mitochondrial membrane, when apoptotic factors are released from the mitochondria (see chapter I.2.2). This triggering of the apoptotic program by mitochondria is a central element in the reaction to many cytotoxic stimuli (82, 83, 157). The mitochondrial activation of the apoptotic program is induced by the release of several factors from the mitochondrial intermembrane space, and this release is inhibited by antiapoptotic proteins of the Bcl-2 family, such as Bcl-x_L and Bcl-2 (35, 154, 155, 156).

Death receptor stimulation induces the autoactivation of procaspases-8 or -2 with subsequent activation of the entire cascade (see above), which theoretically should not require the involvement of mitochondrial reactions to the apoptosis. The test, whether a certain apoptotic reaction can be blocked by overexpression of Bcl-x_L or Bcl-2, is considered as an indicator of such a mitochondrial involvement. This test yielded controversial data on the involvement of Bcl-2 sensitive steps in death receptor induced apoptosis, and the grouping of cells into type I and type II cells was proposed on the basis of this test (127, 133). In type-I cells, the DISC-mediated activation of procaspase-8 and the subsequent activation of the effector caspase-3 is sufficient for activation of the program, which cannot be blocked by Bcl-2-overexpression, as is observed in T lymphocytes (133). In type II cells, death receptors activate only a small amount of caspase-8, and additional contributions from mitochondria are necessary for activation of the program, which is sensitive to blockade by Bcl-2 overexpression, as is observed in hepatocytes or B lymphocytes (133). Consequently, death receptor-induced apoptosis in type II cells can also be modulated by signal cascades, which modulate Bcl-functions, such as Ber-Abl (4), MAP kinase (62), PI 3-kinase PKB (55) or PKC (127). Probably, in most tissues the type II regulation of apoptosis prevails, and this involvement of mitochondria in death receptor apoptosis induces the question, how the apoptotic signal is transmitted from the receptor DISCs to the mitochondria. Several interactions between death receptors and mitochondria have been identified, probably contributing to this coupling, which might be mediated by different mechanisms in different tissues.

A "caspase activated factor" or CAF has been identified recently, which induces mitochondrial release of apoptotic signals (152) and which might be identical to a "cytochrome c efflux-inducing factor" or CIF (52, 53) and has some similarities to the caspase-activated Bcl-protein Bid (49). A similar coupling function could also be performed by the death domain containing protein MRIT, which interacts with Bcl-proteins and with caspases (51). Furthermore, a TNF-induced clustering of mitochondria towards the perinuclear region, mediated not by the death domain, but by a proximal region of the cytoplasmic domain of the TNF-R1, has been implicated in apoptosis regulation (34). Furthermore, exogenous TNF not only binds to membrane death receptors, but is also internalized (17) and translocated to the mitochondria, where a TNF-binding protein has been identified (89). At the mitochondria, several TNF-mediated effects have been observed, which could be involved in apoptosis, such as radical leakage, permeability changes and cytochrome c release (58, 59, 72). Finally, activated caspases can directly affect the mitochondria by lowering membrane barrier functions and by contributing to signal release (101, 102).

MYOCARDIAL ACTIONS OF DEATH RECEPTORS

Analyses of myocardial mRNA document that death receptors are synthesized in healthy human myocardium, with a left ventricular mRNA concentration for DcR1 of 0.2 amol/µg RNA, for Fas of 0.9, for DR5 of 1.0, DR4 of 11, DR6 of ≈ 2000 and for TNF-R1 of 5000 amol/µg RNA, respectively, while DcR2 and DR3 are not expressed at measurable amounts (data from our laboratory). Together with Fas mRNA, the splice variants of several soluble Fas isoforms are also expressed in the myocytes of healthy human myocardium (H. Schuman, unpublished). Data on the protein expression of death receptors on ventricular myocytes are only available for Fas (42, 94, 184) and TNF receptors (165). TNF-induced myocyte apoptosis in isolated myocytes (84) cannot indicate the effects of TNF (or another death receptor ligand) in the intact organ, since anoikis of the isolated cells might have altered their antiapoptotic control mechanisms (see: Introduction).

In terminal heart failure with enhanced apoptosis of myocytes, the mRNA expression of these soluble Fas antagonists is downregulated (140), and cardiac unloading by cardiac assist devices (i.e.: "artificial hearts" working in parallel to the failing ventricle) induce a time-dependent reexpression of the soluble Fas antagonists and a reduction in myocyte apoptosis (9). However, there is no proof for a FasL/Fas mediated myocardial apoptosis, nor for a causal relationship between the reduced myocardial expression of Fas antagonists and enhanced apoptosis, or vice versa. In adult mouse myocytes, Fas activation (by agonistic antibodies or by perforin-deficient cytotoxic lymphocytes) does not induce apoptosis, but causes depression of contraction, action potential alterations and enhanced arrhythmogenic activity (42), again stressing the importance of nonapoptotic signal cascades in death receptor actions. Similarly, exogenous TNF in pathophysiologically relevant concentrations induces negative inotropic actions and dilatory ventricular remodelling in rats, but no clear signs of apoptosis (16), although transfection-induced overexpression of TNF in the myocardium results in a cardiac pathology like dilatative cardiomyopathy with pronounced apoptosis (85-87). This is highly suggestive for a pathological role of myocardial death receptors in myocarditis associated myocyte apoptosis, but any definitive proof for this assumption is not available.

Thus, our knowledge on the pathophysiological role of death receptors in the myocardium is similar as in other organs (except for the immune system): a plethora of data on molecules and signal cascades contrasts with a deficit of data illustrating the functional role of these receptors in the intact organism.

References

1. Adam, D., K. Wiegman, S. Adam-Klages, A. Ruff, and M. Krönke. A novel cytoplasmic domain of the p55 TNF receptor initiates the neutral sphingomyelinase pathway. *J Biol Chem* 271: 14617-14622, 1996.

2. Adam-Klages, S., D. Adam, K. Wiegmann, S. Struve, W. Kolanus, J. Schneider-Mergener, and M. Kronke. Fan, a novel WD-repeat protein, couples the p55 TNF-receptor to neutral sphingomyelinase. *Cell* 86: 937-947, 1996.

3. Aderka, D., H. Engelmann, Y. Maor, C. Brakebusch, and D. Wallach. Stabilization of the bioactivity of tumor necrosis factor by its soluble receptors. *J Exp Med* 175: 323-329, 1992.

4.   Amarante-Mendes, G. P., A. J. McGahon, W. K. Nishioka, D. E. Afar, O. N. Witte, and D. R. Green. Bcl-2-independent Bcr-Abl-mediated resistance to apoptosis: protection is correlated with upregulation of Bcl-x_L. *Oncogene* 16: 1383-1390, 1998.
5.   Anderson, D. M., E. Maraskovsky, W. L. Billingsley, W. C. Dougall, M. E. Tometsko, E. R. Roux, M. C. Teepe, R. F. DuBose, D. Cosman, and L. Galibert. A homologue of the TNF receptor and its ligand enhance T-cell growth and dendritic-cell function. *Nature* 390: 175-179, 1997.
6.   Ashkenazi, A., and V. M. Dixit. Death receptors: signaling and modulation. *Science* 281: 1305-1308, 1998.
7.   Baeuerle, P. A., and D. Baltimore. NF-κB: ten years after. *Cell* 87: 13-21, 1996.
8.   Barrett, G. L., and A. Georgiu. The low-affinity nerve growth factor receptor p75[NGFR] mediates death of PC12 cells after nerve growth factor withdrawal. *J Neurosci Res* 45: 117-128, 1996.
9.   Bartling, B., H. Milting, H. Schumann, A. El-Banayosy, M. Koerner, R. Koerfer, D. Darmer, J. Holtz, and H. R. Zerkowski. Improved myocardial expression of anti-apoptotic genes under support by ventricular assist devices (VAD) in terminal heart failure (abstr). *Circulation* 98 (supll): I-200, 1998.
10. Becker, K., P. Schneider, K. Hofmann, C. Mattmann, and J. Tschopp. Interaction of Fas (Apo-1/CD95) with proteins implicated in the ubiquitination pathway. *FEBS Lett* 412: 102-106, 1997.
11. Beg, A. A., and D. Baltimore. An essential role for NF-κB in preventing TNF-α-induced cell death. *Science* 274: 782-784, 1996.
12. Beutler, B., I. W. Milsark, and A. Cerami. Cachectin/tumor necrosis factor: production, distribution and metabolic fate in vivo. *J Immunol* 135: 3972-3977, 1985.
13. Bigda, J., I. Beletsky, C. Brakebusch, Y. Vasfolomeev, H. Engelmann, J. Bigda, H. Holtmann, and D. Wallach. Dual role of the p75 tumor necrosis factor (TNF) receptor in TNF cytotoxicity. *J Exp Med* 180: 445-460, 1994.
14. Black, R. A., C. T. Rauch, C. J. Kozlosky, J. L. Peschon, J. L. Slack, M. F. Wolfson, B. J. Castner, K. L. Stocking, P. Reddy, S. Srinivasan, N. Nelson, N. Boiani, K. A. Schooley, M. Gerhart, R. Davis, J. N. Fitzner, R. S. Johnson, R. J. Paxton, C. J. March, and D. P. Cerretti. A metalloproteinase disintegrin that releases tumor-necrosis factor-α from cells. *Nature* 385: 729-733, 1997.
15. Bodmer, J. L., K. Burns, P. Schneider, K. Hofmann, V. Steiner, M. Thome, T. Bornand, M. Hahne, M. Schroeter, K. Becker, A. Wilson, L. E. French, J. L. Browning, H. R. MacDonald, and J. Tschopp. TRAMP, a novel apoptosis-mediating receptor with sequence homology to tumor necrosis factor receptor 1 and Fas (APO-1/CD95). *Immunity* 6: 79-88, 1997.
16. Bozkurt, B., S. B. Kribbs, F. J. Clubb, L. H. Michael, V. V. Didenko, P. J. Hornsby, Y. Seta, H. Oral, F. G. Spinale, and D. L. Mann. Pathophysiologically relevant concentrations of tumor necrosis factor-α promote progressive left ventricular dysfunction and remodeling in rats. *Circulation* 97: 1382-1391, 1998.
17. Bradley, J. R., D. R. Johnson, and J. S. Pober. Four different classes of inhibitors of receptor-mediated endocytosis decrease tumor necrosis factor-induced gene expression in human endothelial cells. *J Immunol* 150: 5544-5555, 1993.
18. Brooks, P. C., and A. L. Et. Integrin αvβ3 antagonists promote tumor-regression by inducing apoptosis of angiogenic blood-vessels. *Cell* 79: 1157-1164, 1994.
19. Buckley, C. D., D. Pilling, N. V. Henriquez, G. Parsonage, K. Threlfall, D. Scheel-Toellner, D. L. Simmons, A. N. Akbar, J. M. Lord, and M. Salmon. RDG peptides induce apoptosis by direct caspase-3 activation. *Nature* 397: 534-539, 1999.
20. Burns, K., F. Martinon, C. Esslinger, H. Pahl, P. Schneider, J. L. Bodmer, F. Di Marco, L. French, and J. Tschopp. MyD88, an adapter protein involved in interleukin-1 signaling. *J Biol Chem* 273: 12203-12209, 1998.
21. Cascino, I., G. Papoff, R. De Maria, R. Testi, and G. Ruberti. Fas/Apo-1 (CD95) receptor lacking the intracytoplasmic signaling domain protects tumor cells from Fas-mediated apoptosis. *J Immunol* 156: 13-17, 1996.
22. Chang, H. Y., H. Nishitoh, X. Yang, H. Ichijo, and D. Baltimore. Activation of apoptosis signal-regulating kinase 1 (ASK1) by the adapter protein Daxx. *Science* 281: 1860-1863, 1998.
23. Chaudhary, P. M., M. Eby, A. Jasmin, A. Bookwalker, J. Murray, and L. Hood. Death receptor 5, a new member of TNFR family, and DR4 induce FADD-dependent apoptosis and activate the NF-κB pathway. *Immunity* 7: 821-830, 1997.

24. Cheema, S. S., G. L. Barrett, and P. F. Bartlett. Reducing p75 nerve growth factor receptor levels using antisense oligonucleotides prevents the loss of axotomized sensory neurons in the dorsal root ganglia of newborn rats. *J Neurosci Res* 46: 239-245, 1996.

25. Chen, C. S., M. Mrksich, S. Huang, G. M. Whitesites, and D. E. Ingber. Geometric control of cell life and death. *Science* 276: 1425-1428, 1997.

26. Cheng, J., C. Liu, W. J. Koopman, and J. D. Mountz. Characterization of human Fas gene: exon/intron organization and promoter region. *J Immunol* 154: 1239-1245, 1995.

27. Chicheportiche, Y., P. R. Bourdon, H. Xu, Y. M. Hsu, H. Scott, C. Hession, I. Garcia, and J. L. Browning. TWEAK, a new secreted ligand in the tumor necrosis factor family that weakly induces apoptosis. *J Biol Chem* 272: 32401-32410, 1997.

28. Chinnaiyan, A. M., O. R. K, G. L. Yu, R. H. Lyons, M. Garg, D. R. Duan, L. Xing, R. Gentz, J. Ni, and V. M. Dixit. Signal transduction by DR3, a death domain-containing receptor related to TNFR-1 and CD95. *Science* 274: 990-992, 1996.

29. Choi, K. B., F. Wong, J. M. Harlan, P. M. Chaudhary, L. Hood, and A. Karsan. Lipopolysaccharide mediates endothelial apoptosis by a FADD-dependent pathway. *J Biol Chem* 273: 20185-20188, 1998.

30. Chou, J. J., H. Matsuo, H. Duan, and G. Wagner. Solution structure of the RAIDD CARD and model for CARD/CARD interaction in caspase-2 and caspase-9 recruitment. *Cell* 94: 171-180, 1998.

31. Chu, K. T., X. H. Niu, and L. T. Williams. A Fas-associated protein factor, FAF1, potentiates Fas-mediated apoptosis. *Proc Natl Acad Sci* 92: 11894-11898, 1995.

32. Crowe, P. D., B. N. Walter, K. M. Mohler, C. Otten-Evans, R. A. Black, and C. F. Ware. A metalloprotease inhibitor blocks shedding of the 80-kD TNF receptor and TNF processing in T lymphocytes. *J Exp Med* 181: 1205-1208, 1995.

33. De Groote, D., G. E. Grau, I. Dehart, and P. Franchimont. Stabilization of functional tumor necrosis factor-α by its soluble TNF receptors. *Eur Cytokine Netw* 4: 359-362, 1993.

34. De Vos, K., V. Goossens, E. Boone, D. Vercammen, K. Vancompernolle, P. Vandenabeele, G. Haegeman, W. Fiers, and J. Grooten. The 55-kDa tumor necrosis factor receptor induces clustering of mitochondria through its membrane-proximal region. *J Biol Chem* 273: 9673-9680, 1998.

35. Decaudin, D., S. Geley, R. Hirsch, M. Castedo, P. Marchetti, A. Macho, R. Kofler, and G. Kroemer. Bcl-2 and Bcl-x$_L$ antagonize the mitochondrial dysfunction preceding nuclear apoptosis induced by chemotherapeutic agents. *Cancer Res* 57: 62-67, 1997.

36. Degli-Esposti, M. A., W. C. Dougall, P. J. Smolak, J. Waugh, C. A. Smith, and R. G. Goodwin. The novel receptor TRAIL-R4 induces NF-kB and protects against TRAIL-mediated apoptosis, yet retains an incomplete death domain. *Immunity* 7: 813-820, 1997.

37. Degli-Esposti, M. A., P. J. Smolak, H. Walczak, J. Waugh, C. P. Huang, R. F. DuBose, R. G. Goodwin, and C. A. Smith. Cloning and characterization of TRAIL-R3, a novel member of the emerging TRAIL receptor family. *J Exp Med* 186: 1165-1170, 1997.

38. Duan, H., and V. M. Dixit. Raidd is a new 'death' adapter molecule. *Nature* 385: 86-89, 1997.

39. Ellis, R. E., J. Yuan, and H. R. Horvitz. Mechanisms and functions of cell death. *Annu Rev Cell Biol* 7: 663-698, 1991.

40. Emery, J. G., P. McDonnell, M. B. Burke, K. C. Deen, S. Lyn, C. Silverman, E. Dul, E. R. Appelbaum, C. Eichman, R. DiPrinzio, R. A. Dodds, I. E. James, M. Rosenberg, J. C. Lee, and P. R. Young. Osteoprotegerin is a receptor for the cytotoxic ligand TRAIL. *J Biol Chem* 273: 14363-14367, 1998.

41. Engelmann, H., D. Novick, and D. Wallach. Two tumor necrosis factor-binding proteins purified from human urine: evidence for immunological cross-reactivity with cell surface tumor necrosis factor receptors. *J Biol Chem* 1990: 1531-1536, 1990.

42. Felzen, B., M. Shilkrut, H. Less, I. Sarapov, G. Maor, R. Coleman, R. B. Robinson, G. Berke, and O. Binah. Fas (CD95/Apo-1)-mediated damage to ventricular myocytes induced by cytotoxic T lymphocytes from perforin-deficient mice: a major role for Inositol 1, 4, 5-Triphosphate. *Circ Res* 82: 438-450, 1998.

43. Frade, J. M., A. Rodrígez-Tebar, and Y. A. Barde. Induction of cell death by endogenous nerve growth factor through its p75 receptor. *Nature* 383: 166-168, 1996.

44. Frisch, S. M., and E. Ruoslahti. Integrins and anoikis. *Curr Opin Cell Biol* 9: 701-706, 1997.

45. Goltsev, Y. V., A. V. Kovalenko, E. Arnold, E. E. Varfolomeev, V. M. Brodianskii, and D. Wallach. CASH, a novel caspase homologue with death effector domains. *J Biol Chem* 272: 19641-19644, 1997.

46. Gong, L., T. Kamitani, K. Fujise, L. S. Caskey, and E. T. Yeh. Preferential interaction of sentrin with a ubiquitin-conjugating enzyme, Ubc9. *J Biol Chem* 272: 28198-28201, 1997.

47. Grell, M., E. Douni, H. Wajant, M. Löhden, M. Clauss, B. Baxeiner, S. Georgopoulos, W. Lesslauer, G. Kollias, K. Pfizenmaier, and P. Scheurich. The transmembrane form of tumor necrosis factor is the prime activating ligand of the 80 kDa tumor necrosis factor receptor. *Cell* 83: 793-802, 1995.

48. Griffith, T. S., and D. H. Lynch. TRAIL: a molecule with multiple receptors and control mechanisms. *Curr Opin Immunol* 10: 559-563, 1998.

49. Gross, A., X. M. Yin, K. Wang, M. C. Wei, J. Jockel, C. Milliman, H. Erdjument-Bromage, P. Tempst, and S. J. Korsmeyer. Caspase cleaved BID targets mitochondria and is required for cytochrome c release, while BCL-XL prevents this release but not tumor necrosis factor-R1/Fas death. *J Biol Chem* 274: 1156-1163, 1999.

50. Gruss, H. J. Molecular, structural, and biological characteristics of the tumor necrosis factor ligand superfamily. *Int J Clin Lab Res* 26: 143-159, 1996.

51. Han, D. K. M., P. M. Chaudhary, M. E. Wright, C. Friedman, B. J. Trask, R. T. Riedel, D. G. Baskin, S. M. Schwartz, and L. Hood. MRIT, a novel death-effector domain-containing protein, interacts with caspases and Bcl-x$_L$ and initiates cell death. *Proc Natl Acad Sci* 94: 11333-11338, 1997.

52. Han, Z., K. Bhalla, P. Pantazis, E. A. Hendrickson, and J. H. Wyche. Cif (Cytochrome c efflux-inducing factor) activity is regulated by Bcl-2 and caspase and correlates with the activation of Bid. *Mol Cell Biol* 19: 1381-1389, 1999.

53. Han, Z., G. Li, T. A. Bremner, T. S. Lange, G. Zhang, R. Jemmerson, J. H. Wyche, and E. A. Hendrickson. A cytosolic factor is required for mitochondrial cytochrome c efflux during apoptosis. *Cell Death Diff* 5: 469-479, 1998.

54. Hardimann, G., F. L. Rock, S. Balasubramanian, R. A. Kastelein, and J. F. Bazan. Molecular characterization and modular analysis of human MyD88. *Oncogene* 13: 2467-2475, 1996.

55. Häusler, P., G. Papoff, A. Eramo, K. Reif, C. D. A., and G. Ruberti. Protection of CD95-mediated apoptosis by activation of phosphatidylinositide 3-kinase and protein kinase B. *Eur J Immunol* 28: 57-69, 1998.

56. Hengartner, M. O. CED-4 is a stranger no more. *Nature* 388: 714-715, 1997.

57. Hengartner, M. O., and H. R. Horvitz. Programmed cell death in Caenorhabditis elegans. *Curr Opin Genet Dev* 4: 581-?, 1994.

58. Hennet, T., C. Richter, and E. Peterhans. Tumour necrosis factor-α induces superoxide anion generation in mitochondria of L929 cells. *Biochem J* 289: 587-592, 1993.

59. Higuchi, M., R. J. Proske, and E. T. H. Yeh. Inhibition of mitochondrial respiration chain complex I by TNF results in cytochrome c release, membrane permeability transition, and apoptosis. *Oncogene* 17: 2515-2524, 1998.

60. Hofmann, K., P. Bucher, and J. Tschopp. The CARD domain: a new apoptotic signalling motif. *Trends Biochem Sci* 22: 155-156, 1997.

61. Hohmann, H. P., R. Remy, M. Brockhaus, and A. P. Van Loon. Two different cell types have different major receptors for human tumor necrosis factor (TNF alpha). *J Biol Chem* 264: 14927-14934, 1989.

62. Holmstrom, T. H., S. C. Chow, I. Elo, E. T. Coffey, S. Orrenius, L. Sistonen, and J. E. Eriksson. Suppression of Fas/APO-1-mediated apoptosis by mitogen-activated kinase signaling. *J Immunol* 160: 2626-2636, 1998.

63. Hu, S., C. Vincenz, J. Ni, R. Gentz, and V. M. Dixit. I-FLICE, a novel inhibitor of tumor necrosis factor receptor-1- and CD-95-induced apoptosis. *J Biol Chem* 272: 17255-17257, 1997.

64. Inohara, N., L. del Peso, T. Koseki, S. Chen, and G. Núñez. RICK, a novel protein kinase containing a caspase recruitment domain, interacts with CLARP and regulates CD95-mediated apoptosis. *J Biol Chem* 273: 12296-12300, 1998.

65. Inohara, N., T. Koseki, Y. Hu, S. Chen, and Núñez, G. CLARP, a death effector domain-containing protein interacts with caspase-8 and regulates apoptosis. *Proc Natl Acad Sci* 94: 10717-10722, 1997.

22

DEATH RECEPTORS AND THEIR LIGANDS

66. Irmler, M., M. Thome, M. Hahne, P. Schneider, K. Hofmann, V. Steiner, J. L. Bodmer, M. Schroeter, K. Burns, C. Mattmann, D. Rimoldi, L. E. French, and J. Tschopp. Inhibition of death receptor signals by cellular FLIP. *Nature* 388: 190-195, 1997.

67. Itoh, N., and S. Nagata. A novel protein domain required for apoptosis: mutational analysis of human Fas antigen. *J Biol Chem* 268: 10932-10937, 1993.

68. Itoh, N., S. Yonehara, A. Ishii, M. Yonehara, S. Mizushima, M. Sameshima, A. Hase, Y. Seto, and S. Nagata. The polypeptide encoded by the cDNA for human surface antigen Fas can mediate apoptosis. *Cell* 66: 233-243, 1991.

69. Jaattela, M., H. Mouritzen, F. Elling, and L. Bastholm. A20 zinc finger protein inhibits TNF and IL-1 signaling. *J Immunol* 156: 1166-1173, 1996.

70. Jaunin, F., K. Burns, J. Tschopp, T. E. Martin, and S. Fakan. Ultrastructural distribution of the death-domain-containing MyD88 protein in HeLa cells. *Exp Cell Res* 243: 67-75, 1998.

71. Jiang, Y., J. D. Woronicz, and D. V. Goeddel. Prevention of constitutive TNF receptor signaling by silencer of death domains. *Science* 283: 543-546, 1999.

72. Kagan, B. L., R. L. Baldwin, D. Munoz, and B. J. Wisnieski. Formation of ion-permeable channels by tumor necrosis factor-α. *Science* 257: 1427-1430, 1993.

73. Kamitani, T., K. Kito, H. P. Nguyen, H. F.-K. Wada, T., and E. T. Yeh. Identification of three sentrinization sites in PML. *J Biol Chem* 273: 26675-26682, 1998.

74. Kamitani, T., H. P. Nguyen, and E. T. Yeh. Preferential modification of nuclear proteins by a novel ubiquitin-like molecule. *J Biol Chem* 272: 14001-14004, 1997.

75. Kekelar, A., and C. B. Thompson. Bcl-2-family proteins: the role of the BH3 domain in apoptosis. *Trends Cell Biol* 8: 324-330, 1998.

76. Kerr, J. F. R. Shrinkage necrosis: a distinct mode of cellular death. *J Pathol* 105: 13-20, 1971.

77. Kerr, J. F. R., A. H. Wyllie, and A. R. Currie. Apoptosis: a basic biological phenomenon with wide-ranging implications in tissue kinetics. *Br J Cancer* 26: 239-257, 1972.

78. Kiriakidou, M., D. A. Driscoll, J. M. Lopez-Guisa, and J. F. Strauss. Cloning and expression of primate Daxx cDNAs and mapping of the human gene to chromosome 6p21.3 in the MHC region. *DNA Cell Biol* 16: 1289-1298, 1997.

79. Kischkel, F. C., S. Hellbardt, I. Behrmann, M. Germer, M. Pawlita, P. H. Krammer, and M. E. Peter. Cytotoxicity-dependent APO-1 (Fas/CD95)-associated proteins form a death-inducing signaling complex (DISC) with the receptor. *Embo J* 14: 5579-5588, 1995.

80. Kitson, J., T. Raven, Y. P. Jiang, D. V. Goeddel, K. M. Giles, K. T. Pun, C. J. Grinham, R. Brown, and S. N. Farrow. A death-domain-containing receptor that mediates apoptosis. *Nature* 384: 372-375, 1996.

81. Kolesnick, R. N., and M. Krönke. Regulation of ceramide production and apoptosis. *Ann Rev Physiol* 60: 643-665, 1998.

82. Kroemer, G., B. Dallaporta, and M. Resche-Rigon. The mitochondrial death/life regulator in apoptosis and necrosis. *Ann Rev Physiol* 60: 619-642, 1998.

83. Kroemer, G., N. Zamzami, and S. A. Susin. Mitochondrial control of apoptosis. *Immunol Today* 18: 44-51, 1997.

84. Krown, K. A., M. T. Page, C. Nguyen, D. Zechner, V. Gutierrez, K. L. Comstock, C. C. Glembotski, P. J. E. Quintana, and R. A. Sabbadini. Tumor necrosis factor alpha-induced apoptosis in cardiac myocytes - Involvement of the sphingolipid signaling cascade in cardiac cell death. *J Clin Invest* 98: 2854-2865, 1996.

85. Kubota, T., C. F. McTiernan, C. S. Frye, A. J. Demetris, and A. M. Feldman. Cardiac-specific overexpression of tumor necrosis factor-alpha causes lethal myocarditis in transgenic mice. *J Card Fail* 3: 117-24, 1997.

86. Kubota, T., C. F. McTiernan, C. S. Frye, S. E. Slawson, B. H. Lemster, A. P. Koretsky, A. J. Demetris, and A. M. Feldman. Dilated cardiomyopathy in transgenic mice with cardiac-specific overexpression of tumor necrosis factor-alpha. *Circ Res* 81: 627-35, 1997.

87. Kubota, T., M. Miyagishima, G. S. Bounutas, C. F. McTiernan, and A. M. Feldman. Overexpression of tumor necrosis factor-α activates the expression of multiple members of the apoptosis pathway in transgenic mice. *Circulation* 98: I-462, 1998.

88. Lacey, D. L., E. Timms, H. L. Tan, M. J. Kelley, C. R. Dunstan, T. Burgess, R. Elliott, A. Colombero, G. Elliott, S. Sully, and A. L. Et. Osteoprotegerin ligand is a cytokine that regulates osteoclast differentiation and activation. *Cell* 93: 165-176, 1998.

89. Ledgerwood, E. C., J. B. Prins, N. A. Bright, D. R. Johnson, K. Wolfreys, J. S. Pober, S. O'Rahily, and J. R. Bradley. Tumor necrosis factor is delivered to mitochondria where a tumor necrosis factor-binding protein is localized. *Lab Invest* 78: 1583-1589, 1998.

90. Lee, S. Y., S. Y. Lee, and Y. Choi. TRAF-interacting protein (TRIP): a novel component of the tumor necrosis factor receptor (TNFR)- and CD30-TRAF signaling complexes that inhibits TRAF2-mediated NF-κB activation. *J Exp Med* 185: 1275-1285, 1997.

91. Liang, H., and S. W. Fesik. Three-dimensional structures of proteins involved in programmed cell death. *J Mol Biol* 274: 291-302, 1997.

92. Liepinsh, E., L. L. Ilag, G. Otting, and C. F. Ibanez. NMR structure of the death domain of the p75 neurotrophin receptor. *EMBO J* 16: 4999-5005, 1997.

93. Liu, C., J. Cheng, and J. D. Mountz. Differential expression of human Fas mRNA species upon peripheral blood mononuclear cell activation. *Biochem J* 310: 957-963, 1995.

94. Liu, Y., E. Cigola, W. Cheng, J. Kajastura, G. Olivetti, T. H. Hintze, and P. Anversa. Myocyte nuclear mitotic division and programmed myocyte cell death characterize the cardiac myopathy induced by rapid ventricular pacing in dogs. *Lab Invest* 73: 771-787, 1995.

95. Liu, Z.-G., H. Hsu, D. Goeddel, and M. Karin. Dissection of TNF receptor 1 effector functions: JNK activation is not linked to apoptosis while NF-κB activation prevents cell death. *Cell* 87: 565-576, 1996.

96. MacFarlane, M., M. Ahmad, S. M. Srinivasula, T. Fernandes-Alnemri, G. M. Cohen, and E. S. Alnemri. Identification and molecular cloning of two novel receptors for the cytotoxic ligand TRAIL. *J Biol Chem* 272: 25417-25420, 1997.

97. Malinin, N. L., M. P. Boldin, A. V. Kovalenko, and D. Wallach. MAP3K-related kinase involved in NF-κB induction by TNF, CD95 and IL-1. *Nature* 385: 540-544, 1997.

98. Marsters, S. A., J. P. Sheridan, C. J. Donahue, R. M. Pitti, C. L. Gray, A. D. Goddard, K. D. Bauer, and A. Ashkenazi. Apo-3, a new member of the tumor necrosis factor receptor family, contains a death domain and activates apoptosis and NF-κB. *Current Biol* 6: 1669-1676, 1996.

99. Marsters, S. A., J. P. Sheridan, R. M. Pitti, J. Brush, A. Goddard, and A. Ashkenazi. Identification of a ligand for the death-domain-containing receptor Apo-3. *Curr Biol* 8: 525-528, 1998.

100. Marsters, S. T., J. P. Sheridan, R. M. Pitti, A. Huang, M. Skubatch, D. Baldwin, J. Yuan, A. Gurney, A. D. Goddard, P. Godowski, and A. Ashkenazi. A novel receptor for Apo-2L/TRAIL contains a truncated death domain. *Curr Biol* 7: 1003-1006, 1997.

101. Marzo, I., C. Brenner, N. Zamzami, S. A. Susin, G. Beutner, D. Brdiczka, R. Remy, Z.-H. Xie, J. C. Reed, and G. Kroemer. The permeability pore complex: A target for apoptosis regulation by caspases and Bcl-2-related proteins. *J Exp Med* 187: 1261-1271, 1998.

102. Marzo, I., S. A. Susin, P. X. Petit, and L. Ravagnan. Caspases disrupt mitochondrial membrane barrier function. *FEBS Lett* 427: 198-202, 1998.

103. Meakin, S. O., and E. M. Shooter. The nerve growth factor family of receptors. *Trends Neurosci* 15: 323-331, 1992.

104. Medema, J. P., C. Scaffidi, F. C. Hischkel, A. Shevchenko, M. Mann, P. H. Krammer, and M. E. Peter. FLICE is activated by association with the CD95 death-inducing signaling complex (DISC). *Embo J* 16: 2794-2804, 1997.

105. Meredith, J. E., and M. A. Schwartz. Integrins, adhesion and apoptosis. *Trends Cell Biol* 7: 146-150, 1997.

106. Mohler, K. M., D. S. Torrance, C. A. Smith, R. G. Goodwin, K. E. Stremler, V. F. Fung, H. Madami, and M. B. Widmer. Soluble tumor necrosis factor (TNF) receptors are effective therapeutic agents in lethal endotoxemia and function simultaneously as both TNF carriers and TNF antagonists. *J Immunol* 151: 1548-1561, 1993.

107. Mongkolsapaya, J., A. E. Cowper, X. N. Xu, G. Morris, A. J. McMichael, J. J. Bell, and G. R. Screaton. Lymphocyte inhibitor of TRAIL (TNF-related apoptosis-inducing ligand): a new receptor protecting lymphocytes from the death ligand TRAIL. *J Immunol* 160: 3-6, 1997.

108. Morinaga, T., N. Nakagawa, T. Yasuda, E. Tsuda, and K. Higashio. Cloning and characterization of the gene encoding human osteoprotegerin/osteoclastogenesis-inhibitory factor. *Eur J Biochem* 254: 685-691, 1998.

109. Moss, M. L., S. L. C. Jin, M. E. Milla, H. Burkhart, H. L. Carter, W. J. Chen, W. C. Clay, J. R. Didsbury, D. Hassler, C. R. Hoffman, T. A. Kost, M. H. Lambert, M. A. Leesnitzer, P. McCauley, G. McGeehan, J. Mitchell, M. Moyer, G. Pahel, W. Rocque, L. K. Overton, F. Schoenen, T.

Seaton, J. L. Su, J. Warner, D. Willard, and J. D. Becherer. Cloning of a disintegrin metalloproteinase that processes precursor tumour-necrosis factor-α. *Nature* 385: 733-736, 1997.

110. Muellberg, J., F. H. Durie, C. Otten-Evans, M. R. Alderson, S. Rose-John, D. Cosman, R. A. Black, and K. M. Mohler. A metalloprotease inhibitor blocks shedding of the IL-6 receptor and the p60 TNF receptor. *J Immunol* 155: 5198-5205, 1995.

111. Muzio, M., J. Ni, P. Feng, and V. M. Dixit. IRAK (Pelle) family member IRAK-2 and MyD88 as proximal mediators of IL-1 signaling. *Science* 278: 1612-1615, 1997.

112. Nagata, S. Fas and Fas ligand: a death factor and its receptor. *Adv Immunol* 57: 129-?, 1994.

113. Nagata, S., and P. Golstein. The Fas death factor. *Science* 267: 1449-1456, 1995.

114. Nagato, S. Apoptosis by death factor. *Cell* 88: 355-365, 1997.

115. Newton, K., A. H. Harris, M. L. Barth, K. G. C. Smith, and A. Strasser. A dominant interfering mutant of FADD/MORT1 enhances deletion of autoreactive thymocytes and inhibits proliferation of mature T lymphocytes. *EMBO J* 18: 706-718, 1998.

116. Oehm, A., I. Behrmann, W. Falk, M. Pawlita, G. Maier, C. Klas, M. Li-Weber, S. Richards, J. Dhein, B. C. Trauth, H. Ponstingl, and P. H. Krammer. Purification and molecular cloning of the APO-1 cell surface antigen, a new member of the TNF/NGF receptor superfamily: sequence identity with the Fas antigen. *J Biol Chem* 267: 10709-10715, 1992.

117. Okura, T., L. Gong, T. Kamitani, T. Wada, I. Okura, C. F. Wei, H. M. Chang, and E. T. Yeh. Protection against Fas/Apo-1- and tumor necrosis factor-mediated cell death by a novel protein, sentrin. *J Immunol* 15: 4277-4288, 1996.

118. Opipari, A. W., H. M. Hu, R. Yabkowitz, and V. M. Dixit. The A20 zinc finger protein protects cells from tumor necrosis factor cytotoxicity. *J Biol Chem* 267: 12424-12427, 1992.

119. Orlinick, J. R., A. Vaishnaw, K. B. Elkon, and M. v. Chao. Requirement of cysteine-rich repeats of the Fas receptor for binding the Fas ligand. *J Biol Chem* 272: 28889-28894, 1997.

120. Pan, G., J. H. Bauer, V. Haridas, S. Wang, D. Liu, G. Yu, C. Vincenz, B. B. Aggarwal, J. Ni, and V. M. Dixit. Identification and functional characterization of DR6, a novel death domain-containing TNF receptor. *FEBS Lett* 431: 351-356, 1998.

121. Pan, G., J. Ni, Y. F. Wei, Q. L. Yu, R. Gentz, and V. M. Dixit. An antagonist decoy receptor and a death domain-containing receptor for TRAIL. *Science* 277: 815-818, 1997.

122. Pan, G., J. Ni, G. L. Yu, Y. F. Wei, and V. M. Dixit. TRUNDD, a new member of the TRAIL receptor family that antagonizes TRAIL signalling. *FEBS Lett* 424: 41-45, 1998.

123. Pan, G., K. O'Rourke, A. M. Chinnaiyan, R. Gentz, R. Ebner, J. Ni, and V. M. Dixit. The receptor for the cytotoxic ligand TRAIL. *Science* 276: 111-113, 1997.

124. Pan, G. H., K. O'Rourke, and V. M. Dixit. Caspase-9, Bcl-xL, and Apaf-1 form a ternary complex. *J Biol Chem* 273: 5841-5845, 1998.

125. Papoff, G., I. Cascino, A. Eramo, G. Starace, D. H. Lynch, and G. Ruberti. An N-terminal domain shared by Fas/Apo-1 (CD95) soluble variants prevents cell death in vitro. *J Immunol* 156: 4622-4630, 1996.

126. Pasqualini, R., E. Koivunen, and E. Ruoslahti. A peptide isolated from phage display libraries is a structural and functional mimic of an RGD-binding site on integrins. *J Cell Biol* 130: 1189-1196, 1995.

127. Peter, M. E., and P. E. Krammer. Mechanisms of CD95 (APO-1/Fas)-mediated apoptosis. *Curr Opin Immunol* 10: 545-551, 1998.

128. Pitti, R. M., S. A. Marsters, D. A. Lawrence, M. Roy, F. C. Kischkel, P. Dowd, A. Huang, C. J. Donahue, S. W. Sherwood, A. L. Gurney, K. J. Hillan, R. L. Cohen, A. D. Goddard, D. Botstein, and A. Ashkenazi. Genomic amplification of a decoy receptor for Fas ligand in lung and colon cancer. *Nature* 396: 699-703, 1998.

129. Pitti, R. M., S. A. Marsters, S. Ruppert, C. J. Donahue, A. Moore, and A. Ashkenazi. Induction of apoptosis by Apo-2 ligand, a new member of the tumor necrosis factor cytokine family. *J Biol Chem* 271: 12687-12690, 1996.

130. Ruoslahti, E. RGD and other recognition sequences for integrins. *Ann Rev Cell Dev Biol* 12: 697-715, 1996.

131. Ruoslahti, E., and J. Reed. New way to activate caspases. *Nature* 397: 479-480, 1999.

132. Sato, T., S. Irie, S. Kitada, and J. C. Reed. FAP-1: a protein tyrosine phosphatase that associates with Fas. *Science* 268: 411-415, 1995.

133. Scaffidi, C., S. Fulda, A. Srinivasan, C. Friesen, F. Li, K. J. Tomaselli, K. M. Debatin, P. H. Krammer, and M. E. Peter. Two CD95 (APO-1/Fas) signaling pathways. *EMBO J* 17: 1675-1687, 1998.

134. Schall, T. J., M. Lewis, K. J. Koller, A. Lee, G. C. Rice, G. H. W. Wong, T. Gatanaga, G. A. Granger, R. Lentz, H. Raab, W. J. Kohr, and D. V. Goeddel. Molecular cloning and expression of a receptor for human tumor necrosis factor. *Cell* 61: 361-370, 1990.
135. Schneider, P., J. L. Bodmer, M. Thome, K. Hofmann, N. Holler, and J. Tschopp. Characterization of two receptors for TRAIL. *FEBS Lett* 416: 329-334, 1997.
136. Schneider, P., M. Thome, K. Burns, J. L. Bodmer, K. Hofmann, T. Kataoka, N. Holler, and J. Tschopp. TRAIL receptors 1 (DR4) and 2 (DR5) signal FADD-dependent apoptosis and activate NF-κB. *Immunity* 7: 831-836, 1997.
137. Schreck, R., K. Albermann, and P. A. Baeuerle. Nuclear factor kappa B: an oxidative stress-response transcription factor of eukaryotic cells. *Free Rad Res Comm* 17: 221-227, 1992.
138. Schuchmann, M., S. Hess, P. Bufler, C. Brakebusch, D. Wallach, A. Porter, G. Riethmueller, and H. Engelmann. Functional discrepancies between tumor necrosis factor and lymphotoxin α explained by trimer stability and distinct receptor interactions. *Eur J Immunol* 25: 2183-2189, 1995.
139. Schulze-Osthoff, K., D. Ferrari, M. Los, S. Wesselborg, and M. E. Peter. Apoptosis signaling by death receptors. *Eur J Biochem* 254: 439-459, 1998.
140. Schumann, H., H. Morawietz, K. Hakim, H. R. Zerkowski, T. Eschenhagen, J. Holtz, and D. Darmer. Alternative splicing of the primary Fas transcript generating soluble Fas antagonists is suppressed in the failing human ventricular myocardium. *Biochem Biophys Res Comm* 239: 794-798, 1997.
141. Screaton, G. R., J. Monkolsapaya, X. N. Xu, A. E. Cowper, A. J. McMichael, and J. L. Bell. TRICK2, a new alternatively spliced receptor that transduces the cytotoxic signal from TRAIL. *Curr Biol* 7: 693-696, 1997.
142. Screaton, G. R., X. N. Xu, A. L. Olsen, A. E. Cowper, R. Tan, A. J. McMichael, and J. I. Bell. LARD: a new lymphoid-specific death domain containing receptor regulated by alternative premRNA splicing. *Proc Natl Acad Sci* 94: 4615-4619, 1997.
143. Sheridan, J. P., S. A. Marsters, R. M. Pitti, A. Gurney, M. Skubatch, D. Baldwin, L. Ramakrishnan, C. L. Gray, K. Baker, W. I. Wood, A. D. Goddard, P. Godowski, and A. Ashkenazi. Control of TRAIL-induced apoptosis by a family of signaling and decoy receptors. *Science* 277: 818-821, 1997.
144. Shu, H. B., D. R. Halpin, and D. V. Goeddel. Casper is a FADD- and caspase-related inducer of apoptosis. *Immunity* 6: 751-763, 1997.
145. Shu, H. B., M. Takeuchi, and D. V. Goeddel. The tumor necrosis factor receptor 2 signal transducers TRAF2 and cIAP1 are components of the tumor necrosis factor 1 signaling complex. *Proc Natl Acad Sci* 93: 13973-13978, 1996.
146. Siegel, R. M., D. A. Martin, L. Zheng, S. Y. Ng, J. Bertin, J. Cohen, and M. J. Lenardo. Death-effector filaments: novel cytoplasmic structures that recruit caspases and trigger apoptosis. *J Cell Biol* 141: 1243-1253, 1998.
147. Simonet, W. S., D. L. Lacey, C. R. Dunstan, M. Kelley, M. S. Chang, R. Luthy, H. Q. Nguyen, S. Wooden, L. Bennett, T. Boone, G. Shimamoto, M. DeRose, R. Elliott, A. Colombero, H. L. Tan, G. Trail, J. Sullivan, E. Davy, N. Bucay, L. Renshaw-Gegg, T. M. Hughes, D. Hill, W. Pattison, P. Campbell, S. Sander, G. Van, J. Tarpley, P. Derby, R. Lee, A. E. Program, and W. J. Boyle. Osteoprotegerin: a novel secreted protein involved in the regulation of bone density. *Cell* 89: 309-319, 1997.
148. Smith, C. A., T. Davis, D. Anderson, L. Solam, M. P. Beckmann, R. Jerzy, S. K. Dower, D. Cosman, and R. G. Goodwin. A receptor for tumor necrosis factor defines an unusual family of cellular and viral proteins. *Science* 248: 1019-1023, 1990.
149. Song, H. Y., J. D. Dunbar, and D. B. Donner. Aggregation of the intracellular domain of the type 1 tumor necrosis factor receptor defined by the two-hybrid system. *J Biol Chem* 269: 22492-22495, 1994.
150. Srinivasula, S. M., M. Ahmad, S. Ottilie, F. Bullrich, S. Banks, T. Fernandes-Alnemri, C. M. Croce, G. Litwack, K. J. Tomaselli, R. C. Armstrong, and E. S. Alnemeri. FLAME-1, a novel FADD-like anti-apoptotic molecule that regulates Fas/TNFR1-induced apoptosis. *J Biol Chem* 272: 18542-18545, 1997.
151. Stankovski, I., and D. Baltimore. NF-κB activation: the IκB kinase revealed? *Cell* 91: 299-302, 1997.
152. Steemans, M., V. Goossens, M. Van de Craen, F. Van Hereweghe, K. Vancompernolle, K. De Vos, P. Vandenabeele, and J. Groten. A caspase-activated factor (CAF) induces mitochondrial

membrane depolarization and cytochrome c release by a nonproteolytic mechanism. *J Exp Med* 188: 2193-2198, 1998.

153. Suda, T., T. Takahashi, P. Goldstein, and S. Nagata. Molecular cloning and expression of the Fas ligand, a novel member of the tumor necrosis factor family. *Cell* 75: 1169-1178, 1993.

154. Susin, S. A., H. K. Lorenzo, N. Zamzami, I. Marzo, C. Brenner, N. Larochette, M. C. Prévost, P. M. Alzari, and G. Kroemer. Mitochondrial release of caspase-2 and -9 during the apoptotic process. *J Exp Med* 189: 381-393, 1999.

155. Susin, S. A., H. K. Lorenzo, N. Zamzami, I. Marzo, B. E. Snow, G. M. Brothers, J. Mangion, E. Jacotot, P. Costantini, M. Loeffler, N. Larochette, D. R. Goodletti, R. Aebersold, D. P. Siderovski, J. M. Penninger, and G. Kroemer. Molecular characterization of mitochondrial apoptosis-inducing factor. *Nature* 397: 441-446, 1999.

156. Susin, S. A., N. Zamzami, M. Castedo, T. Hirsch, P. Marchetti, A. Macho, E. Daugas, M. Geuskens, and G. Kroemer. Bcl-2 inhibits the mitochondrial release of an apoptogenic protease. *J Exp Med* 184: 1331-1341, 1996.

157. Susin, S. A., N. Zamzami, and G. Kroemer. Mitochondrial regulation of apoptosis: doubt no more. *Biochim Biophys Acta* 1366: 151-165, 1998.

158. Tanaka, M., H. Ino, K. Ohno, K. Hattori, W. Sato, T. Ozawa, T. Tanaka and S. Itoyama. Mitochondrial mutation in fatal infantile cardiomyopathy. *Lancet* 336: 1452, 1990.

159. Tanaka, M., T. Itai, M. Adachi, and S. Nagata. Downregulation of Fas ligand by shedding. *Nature Med* 4: 31-36, 1998.

160. Tartaglia, A. T., D. Pennica, and D. V. Goeddel. Ligand passing the 75-kDa tumor necrosis factor (TNF) receptor recruits TNF for signaling by the 55-kDa TNF receptor. *J Biol Chem* 268: 18542-18548, 1993.

161. Tartaglia, L. A., T. M. Ayres, G. H. W. Wong, and D. V. Goeddel. A novel domain within the 55 kD TNF receptor signals cell death. *Cell* 74: 845-853, 1993.

162. Tartaglia, L. A., M. Rothe, Y. F. Hu, and D. V. Goeddel. Tumor necrosis factor's cytotoxic activity is signaled by the p55 TNF receptor. *Cell* 73: 213-216, 1993.

163. Thoma, B., M. Grell, K. Pfizenmaier, and P. Scheurich. Identification of a 60 kDa tumor necrosis factor (TNF) receptor as the major signal transducing component in TNF responses. *J Exp Med* 172: 1019-1023, 1990.

164. Thornberry, N. A., and Y. Lazebnik. Caspases: enemies within. *Science* 281: 1313-1316, 1998.

165. Torre-Amione, G., S. Kapadia, J. Lee, J. B. Durand, R. D. Bies, J. B. Young, and D. L. Mann. Tumor necrosis factor-α and tumor necrosis factor receptors in the failing human heart. *Circulation* 93: 704-711, 1996.

166. Trauth, B. C., C. Klas, A. M. J. Peters, S. Matzku, P. Moeller, W. Falk, K. M. Debatin, and P. H. Krammer. Monoclonal antibody-mediated tumor regression by induction of apoptosis. *Science* 245: 301-305, 1989.

167. Tsuda, E., M. Goto, S. I. Mochiguzi, K. Yano, F. Kobayashi, T. Morinaga, and K. Higashio. Isolation of a novel cytokine from human fibroblasts that specifically inhibits osteoclastogenesis. *Biochem Biophys Res Comm* 234: 137-142, 1997.

168. Uren, A. G., M. Pakusch, C. J. Hawkins, K. L. Puls, and D. L. Vaux. Cloning and expression of apoptosis inhibitory protein homologs that function to inhibit apoptosis and/or bind tumor necrosis factor receptor-associated factors. *Proc Natl Acad Sci* 93: 4974-4978, 1996.

169. Uren, A. G., and D. L. Vaux. Viral inhibitors of apoptosis. *Vitam Horm* 53: 175-193, 1997.

170. Van Antwerp, D. J., S. J. Martin, T. Kafri, D. R. Green, and I. M. Verma. Suppression of TNF-α-induced apoptosis by NF-κB. *Science* 274: 787-789, 1996.

171. Walczak, H., M. A. Degli-Esposti, R. S. Johnson, P. J. Smolak, J. Y. Waugh, N. Bioani, M. S. Timour, M. J. Gerhart, K. A. Schooley, C. A. Smith, R. G. Goodwin, and C. T. Rauch. TRAIL-R2: a novel apoptosis-mediating receptor for TRAIL. *Embo J* 16: 5386-5397, 1997.

172. Wallach, D., A. V. Kovalenko, E. E. Vasfolomeev, and M. P. Boldin. Death-inducing functions of ligands of the tumor necrosis factor family: a Sanhedrin verdict. *Curr Opin Immunol* 10: 279-288, 1998.

173. Wang, C. Y., M. W. Mayo, and A. S. Baldwin. TNF- and cancer therapy-induced apoptosis: potentiation by inhibition of NF-κB. *Science* 274: 784-787, 1996.

174. Warzowa, K., P. Ribeiro, C. Charlot, N. Renard, B. Coiffier, and G. Salles. A new death receptor 3 isoform: expression in human lymphoid cell lines and non-Hodgkin's lymphomas. *Biochem Biophys Res Comm* 242: 376-379, 1998.

175. Weiss, T., M. Grell, K. Siemienski, F. Muhlenbeck, H. Durkop, K. Pfizenmaier, P. Scheurich, and H. Wajant. TNFR80-dependent enhancement of TNFR60-induced cell death is mediated by TNFR60-associated factor 2 and is specific for TNFR60. *J Immunol* 161: 3136-3142, 1998.
176. Wiegmann, K., S. Schuetze, T. Machleidt, D. Witte, and M. Kroenke. Functional dichotomy of neutral and acidic sphingomyelinases in tumor necrosis factor signaling. *Cell* 78: 1005-1015, 1994.
177. Wiley, S. R., K. Schooley, P. J. Smolak, W. S. Din, C. P. Huang, J. K. Nicholl, G. R. Sutherland, T. D. Smith, C. Rauch, C. A. Smith, and R. G. Goodwin. Identification and characterization of a new member of the TNF family that induces apoptosis. *Immunity* 3: 673-682, 1995.
178. Wong, B. R., J. Rho, J. Arron, E. Robinson, J. Orlinick, M. Chao, S. Kalachikov, E. Cayani, F. S. Bartlett, W. N. Frankel, S. Y. Lee, and Y. Choi. TRANCE is a novel ligand of the tumor necrosis factor receptor family that activates c-Jun N-terminal kinase in T cells. *J Biol Chem* 272: 25190-25194, 1997.
179. Wu, G. S., T. F. Burns, E. R. McDonald, W. Jiang, R. Meng, I. D. Krantz, G. Kao, D. D. Gan, J. Y. Zhou, R. Muschel, S. R. Hamilton, N. B. Spinner, S. Markowitz, G. Wu, and W. S. el-Deiry. Killer/DR5 is DNA damage-inducible p53-regulated death receptor gene. *Nature Genet* 17: 141-143, 1997.
180. Yamaguchi, K., M. Kinosaki, M. Goto, F. Kobayashi, E. Tsuda, T. Morinaga, and K. Higashio. Characterization of structural domains of osteoclastogenesis inhibitory factor. *J Biol Chem* 273: 5117-5123, 1998.
181. Yanagisawa, J., M. Takahashi, H. Kanki, H. Yano-Yanagisawa, T. Tazunoki, E. Sawa, T. Nishitoba, M. Kamishohara, E. Kobayashi, S. Kataoka, and T. Sato. The molecular interaction of Fas and FAP-1: a tripeptide blocker of human Fas interaction with FAP-1 promotes Fas-induced apoptosis. *J Biol Chem* 272: 8539-8545, 1997.
182. Yasuda, H., N. Shima, N. Nakagawa, S. I. Mochizuki, K. Yano, N. Fujise, Y. Sato, M. Goto, K. Yamaguchi, M. Kuriyama, T. Kanno, A. Murakami, E. Tsuda, T. Morinaga, and K. Higashio. Identity of osteoclastogenesis inhibitory factor (OCIF) and osteoprotegerin (OPG): a mechanism by which OPG-OCIF inhibits osteoclastogenesis in vitro. *Endocrinology* 139: 1329-1337, 1998.
183. Yonehara, S., A. Ishii, and M. Yonehara. A cell-killing monoclonal antibody (anti-Fas) to a cell surface antigen downregulated with the receptor of tumor necrosis factor. *J Exp Med* 169: 1747-1756, 1989.
184. Yue, T. L., X. L. Ma, X. Wang, A. M. Romanic, G. L. Liu, C. Louden, J. L. Gu, S. Kumar, G. Poste, R. R. Ruffolo, and G. Z. Feuerstein. Possible involvement of stress-activated protein kinase signaling pathway and Fas receptor expression in prevention of ischemia/reperfusion-induced cardiomyocyte apoptosis by carvedilol. *Circ Res* 82: 166-174, 1998.
185. Zornig, M., A. O. Hueber, and G. Evan. p53-dependent impairment of T-cell proliferation in FADD dominant negative transgenic mice. *Curr Biol* 8: 467-470, 1998.

I.1.2
Regulation of apoptosis by CD 137

Herbert Schwarz, Ph.D.
Universität Regensburg, Regensburg, Germany

INTRODUCTION

CD137 (ILA/4-1BB) is a member of the TNF receptor family and was identified in screens for genes induced upon lymphocyte activation (1,2). CD137 is expressed by activated lymphocytes and expression its is strictly activation dependent (3). Expression of CD137 can also be induced in non-immune cells, like chondrocytes (4). In vivo, the highest expression of CD137 has been found in blood vessel walls. Since expresssion and function of CD137 are not yet investigated in the heart, lymphocytes serve as a model. The gene for human CD137 resides on chromosome 1p36, and this chromosomal region is associated with mutations in several malignancies (6).

Soluble forms of CD137 (sCD137) are generated by differential splicing and are present at enhanced concentrations in sera of patients with rheumatoid arthritis. Soluble CD137 is expressed exclusively by activated T lymphocytes and levels of sCD137 correlate with activation induced cell death caused by mitogen overstimulation in these cells (4).

Anti-CD137 antibodies and the CD137 ligand co-stimulate proliferation of activated T cells (7-9), and costimulation through CD137 provides an alternative and synergistic activating signal to that through CD28 (10). Injection of agonistic anti-CD137 antibodies induces a potent anti-tumor TH1 immune response and leads to the elimination of tumors in vivo (11).

The human CD137 ligand is expressed constitutively by monocytes and B cells and its expression is inducible in T lymphocytes (7). The ligands for the TNF receptor family members also form a family of structurally related proteins, known as the TNF ligand family, and they can be expressed as soluble and as cell surface molecules (12). For several members of this family bidirectional signaling has been shown, where also the ligand transduces a signal into the cell it is expressed on. For example, stimulation of dendritic cells by OX40 protein leads to a strong increase in cytokine production and expression of T lymphocyte costimulatory molecules (13). In T lymphocytes, reverse signaling through CD30 ligand enhances cell proliferation (14).

INDUCTION OF T LYMPHOCYTE APOPTOSIS BY CD137 THROUGH REVERSE SIGNALING

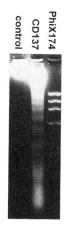

Bidirectional transduction of signals also exists for the CD137 receptor/ligand system. While cross-linking of CD137 activates T lymphocytes (7-9), cross-linking of the CD137 ligand has the opposite effect. This reverse signaling through the CD137 ligand inhibits proliferation of T lymphocytes and reduces the viability of the cells. Analysis of genomic DNA from these lymphocytes revealed the induction of nucleosomal DNA fragmentation, a hallmark of apoptosis (figure 1), and the cells displayed morphological changes indicative of apoptosis. For these activities, immobilization of the CD137 protein is essential, indicating that the CD137 receptor protein needs to crosslink a corresponding ligand/coreceptor expressed on T lymphocytes. No sequence motif known to mediate apoptosis is present in the cytoplasmic domain of the human CD137 ligand (7). Therefore, apoptosis has to be induced through a novel, unknown pathway, or other ligands for CD137 must exist. A similar situation has been found for CD95, where the receptor, as well as the ligand is expressed on CD8 positive T lymphocytes. And while the signal through the CD95 induces apoptosis, the

Figure 1 CD137 induces internucleosomal DNA fragmentation. Lymphocytes were cultured for 24 h on glutaraldehyde-fixed CHO cells transfected with an empty vector (control) and a vector expressing CD137. DNA of the lymphocytes was isolated and separated on a 2% agarose gel.

signal through CD95 ligand stimulates proliferation (15). For both, CD95 and CD137 the physiological significance of this bidirectional signaling with opposing effects for the cells have not yet been elucidated.

Though, many members of the TNF receptor family are involved in induction of apoptosis, CD137 is unique in the sense that cross-linking of the ligand by the receptor provides the death signal and that the ligand-bearing cell is the one which dies (9). This is the opposite situation compared to CD95 or the p55 TNF receptor, where the receptor-bearing cell is the one which undergoes apoptosis (figure 2), (16-18). However, since in the TNF receptor family the receptors as well as the ligands are expressed at the cell surface, transmission of signals through the ligands is possible and the distinction between which molecule serves as receptor or as ligand becomes blurred. A third mechanism is found in the case of the p75 nerve growth factor receptor, where apoptosis can be induced by the unoccupied receptor and this activity is suppressed by binding of the ligand to the receptor (figure 2), (19).

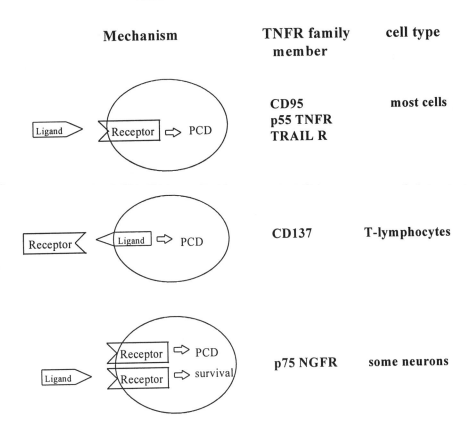

| Mechanism | TNFR family member | cell type |

Figure 2 Schematic representation of the three different mechanisms by which TNF receptor family members are able to induce apoptosis. PCD: programmed cell death = apoptosis.

CD137 INDUCES EXPRESSION OF CD95 IN T LYMPHOCYTES

In order to identify mechanisms of CD137-mediated apoptosis in lymphocytes, the regulation of known apoptosis-associated genes by CD137 was investigated. Immobilized CD137 significantly induced expression of CD95 in resting, total lymphocytes (figure 3). CD95 expression was increased in CD4 and CD8 positive T lymphocytes 3.8 and 2.4 fold, respectively. Fitting nicely to induction of CD95 expression, CD137 also reduced levels of the anti-apoptotic bcl-2 by about half.

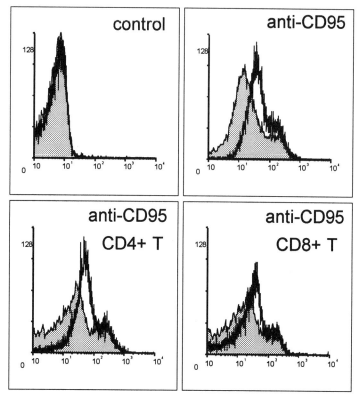

Figure 3 CD137 induces expression of CD95. Primary resting lymphocytes were cultured on tissue culture plates coated with 5 μg/ml Fc (gray) or CD137-Fc protein (white), respectively. CD95 expression was determined by flow cytometry after two days. Upper panel: Total lymphocytes stained with anti-CD95 and an isotype control antibody, respectively. Lower panel: CD4+ and CD8+ T lymphocytes were stained for CD95 expression.

CD137-INDUCED APOPTOSIS IS INDEPENDENT OF CD95

Since CD137 as well as CD95 are involved in induction of apoptosis in lymphocytes, and CD95 expression is induced by CD137, we speculated that CD137 may induce apoptosis via the CD95 pathway. CD137 increased the percentage of apoptotic cells among anti-CD3 activated lymphocytes from 26 to 49 % (figure 4). This increase in apoptosis is of the same magnitude as the one induced by anti-CD95. Antagonistic F(ab')₂ anti-CD95 fragments did not inhibit CD137 induced apoptosis, thereby discarding the hypothesis that CD137 induced lymphocyte apoptosis is mediated via CD95 (figure 4). No synergistic or additive effect on induction of apoptosis could be observed with the combination of CD137 and anti-CD95, indicating the existence of shared signaling pathways further downstream for the two molecules (figure 4).

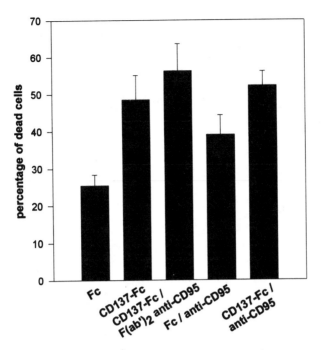

Figure 4 Induction of apoptosis by CD137 is independent of CD95. Lymphocytes were activated for 3 days with immobilized anti-CD3 (5 μg/ml), depleted of dead cells by ficoll gradient centrifugation, and plated on tissue culture plates coated with 5 μg/ml Fc (control) or CD137-Fc protein. Agonistic anti-CD95 (200 ng/ml) and antagonistic F(ab')$_2$ anti-CD95 antibody fragments (200 ng/ml) were added where indicated. The percentages of dead cells were determined by trypan blue staining after two days.

CD137 PROLONGS SURVIVAL OF MONOCYTES

Reverse signaling through CD137 ligand also exists for monocytes and in monocytes it regulates cell survival as well. However, in contrast to T lymphocytes, CD137 ligand delivers is not an apoptosis-promoting signal, rather an activating and apoptosis-inhibiting one (20).

Primary peripheral monocytes cultured on untreated tissue culture plates, or plates coated with Fc protein, attached only slightly and retained a rounded morphology (figure 5). During 10 days of culture the cells died gradually. Survival of the monocytes was substantially prolonged when the cells were grown on tissue culture plates coated with the CD137-Fc fusion protein. CD137-Fc protein induced adherence of monocytes and these cells adapted an irregular shape. This effect was visible from day one onwards. As time of culture progressed, cells spread out, grew in size and developed a more complex morphology. On day 10 of culture, the three basic morphologies of in vitro differentiated monocytes could be identified: elongated ones, rounded ones and branched ones. However, the most significant effect of CD137 protein was that it substantially prolonged the survival of primary, peripheral monocytes.

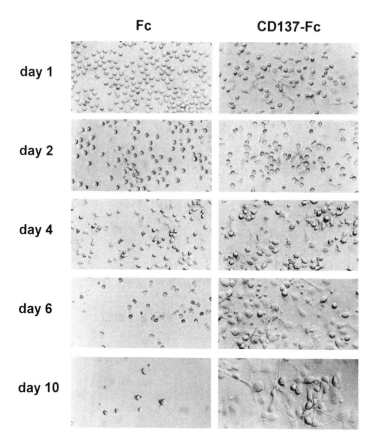

Figure 5 CD137 prolongs survival of peripheral monocytes. Primary monocytes were cultured on immobilized Fc or CD137-Fc protein (1 µg/ml). Photographs were taken at indicated times at a magnification of 400x.

PROLONGATION OF MONOCYTE SURVIVAL BY CD137 IS MEDIATED BY M-CSF

An essential survival factor for monocytes is the hematopoietic growth factor macrophage colony-stimulating factor (M-CSF) (21). It is therefore possible that CD137 promoted monocyte survival via M-CSF and as shown in figure 6, CD137 did in fact induce expression of M-CSF. Here too, immobilization of CD137 protein was necessary as soluble CD137 induced only low levels of M-CSF and did not promote monocyte survival.

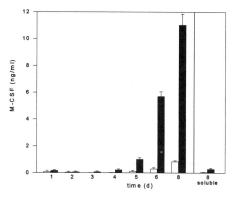

Figure 6 CD137 induces expression of M-CSF. 10^5 primary monocytes were cultured on immobilized Fc or CD137-Fc protein (1 µg/ml). In order to keep CD137-Fc protein (1 µg/ml) soluble (right section), immobilization of CD137-Fc protein was prevented by prior coating of the tissue culture plates with fetal calf serum (1 h at 4°C). Supernatants were harvested at indicated times, and concentrations of M-CSF were determined by ELISA.

M-CSF was not only induced by CD137, but was also essential for CD137 induced monocyte survival. Immobilized CD137 protein or M-CSF at 100 ng/ml enabled the survival of about 80% of the cells for 12 days. The survival enhancing effect of both proteins was abolished by the sequestration of M-CSF by neutralizing antibodies (figure 7).

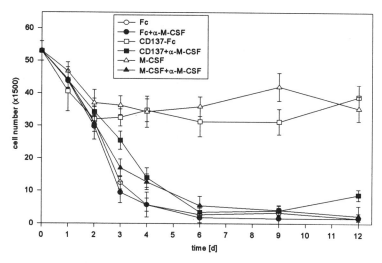

Figure 7 Neutralization of M-CSF inhibits CD137 induced monocyte survival. 10^5 primary monocytes were cultured on immobilized Fc or CD137-Fc protein (1 µg/ml) and neutralizing anti-M-CSF antibody was added at 2 µg/ml. The numbers of living monocytes, treated with Fc or CD137-Fc protein or with 100 ng/ml M-CSF were determined by cell counting. Live cells in four representative fields were counted and the mean and standard deviation of four such countings are depicted.

CD137 IS EXPRESSED STRONGLY IN VESSEL WALLS

Surveying CD137 expression, strong CD137 immunoreactivity was found in the walls of blood vessels, especially in inflamed tissues (figure 8). Since expression of CD137 in non-immune cells is induced by proinflammatory cytokines (3,4), the physiological significance of this finding may be a CD137-mediated facilitation of extravasation and recruitment of monocytes at sites of inflammatory reactions. At the same time monocytes could be further activated by contact with CD137 on vessel walls.

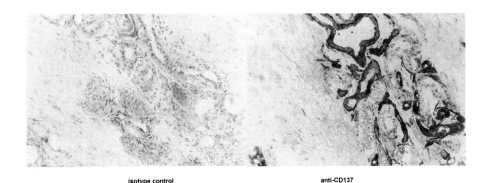

isotype control   anti-CD137

Figure 8 Expression of CD137 in vessel walls. Cryostat section of skin biopsy obtained from a vasculitis patient were stained with anti-CD137 monoclonal antibody (clone BBK-2, Bioscource; right photograph) or MOPC21 (Sigma) as an isotype control (left photograph).

So far a role for CD137 in regulation of apoptosis has been documented for T lymphocytes and monocytes. However, CD137 can also be expressed by non-immune cells, and sites of expression and function of CD137 outside the immune system have been characterized only superficially. But like in the case of the CD95 and TNF receptor/ligand systems, regulation of apoptosis by CD137 receptor and ligand may not be restricted to immune cells.

References

1. Smith CA, Farrah T, Goodwin RG. The TNF receptor superfamily of cellular and viral proteins: Activation, costimulation, and death. Cell 1994;76:959.
2. Lotz M, Setareh M, Von Kempis J, Schwarz H. The nerve growth factor/tumor necrosis factor receptor family. J Leukoc Biol 1996;60:1.
3. Schwarz H, Valbracht J, Tuckwell J, Kempis J, Lotz M. ILA, the human 4-1BB homologue is inducible in lymphoid and other cell lines. Blood 1995;85:1043.
4. von Kempis J, Schwarz H, Lotz M. Differentiation-dependent and stimulus-specific expression of ILA, the human 4-1BB-homologue, in cells of mesenchymal origin. Osteoarthritis Cartilage 1997;5:394-406.

5. Schwarz H, Arden K, Lotz M. CD137, a member of the tumor necrosis factor receptor family is located on chromosome 1p36, in a cluster of related genes, and colocalizes with several malignancies. Biochem Biophys Res Comm 1997;235:699.

6. Michel J, Langstein J, Hofstädter F, Schwarz H. A soluble form of CD137 (ILA/4-1BB) is released by activated lymphocytes and is detectable in sera of patients with rheumatoid arthritis. Eur J Immunol 1998; 28:290.

7. Alderson MR, Smith CA, Tough TW, Davis-Smith T, Armitage RJ, Falk B, Roux E, Baker E, Sutherland GR, Din WS, Goodwin RG. Molecular and biological characterization of human 4-1BB and its ligand. Eur J Immunol 1994;24:2219.

8. Pollok KE, Kim YJ, Zhou Z, Hurtado J, Kim KK, Pickard RT Kwon BS. (1993) Inducible T cell antigen 4-1BB. Analysis of expression and function. J Immunol 1993;150:771.

9. Schwarz H, Blanco F, Valbracht J, Kempis J, Lotz M. ILA, A member of the human NGF/TNF receptor family regulates T lymphocyte proliferation and survival. Blood 1996;87:2839.

10. Debenedette MA, Shahinian A, Mak TW, Watts, TH. Costimulation of CD28- T lymphocytes by 4-1BB ligand. J Immunol 1997;158:551.

11. Melero I, Shuford WW, Newby SA, Aruffo A, Ledbetter JA, Hellström KE, Mittler RS, Chen L. Monoclonal antibodies against 4-1BB T cell activation molecule eradicate established tumors. Nat Med 1997;3:682.

12. Beutler B, van Huffel C. Unraveling function in the TNF ligand and receptor families. Science. 1994;264:667-8.

13. Ohshima Y, Tanaka Y, Tozawa H, Takahashi Y, Maliszewski C, Delespesse G. Expression and function of OX40 ligand on human dendritic cells. J Immunol 1997; 159:3838-48.

14. Wiley SR, Goodwin RG, Smith CA. Reverse signaling via CD30 ligand. J Immunol 1996;15:157:3635-9

15. Suzuki I, Fink PJ. Maximal proliferation of cytotoxic T lymphocytes requires reverse signaling through Fas ligand. J Exp Med 1998;187:123-8.

16. Beutler B, Cerami A. The biology of cachectin/TNF - a primary mediator of the host response. Annu Rev Immunol 1989;7:625.

17. Itoh N, Yonehara S, Ishii A, Yonehara M, Mizushima S, Sameshima M, Hase A, Seto Y, Nagata S. The polypeptide encoded by the cDNA for human cell surface antigen Fas can mediate apoptosis. Cell 1991;66:233.

18. Oehm A, Behrmann I, Falk W, Pawlita M, Maier G, Klas C, Li-Weber M, Richards S, Dhein J, Trauth BC, et-al. (1992) Purification and molecular cloning of the APO-1 cell surface antigen, a member of the tumor necrosis factor/nerve growth factor receptor superfamily. Sequence identity with the Fas antigen. J Biol Chem 1992;267:10709.

19. Rabizadeh S, Oh J, Zhong LT, Yang J, Bitler CM, Butcher LL, Bredesen, DE Induction of apoptosis by the low-affinity NGF receptor. Science 1993;261:345.

20. Langstein J, Michel J, Fritsche J, Kreutz M, Andreesen R, Schwarz H. CD137, (ILA/4-1BB), a member of the TNF receptor family regulates monocyte activation via reverse signaling. J Immunol 1998;160:2488-2494.

21. Brugger W, Kreutz M, Andreesen R. Macrophage colony-stimulating factor is required for human monocyte survival and acts as a cofactor for their terminal differentiation to macrophages in vitro. J Leukoc Biol 1991;49:483-488.

I.1.3
Reactive oxygen species and apoptosis

Rüdiger von Harsdorf, M.D.
Humboldt-Universität zu Berlin, Berlin, Germany

INTRODUCTION

There is an increasing body of evidence suggesting an important role of apoptosis for cardiac development and diseases. This is based on the observation that in animals and humans the ontogenesis of the normal heart is characterized by the appearance of apoptosis peaking in the perinatal period (1) and in specific regions of the heart (2). Furthermore, myocardial infarction has been shown to be associated with apoptosis in rats (3) and humans (4). Additionally, apoptosis is evident in the heart of patients suffering from certain conductance disturbances (2) as well as in human cardiomyopathies, including the arrhythmogenic right ventricular dysplesia (5) and dilated cardiomyopathy (6). Those studies are important not only because of their proof of apoptotic cell death in yet another organ, but particularly because they let us understand that the capacity for apoptotic cell death exists in both mitotic cells and in post-mitotic cells. However, only little information exists regarding the identification of stimuli responsible for the induction of apoptosis in the heart.

Interestingly, apoptosis could be proven to occur during reperfusion following ischemia in several organs, including the heart (7). However, it is not known how reperfusion triggers apoptosis in this event. Experimental studies employing isolated organ preparations or in vivo animal models have demonstrated the generation of reactive oxygen species (ROS) during ischemia and reperfusion (8). Also, there are several clinical procedures which frequently are associated with ischemia and reperfusion injury on one side and production and release of ROS on the other, including clinical bypass surgery (9) , thrombosis (10) , and coronary balloon angioplasty (11). The threat being immanent in ROS even for the ontogenesis of the normal heart was demonstrated recently by the induction of cardiomyopathies and early lethalty in knockout-mice lacking the manganese superoxide dismutase, which acts as an intracellular ROS-scavenger (12). However, in all these cases it remains unclear how ROS induce the pathological phenotype.

Vascular remodeling represents the pathophysiological basis of many diseases, including atherosclerosis, hypertension and restenosis. It is referring to the modulation of the phenotype of vascular smooth muscle cells (VSMCs) which is characterized not only by cell migration and synthesis of extracellular matrix, but also by such contrasting phenomenon as cell proliferation on one hand, and cell death on the other.

Recently, ROS have been found to be related to VSMC proliferation. In vivo studies show that balloon-injured arteries produce increased amounts of ROS (13). Vitamin E, an antioxidant, can attenuate intimal response to balloon injury (14). In vitro studies also demonstrate that ROS can stimulate DNA synthesis in VSMCs (15,16). Since ROS comprise a group of different molecules, including hydrogen peroxide (H_2O_2), superoxide anion (O_2^-) and hydroxyl radical ($\cdot OH$), it would be important to understand the specific role of each of these species for VSMC proliferation.

There is an increasing body of evidence showing that apoptosis of VSMCs participates in the pathogenesis of atherosclerosis, restenosis and hypertension (17-20) , and plays a role in intimal thickening induced by endothelial denudation (21). Furthermore, inflammatory components are important for the induction of apoptosis as indicated by the observation that simultaneous treatment with interferon-γ and TNF-α and/or IL-1-β can trigger apoptosis in cultured human and rat VSMCs (22). While cultured human VSMCs derived from normal vessels undergo apoptosis only upon serum withdrawal, VSMCs from coronary atherosclerotic plaques are much more susceptible to apoptotic stimuli resulting in a significantly elevated rate of apoptosis after serum deprivation (23). Eukaryotic cells continuously produce ROS in physiological levels. The imbalance between their generation and decomposition has been shown to be implicated in many kinds of clinical disorders (24,25). It is therefore conceivable that ROS might participate in inducing apoptosis of VSMCs. However, whether ROS can trigger VSMC apoptosis remains unknown.

The following chapters address the importance of ROS for the induction of apoptosis in the cardiovascular system and summarize our studies performed with cardiomyocytes (26), cardiac fibroblasts (27) and vascular smooth muscle cells (28-30).

WHAT ARE REACTIVE OXYGEN SPECIES (ROS)?

ROS are extremely unstable and highly reactive oxygen compounds with atoms carrying one or more unpaired electrons. The family of molecules to which the specification of ROS applies includes superoxide anion (O_2^-), hydrogen peroxide (H_2O_2), hydroxyl radicals ($OH\cdot$), and nitrogen oxides (NO, $ONOO^-$). These ROS are produced either by the mitochondrial respiratory chain (cytochrome-oxidase complex containing ubiquinone and NADH-dehydrogenase), or by metabolism of arachidonic acid (COX), membrane bound oxidases (NADPH), xanthine oxidase, or phospholipases.

WHERE DO REACTIVE OXYGEN SPECIES ORIGINATE?

This means, that basically any cell is able to generate ROS intracellularly as long as it contains mitochondria (this applies particularly to the heart) or enzymes involved in redox processes.

However, ROS released into the extracellular environment play an important role probably as an evolutionary conserved mechanism in order to fight infectious agents in our blood, which applies to activated leukocytes, macrophages, and endothelial cells. These ROS also act in a paracrine fashion on cells in the vicinity, which could be vascular smooth muscle cells or cardiomyocytes.

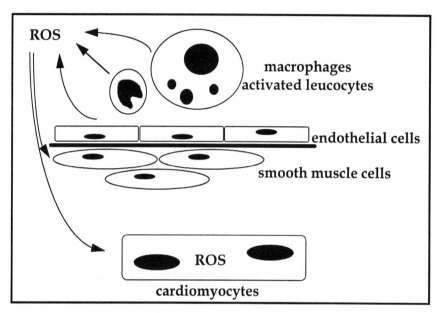

Figure 1 Schematic diagram depicting the origination of ROS relevant to the cardiovascular system. Note, that ROS can act intracellularly as well as extracellularly.

WHY ARE ROS IMPORTANT?

The ubiquitous nature of ROS-generation led to the evolutionary concept of cellular ROS-self-defense systems including several enzymes like superoxide dismutase (SOD 1-3), catalase, or glutathione peroxidase, and molecules like tocopherol, ascorbic acid, retinol, albumin, or bilirubin.

An imbalance between generation and scavenging of ROS causes oxidative stress. The heart is particularly susceptible to such stress due to its high level of energy requirement provided by oxidative phosphorylation, which is reflected by the high concentration of mitochondria in cardiomyocytes.

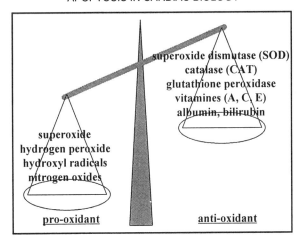

Figure 2 ROS cause cellular dysfunction through the alteration of the intracellular balance between pro-oxidant and anti-oxidant molecules resulting in oxidative stress.

MODE OF ACTION OF ROS

It is known for quite a long time that oxidative stress causes alterations of the structure of cellular components involving lipid peroxidation, protein and enzyme denaturation, and mutagenic damage to nucleic acids. All of this may result in cell death (mainly due to necrosis). However, recent evidence suggests that oxidative stress may directly alter certain cellular functions through its affect on the intracellular redox state. This may lead to a change in DNA-binding activity and/or transactivating activity of redox-sensitive transcription factors leading to a change of gene expression. This may lead to growth responses resulting in proliferation of dividing cells and conceivably in hypertrophy of post-mitotic cells, or the activation of programmed cell death (apoptosis).

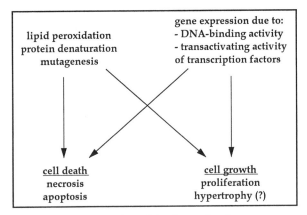

Figure 3 Modes of action of ROS. Note, that cellular damage is only one consequence of exposure to ROS. In contrast, particularly lower doses of intracellularly acting ROS may lead to cellular growth or programmed cell death via the activation of a variety of signaling cascades.

WHAT IS THE RELEVANCE OF ROS TO APOPTOSIS AND CARDIOVASCULAR DISEASES?

There is increasing evidence that most chemical or physical agents inducing apoptosis also evoke oxidative stress: UV-irradiation, γ-radiation, aging, and notably ischemia/reperfusion.

In the heart the generation of ROS during ischemia/reperfusion has been demonstrated unequivocally, which applies to several clinical conditions: angioplasty, thrombolysis, bypass surgery, and heart transplantation. Meanwhile, there is increasing evidence that the generation of ROS has implications for several other cardiovascular diseases including congestive heart failure, arterial hypertension, arteriosclerosis, smoking, and inflammatory processes. In all of these diseases the occurrence of apoptosis has been demonstrated as well. Therefore, ROS mediated apoptosis may affect a variety of cardiovascular diseases in a causative fashion.

ischemia/reperfusion:	angioplasty
	thrombolysis
	bypass surgery
	heart-T_x
congestive heart failure	
hypertension	
arteriosclerosis	
smoking	
inflammation	arteriosclerosis
	myocarditis

Figure 4   List of cardiovascular diseases where the generation of ROS has been demonstrated.

EFFECT OF ROS ON VIABILITY OF CARDIAC CELLS

Taken together, there is enough evidence suggesting that ROS may be important contributors to the development of pathological phenotypes particularly of the heart, but also of the vasculature. Exposure of isolated cardiac cells from neonatal rats to H_2O_2 led to a dose-dependent decrease in cell viability as assessed by MTT-assay (MTT=3-[4,5-dimethyl-thiazol-2-yl] 2,5-diphenyl tetrazolium bromide) (Fig. 5 A). XO plus 0.1 mmol/L xanthine was used to generate O_2^- and again, a dose-dependent decrease in cell viability could be observed (Fig. 5 B). However, since XO/X yields both O_2^- and H_2O_2, the ROS-scavengers superoxide dismutase (SOD), tiron and catalase (CAT) were employed to determine the contribution of each of these ROS in XO/X-induced death of cardiac cells (Fig. 5 C). In the presence of SOD the effect of XO/X on cell viability was partially reversed indicating that the generation of O_2^- contributed to XO/X-induced cell death, a finding which was corroborated by replacing SOD with tiron, a cell membrane permeable scavenger of O_2^-. The presence of CAT had a similar effect on cell viability as SOD. The combination of

CAT with SOD or with tiron resulted in the complete prevention of XO/X-induced cell death.

Taken together, these data suggest that H_2O_2 or O_2^- or both are able to induce death in cardiac cells.

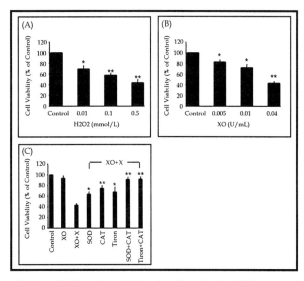

Figure 5 Effect of H_2O_2 or XO/X on the viability of cardiac cells. **A**, MTT-assay, cells were treated for 1 hour with the indicated doses of H_2O_2 plus 0.1 mmol/L $FeSO_4$ and further cultured in ROS-free medium for another 19 hours. **B**, trypan blue exclusion, cells were treated for 1 hour with the indicated doses of XO plus 0.1 mmol/L xanthine and further cultured in ROS-free medium for another 7 hours. **C**, cells were exposed to 0.04 U/ml XO plus 0.1 mmol/L xanthine in the presence of 1000 U/mL superoxide dismutase (SOD), or 500 U/mL catalase (CAT), or 1 mmol/L tiron.

CHARACTERIZATION OF ROS-INDUCED DEATH IN CARDIOMYOCYTES

In order to characterize the death of cardiac cells exposed to ROS, a variety of distinct methods can be employed. Agarose gel electrophoresis revealed that low doses of H_2O_2 or XO/X led to the appearance of a DNA ladder which was replaced by a DNA smear when doses were increased (data not shown). While the latter is a sign of random DNA degradation as occurring during necrotic cell death, the DNA ladder is based on the internucleosomal cleavage of chromosomal DNA by endonucleases as it occurs during the apoptotic type of cell death.

In situ nick-end labeling together with immunofluorescence were employed to further characterize ROS-induced apoptosis. Regarding those cells as apoptotic cardiomyocytes, which simultaneously exhibited positive α-sarcomeric actin staining and TUNEL labeling the amount of apoptotic cells was quantified in cultures exposed to ROS (data not shown). The results show that in contrast to unstimulated control cultures a substantial increase in the percentage of apoptotic cardiomyocytes could be observed when cultures were treated with low doses of H_2O_2. In contrast, the exposure to high doses of H_2O_2 was not associated with a significant number of TUNEL positive cardiomyocytes. Similar results were obtained utilizing low and high doses of XO/X.

Since the TUNEL method and immunofluorescence studies cannot detect apoptotic cells, which as a consequence of their death detach from the surface of the cover slide, a cell death detection ELISA was employed, which specifically detects histone-associated DNA-fragments within the cytoplasmic fraction of stimulated cells and which includes those cells floating in the supernatant of the culture dishes. Additionally, LDH release was assessed as an indicator of cell membrane integrity in order to further differentiate between apoptosis and necrosis.

As can be seen from Fig. 6 A, there was a dose-dependent gradual increase of oligonucleosomes in the cytoplasmic fraction within the lower range of H_2O_2 doses followed by a sharp decline at higher doses of H_2O_2. Moreover, a marked increase in LDH release could be observed when cells were exposed to higher doses of H_2O_2. Similar results were obtained in cells exposed to XO/X (Fig. 6 B). As revealed by the administration of SOD and CAT XO/X-induced DNA fragmentation of cardiomyocytes is triggered by O_2^- or H_2O_2 or both (Fig. 6 C).

Taken together, apoptosis appears to be the predominant form of cell death in cardiomyocytes exposed to low doses of both O_2^- or H_2O_2, whereas signs of necrosis become apparent with higher doses.

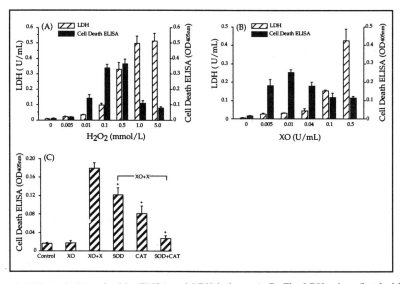

Figure 6 Cell death determined by ELISA and LDH leakage. A, B: The LDH-values (hatched bars) represent the activity of LDH within the culture medium. The histone-associated DNA fragments (black bars) are presented as the optical density at 405 nm. C: Cardiomyocytes were exposed to 0.04 U XO/mL plus 0.1 mmol/L xanthine in the presence of 1000 U/mL superoxide dismutase (SOD) or 500 U/mL catalase (CAT).

EFFECT OF ROS ON CARDIAC FIBROBLASTS

Apoptosis with low doses and necrosis with higher doses: is this a general phenomenon reflecting a stereotyped response of cells exposed to ROS? In order to address this question, cell viability of cardiac fibroblasts exposed to ROS was assessed by trypan blue exclusion. As illustrated in Fig. 7, increasing doses of H_2O_2 led to the induction of cell death. However, as determined by agarose gel electrophoresis and in situ nick-end labeling, there was no evidence showing that H_2O_2 induced death of cardiac fibroblasts occurred by apoptosis (results not shown). XO/X resulted in no apparent reduction of viability of cardiac fibroblasts (Fig. 8 A). In contrast, [^{3}H]-thymidine incorporation and cell counting revealed that XO/X induced proliferation of cardiac fibroblasts (Fig. 8 B and C).

These data indicate that H_2O_2 but not O_2^- causes death of cardiac fibroblasts and that these cells do not undergo apoptosis in response to ROS.

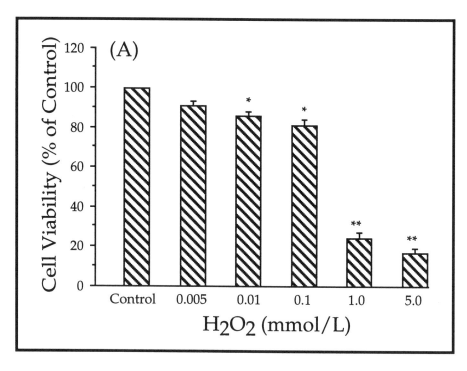

Figure 7 Effect of H_2O_2 on the viability of cardiac fibroblasts assessed by trypan blue exclusion. Cells were treated for 1 hour with different doses of H_2O_2 and further cultured in H_2O_2-free medium for 7 hours. *p<0.05, compared to control.

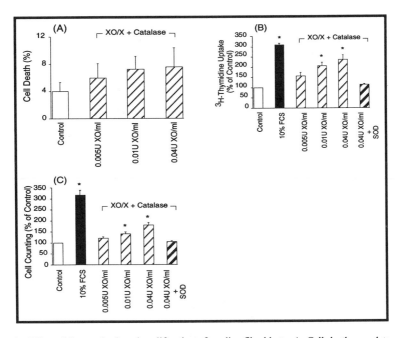

Figure 8 Effect of O_2^- on death and proliferation of cardiac fibroblasts. A: Cell death was determined by trypan blue exclusion after cells were treated for 1 hour with different doses of XO plus 0.1 mM xanthine in the presence of 500 U/ml catalase and further cultured for another 7 hours in the presence of 10% fetal calf serum (FCS). B: [^{3}H]-thymidine incorporation. Cardiac fibroblasts were exposed to different doses of XO plus 0.1 mM xanthine in the presence of 500 U/ml catalase. Superoxide dismutase (SOD) was at 1000 U/ml. Cardiac fibroblasts in 10% FCS served as positive control. *$p<0.05$, compared to control. C: Cell counting. Cell number was counted 6 days after treatment. *$p<0.05$, compared to control.

EFFECT OF ROS ON VASCULAR SMOOTH MUSCLE CELLS

What about vascular smooth muscle cells (VSMCs) and ROS? Although the association between oxidative stress and vascular diseases like hypertension and arteriosclerosis has been demonstrated by a number of investigators, it is yet unclear how ROS contribute to the characteristic vascular phenotype in these instances. Therefore, the effect of ROS on viability of VSMCs was investigated.

A single exposure to H_2O_2 in the presence of 0.1 mmol/L ferrous sulfate resulted in VSMC death in a dose-dependent manner in both growing (10% FCS) and growth-arrested (0.2% FCS) VSMCs isolated from rat aorta (Fig. 9, upper panel). In order to examine, whether H_2O_2 exerts its effect directly or through the formation of hydroxyl radicals ($^{\cdot}$OH) formed by the Fenton reaction, we employed various ROS scavengers (Fig. 9, lower panel). Administration of SOD failed to inhibit H_2O_2 induced cell death.

These data indicate that H_2O_2 induces VSMC death in a dose-dependent manner and exerts its effect predominantly through the formation of $^{\cdot}$OH. Moreover, growth-arrested VSMCs are more susceptible to H_2O_2 treatment than growing VSMCs.

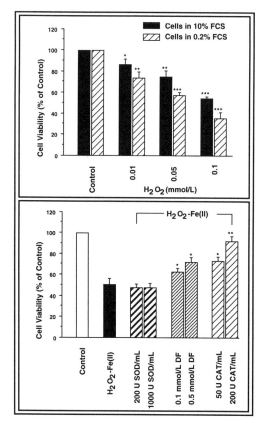

Figure 9 Effect of H_2O_2 on VSMC death analyzed by MTT test. upper panel: Growing (black bars) or growth-arrested (hatched bars) VSMCs were exposed to increasing concentrations of H_2O_2 in the presence of 0.1 mmol/L $FeSO_4$. lower panel: Growing VSMCs were exposed to 0.1 mmol/L H_2O_2 plus 0.1 mmol/L $FeSO_4$ in the presence of superoxide dismutase (SOD), catalase (CAT) or deferoxamine (DF), respectively.

DISTINCT EFFECTS OF O_2^- AND H_2O_2 ON VASCULAR SMOOTH MUSCLE CELLS

A single one hour exposure of growth-arrested VSMCs to XO/X resulted in increases of [^{3}H]-thymidine incorporation (Fig. 10, upper panel) and cell number (Fig. 10, lower panel). Since XO/X yields both O_2^- and H_2O_2, the effect of XO/X in the presence of SOD or CAT was tested. The effect of XO/X was not altered in the presence of CAT. In contrast, the administration of SOD abolished XO/X-induced increases in DNA-synthesis and cell number, resulting in values even below that obtained from unstimulated control cells.

In contrast, three consecutive exposures of growing VSMCs to XO/X conducted every 24 hours led to a gradual and dose-dependent decline of VSMC viability (Fig. 11, upper panel). Interestingly, in growth-arrested VSMCs XO at 0.0025 or 0.005 U/mL continued to induce proliferation after repeated exposures.

REACTIVE OXYGEN SPECIES AND APOPTOSIS

We conclude that XO/X elicits distinct reactions in VSMCs depending on the dose and the frequency of exposure resulting in either proliferation or cell death.

To examine which species of reactive oxygen is responsible for cell death induced by XO/X, SOD and CAT were employed in the treatment of growing VSMCs which were exposed to 0.08 U XO/mL three times (Fig. 11, lower panel). The data show that the administration of SOD augmented cell death after the third exposure to XO/X. This effect of SOD is most likely related to two effects exerted by SOD: the scavenging of O_2^-, which facilitates proliferation rather than death of VSMCs, and an increase in H_2O_2 via SOD-catalyzed dismutation of O_2^-. In contrast, CAT prevented death of VSMCs exposed repeatedly to XO/X.

Taken together, these data suggest that O_2^- and H_2O_2 exert distinct effects on VSMCs with O_2^--inducing proliferation and H_2O_2 triggering cell death.

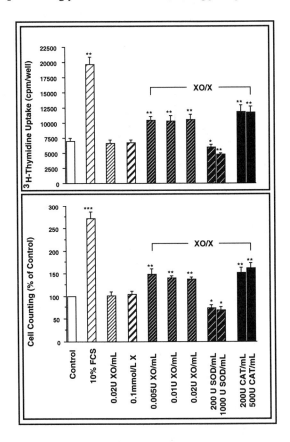

Figure 10 Effect of XO/X on growth-arrested VSMCs. upper panel: [^{3}H]-thymidine incorporation. lower panel: cell counting. VSMCs were exposed to XO in the presence of 0.1 mmol/L xanthine. XO was 0.01 U/mL when superoxide dismutase (SOD) and catalase (CAT) were administrated. VSMCs in 10% fetal calf serum (FCS) served as positive control.

49

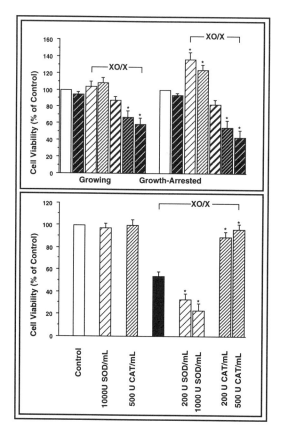

Figure 11 Effect of three exposures to XO/X on VSMCs death assessed by trypan blue exclusion. Cell viability was determined 24 hours after the third exposure to XO/X. **upper panel:** Cell viability of growing and growth-arrested VSMCs exposed to increasing concentrations of XO in the presence of 0.1 mmol/L xanthine. **lower panel:** Effect of antioxidants on viability of growing VSMC exposed to 0.08U XO/mL plus 0.1 mmol/L xanthine.

VSMC DEATH CAUSED BY XO/X OR H_2O_2 OCCURS BY APOPTOSIS

We next determined the nature of VSMC death induced by XO/X and H2O2. The DNA-pattern of growing VSMCs revealed no difference between untreated VSMCs and VSMCs treated once with 0.08 U XO/mL (data not shown). However, a typical "DNA ladder" became evident after the third exposure to 0.08 U XO/mL (data not shown). Additionally, a gradual increase in the formation of the "DNA-ladder" could be obtained by increasing doses of H2O2 (data not shown). Identical results were obtained with growth-arrested VSMCs (data not shown).

Propidium iodide DNA staining was employed together with in situ nick-end labeling (TUNEL method) to characterize apoptosis. Untreated growing VSMCs appear with relatively large and regularly shaped nuclei stained by propidium iodide without being positively labeled by TUNEL. However, condensed and TUNEL-positive nuclei were observed in growing VSMCs 8 hours after the third exposure to

0.08 U XO/mL plus 0.1 mmol/L xanthine (data not shown) and after exposure to 0.1 mmol/L H_2O_2 plus 0.1 mmol/L $FeSO_4$ (data not shown).

The data of the cell death ELISA show that exposure to either XO/X (Fig. 12, left hand side, upper panel) or H_2O_2 (Fig. 12, left hand side, lower panel) led to increases in histone-associated DNA fragments within the cytoplasmic fraction of growing VSMCs as well as growth-arrested VSMCs. The levels of histone-associated DNA fragments were noticeably higher in growth-arrested VSMCs than in growing VSMCs after exposure to H_2O_2 or XO/X. This indicates that growth-arrested VSMCs are more susceptible to ROS-induced apoptosis than growing VSMCs.

Taken together, all these criteria characterizing apoptosis suggest that cell death caused by H_2O_2 or XO/X occurs by apoptosis.

We conclude that there is a great variety of very different cellular responses to ROS involving necrosis or apoptotic death or cell proliferation largely depending on the radical species, the dose, and the affected cell type.

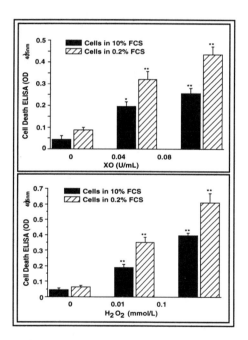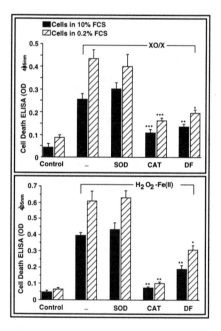

Figure 12 Cell death ELISA determination of the histone-associated DNA fragmentation in VSMCs exposed to XO/X or H_2O_2. **Left hand side:** growing (black bars) or growth-arrested (hatched bars) VSMCs were exposed to increasing concentrations of XO plus 0.1 mmol/L xanthine (upper panel) or to H_2O_2 plus 0.1 mmol/L $FeSO_4$ (lower panel). The ELISA detections were processed 8 hours after the third exposure to XO/X or after treatment with H_2O_2. The histone-associated DNA fragments are presented as the optical density at 405 nm. **Right hand side:** effect of antioxidants on the formation of the histone-associated DNA fragmentation in VSMCs. Superoxide dismutase (SOD) was 1000 U/mL, catalase (CAT) was 500 U/mL, deferoxamine (DF) was 0.5 mmol/L. VSMCs were exposed to **A:** 0.08 U XO/mL in the presence of 0.1 mmol/L xanthine or to **B:** 0.1 mmol/L H_2O_2 in the presence of 0.1 mmol/L $FeSO_4$.

EFFECT OF ROS ON EXPRESSION OF APOPTOSIS-RELATED FACTORS IN CARDIOMYOCYTES

Now, the question is why do we see such different responses? What is the molecular basis for this behavior. Certainly, it has to do with the intracellular signaling cascade activated by ROS.

The induction of apoptosis is associated with the expression and/or activation of specific proteins resulting in the execution of the apoptotic program within the affected cells. In general, there is a plethora of different signaling pathways possible to be involved in apoptosis depending on the stimulus and/or type of cells affected. In order to specify the signaling pathway in ROS-induced apoptosis in cardiomyocytes, we first determined the protein levels of well known apoptosis related factors like Bcl-2, Bax, Bad and p53 (Fig. 13).

Cardiomyocytes were treated with H_2O_2 or XO/X plus CAT to yield O_2^-. Both H_2O_2 and O_2^- induced the expression of p53 which was apparent already 1 to 2 hours after treatment. However, H_2O_2, but not O_2^- was able to induce the expression of Bad. Surprisingly, neither H_2O_2, nor O_2^- led to detectable changes in protein levels of Bcl-2 or Bax throughout the investigated time interval of 8 hours.

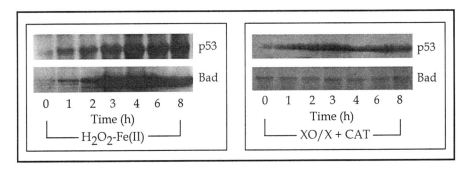

Figure 13 Western blot analysis of p53 and Bad expression in cardiomyocytes exposed to 0.1 mmol/L H_2O_2 plus 0.1 mmol/L $FeSO_4$ or 0.04 U/ml XO plus 0.1 mmol/L xanthine in the presence of 500 U/ml CAT. Cells were treated for 1 hour and further cultured in normal culture medium until the indicated time.

DIFFERENTIAL EFFECT OF H_2O_2 AND O_2^- ON CYTOCHROME C RELEASE AND CASPASE ACTIVATION

Since increasing evidence has recently indicated an important role of mitochondrial cytochrome c release and subsequent CPP32 activation for the execution of apoptosis in a number of different cell types, we next determined the distribution of cytochrome c in cardiomyocytes stimulated with either H_2O_2 or O_2^- (Fig. 14).

At 1-2 hours after exposure to H_2O_2 cytochrome c appeared in the cytosol of cultured cardiomyocytes. In order to exclude the possibility of a significant contamination of our cytosolic fraction with mitochondria, we reprobed our blots with an antibody directed against mitochondrial cytochrome oxidase. Cytochrome oxidase was nearly undetectable throughout the investigated time interval. Release of cytochrome c may lead to the activation of CPP32 (caspase 3), which can be detected by its cleavage from the inactive pro-CPP32 to the active 17 kDa product as we observed it at 3 hours after exposure to H_2O_2. A 85 kDa fragment of PARP also indicating CPP32 activation became visible at 3 hours after H_2O_2 treatment.

These data indicate, that mitochondrial release of cytochrome c with subsequent activation of caspase CPP32 are involved in H_2O_2-induced cardiomyocyte apoptosis.

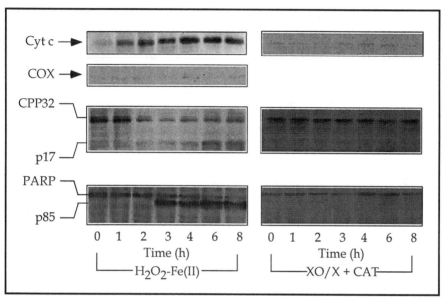

Figure 14 Involvement of cytochrome c release and CPP32 activation in ROS-induced apoptosis. Depicted are levels of cytochrome c (cyt c) and cytochrome oxidase (cox) in cytosolic fractions, CPP32 activation and PARP cleavage as detected by immunoblot analysis. Cardiomyocyte cultures were exposed to 0.1 mmol/L H_2O_2 plus 0.1 mmol/L $FeSO_4$ or to 0.04 U/ml XO plus 0.1 mmol/L xanthine in the presence of 500 U/ml CAT. Cells were treated for 1 hour and further cultured in normal culture medium until the indicated time.

Intriguingly, O_2^--induced cardiomyocyte apoptosis was not accompanied by the release of cytochrome c, activation of CPP32 and cleavage of PARP. However, Z-VAD-fmk, a pan-caspase inhibitor, could significantly inhibit O_2^--induced histone-associated DNA fragmentation (Fig. 15 A). This indicates that O_2^- utilizes caspase pathways other than CPP32 to induce apoptosis in cardiomyocytes. Using anti-Mch2α (caspase 6) antibody revealed that Mch2α was activated as indicated by the formation of p20, the active form of Mch2α, 2 hours after stimulation of cardiomyocytes with XO/X plus CAT (Fig. 15 B). At the same time point lamin A, which is a substrate of Mch2a, was cleaved into a 46 kDa fragment in cardiomyocytes treated with XO/X plus CAT (Fig. 15 C). Z-VAD-fmk could inhibit Mch2α processing, thereby preventing the cleavage of lamin A. In addition, treatment with tiron prevented Mch2α activation and lamin A cleavage.

Thus, it appears that O_2^- utilizes Mch2α to promote the apoptotic pathway involving the cleavage of lamin A.

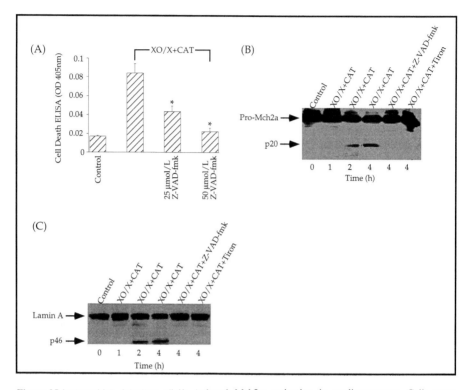

Figure 15 Immunoblot detection of O_2^--induced Mch2α activation in cardiomyocytes. Cells were exposed to 0.04 U XO/mL plus 0.1 mmol/L xanthine in the presence of 500 U/mL. **A**, DNA fragmentation was assessed by Cell Death ELISA. Z-VAD-fmk was added at the indicated doses 2 hours before and immediately after treatment. **B**, immunoblot analysis of Mch2α and its active form p20, and **C**, of lamin A and its cleavage product p46, tiron was at 1 mmol/L, Z-VAD-fmk was at 50 μmol/L.

H_2O_2 INDUCES TRANSLOCATION OF BAX AND BAD FROM CYTOSOL TO MITOCHONDRIA AND THEIR INTERACTION WITH BCL-2

We prepared subcellular fractions before and after treatment with ROS containing either cytosol, or mitochondria enriched heavy membranes (HM), or light membranes (LM). The subcellular localization of Bad, Bax and Bcl-2 all of which are known to be involved in the regulation of cytochrome c release from mitochondria in apoptosis was determined (Fig. 16). Before H_2O_2 treatment, Bad and Bax were found predominantly in the cytosolic fractions with only faint signals in mitochondria-enriched HM, and were undetectable in LM. At 1 hour after H_2O_2 treatment, both Bad and Bax translocated from the cytosol to HM, but not to LM. Before and after H_2O_2 treatment, Bcl-2 could be observed only in HM, but not in the cytosolic or LM fractions. In contrast to H_2O_2, O_2^- did not change the subcellular localization patterns of Bad, Bax or Bcl-2 (data not shown).

In order to determine, whether the translocation of Bad and Bax to the mitochondria involves the interaction of these two factors with Bcl-2, a factor which has been shown to inhibit apoptosis by preventing cytochrome c release immunoprecipitates of Bad or Bax were blotted against an anti-Bcl-2 antibody (Fig. 16). Both Bad and Bax appeared in Bcl-2 complexes in cardiomyocytes at 1 hour after stimulation with H_2O_2. As expected, no dimerization could be observed in cardiomyocytes stimulated by O_2^- (data not shown).

These data indicate that cytochrome c release in cardiomyocytes exposed to H_2O_2 is paralleled by the translocation of Bad and Bax from the cytosol to the mitochondria where they form heterodimers with the anti-apoptotic Bcl-2 suggesting a functional role of these two factors in apoptosis-related cytochrome c release. The lack of their translocation to the mitochondria in O_2^--induced apoptosis may explain why we could not observe cytochrome c release in O_2^--stimulated cardiomyocytes. The effect of ROS on apoptotic signaling in cardiomyocytes is summarized in Fig. 17.

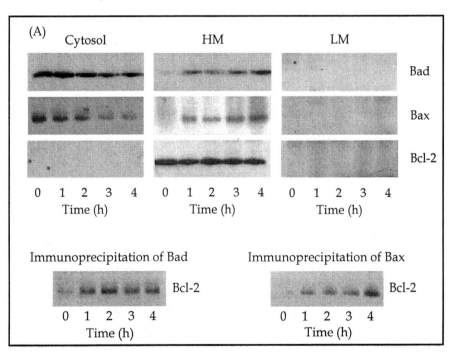

Figure 16 Subcellular distribution of Bad, Bax, and Bcl-2 and the interaction of Bad or Bax with Bcl-2 in cardiomyocytes treated for 1 hour with 0.1 mmol/L H_2O_2 plus 0.1 mmol/L $FeSO_4$ and further cultured in normal culture medium until the indicated time. Following preparations of subcellular fractions Bad, Bax, and Bcl-2 were immunoprecipitated by their specific antibodies and then subjected to SDS-PAGE for immunoblot detection. Immunoprecipitations of Bad or Bax were carried out in heavy membrane fractions and the immunoprecipitated samples were analyzed by immunoblot with anti-Bcl-2 antibody.

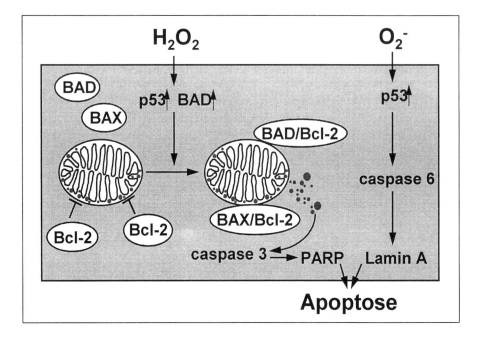

Figure 17 Schematic diagram of the effect of ROS on apoptotic signaling in cardiomyocytes.

MODEL OF FUNCTION OF ROS IN CARDIOVASCULAR CELLS

I would like to end this chapter by outlining a simplified model of function of ROS on cardiomyocytes and probably VSMCs (Fig. 18).

ROS are produced by activated blood cells and endothelial cells and released into the extracellular environment acting in a paracrine fashion on target cells like VSMCs or cardiomyocytes. There they diffuse into the cell or directly stimulate other second messenger systems. Depending on the reactive oxygen species, the dose, and the type of the target cell they elicit distinct intracellular pathways resulting in different cellular responses including programmed cell death and proliferation and thus are able to modulate the phenotype of the affected organ system through multiple pathways.

Additionally, ROS may serve as an independent second messenger system where they are involved in signal transduction leading to cell death or cell proliferation. In this case ROS are generated intracellularly usually as a consequence of stimulation by growth signals (hormones or physical stress). This may involve the production of ROS by membrane bound oxidases or an increased mitochondrial respiration.

Therefore, we have to understand that ROS are important contributors to the development of pathological phenotypes in the heart as well as in the vasculature by acting through multiple pathways.

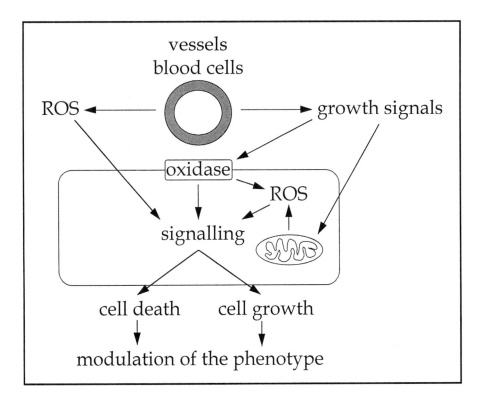

Figure 18 Model of action of ROS on cardiovascular cells.

References

1. Kajstura J, Mansukhani M, Cheng W, Reiss K, Krajewski S, Reed JC, Quaini F, Sonnenblick EH, Anversa P. Programmed cell death and expression of the protooncogene bcl-2 in myocytes during postnatal maturation of the heart. *Exp Cell Res*. 1995;219:110-121.
2. James TN. Normal and abnormal consequences of apoptosis in the human heart. From postnatal morphogenesis to paroxysmal arrhythmias. *Circulation*. 1994;90:556-573.
3. Kajstura J, Cheng W, Reiss K, Clark WA, Sonnenblick EH, Krajewski S, Reed JC, Olivetti G, Anversa P. Apoptotic and necrotic myocyte cell deaths are independent contributing variables of infarct size in rats. *Lab Invest*. 1996;74:86-107.
4. Itoh G, Tamura J, Suzuki M, Suzuki Y, Ikeda H, Koike M, Nomura M, Jie T, Ito K. DNA fragmentation of human infarcted myocardial cells demonstrated by the nick end labeling method and DNA agarose gel electrophoresis. *Am J Pathol*. 1995;146:1325-1331.
5. Mallat Z, Tedgui A, Fontaliran F, Frank R, Durigon M, Fontaine G. Evidence of apoptosis in arrhythmogenic right ventricular dysplasia. *N Engl J Med*. 1996;335:1190-1196.
6. Narula J, Haider N, Virmani R, DiSalvo T, Kolodgie F, Hajjar R, Schmidt U, Semigran M, Dec G, Khaw B. Apoptosis in myocytes in end-stage heart failure. *N Engl J Med*. 1996;335:1182-1189.
7. Gottlieb RA, Burleson KO, Kloner RA, Babior BM, Engler RL. Reperfusion injury induces apoptosis in rabbit cardiomyocytes. *J Clin Invest*. 1994;94:1621-1628.
8. Zweier JL, Flaherty JT, Weisfeldt ML. Direct measurement of free radical generation following reperfusion of ischemic myocardium. *Proc Natl Acad Sci U S A*. 1987;84:1404-1407.
9. Krukenkamp IB, Burns P, Caldarone C, Levitsky S. Perfusion and cardioplegia. *Curr Opin Cardiol*. 1994;9:247-253.

10. Davies SW, Ranjadayalan K, Wickens DG, Dormandy TL, Timmis AD. Lipid peroxidation associated with successful thrombolysis. *Lancet.* 1990;335:741-743.
11. Roberts MJ, Young IS, Trouton TG, Trimble ER, Khan MM, Webb SW, Wilson CM, Patterson GC, Adgey AA. Transient release of lipid peroxides after coronary artery balloon angioplasty. *Lancet.* 1990;336:143-145.
12. Li Y, Huang TT, Carlson EJ, Melov S, Ursell PC, Olson JL, Noble LJ, Yoshimura MP, Berger C, Chan PH, Wallace DC, Epstein CJ. Dilated cardiomyopathy and neonatal lethality in mutant mice lacking manganese superoxide dismutase. *Nat Genet.* 1995;11:376-381.
13. Ferns GA, Forster L, Stewart Lee A, Konneh M, Nourooz Zadeh J, Anggard EE. Probucol inhibits neointimal thickening and macrophage accumulation after balloon injury in the cholesterol-fed rabbit. *Proc Natl Acad Sci U S A.* 1992;89:11312-11316.
14. Konneh MK, Rutherford C, Li SR, Anggard EE, Ferns GA. Vitamin E inhibits the intimal response to balloon catheter injury in the carotid artery of the cholesterol-fed rat. *Atherosclerosis.* 1995;113:29-39.
15. Rao GN, Berk BC. Active oxygen species stimulate vascular smooth muscle cell growth and proto-oncogene expression. *Circ Res.* 1992;70:593-599.
16. Baas AS, Berk BC. Differential activation of mitogen-activated protein kinases by H2O2 and O2- in vascular smooth muscle cells. *Circ Res.* 1995;77:29-36.
17. Isner JM, Kearney M, Bortman S, Passeri J. Apoptosis in human atherosclerosis and restenosis [see comments]. *Circulation.* 1995;91:2703-2711.
18. Geng YJ, Libby P. Evidence for apoptosis in advanced human atheroma. Colocalization with interleukin-1 beta-converting enzyme. *Am J Pathol.* 1995;147:251-266.
19. Han DK, Haudenschild CC, Hong MK, Tinkle BT, Leon MB, Liau G. Evidence for apoptosis in human atherogenesis and in a rat vascular injury model. *Am J Pathol.* 1995;147:267-277.
20. Hamet P, Richard L, Dam TV, Teiger E, Orlov SN, Gaboury L, Gossard F, Tremblay J. Apoptosis in target organs of hypertension. *Hypertension.* 1995;26:642-648.
21. Bochaton Piallat ML, Gabbiani F, Redard M, Desmouliere A, Gabbiani G. Apoptosis participates in cellularity regulation during rat aortic intimal thickening. *Am J Pathol.* 1995;146:1059-1064.
22. Geng YJ, Wu Q, Muszynski M, Hansson GK, Libby P. Apoptosis of vascular smooth muscle cells induced by in vitro stimulation with interferon-gamma, tumor necrosis factor-alpha, and interleukin-1 beta. *Arterioscler Thromb Vasc Biol.* 1996;16:19-27.
23. Bennett MR, Evan GI, Schwartz SM. Apoptosis of human vascular smooth muscle cells derived from normal vessels and coronary atherosclerotic plaques. *J Clin Invest.* 1995;95:2266-2274.
24. Jamieson D. Oxygen toxicity and reactive oxygen metabolites in mammals. *Free Radic Biol Med.* 1989;7:87-108.
25. Kehrer JP. Free radicals as mediators of tissue injury and disease. *Crit Rev Toxicol.* 1993;23:21-48.
26. von Harsdorf R, Li PF, Dietz R. Signaling pathways in reactive oxygen species-induced cardiomyocyte apoptosis. *Circulation.* 1999;99:2934-2941.
27. Li PF, Dietz R, von Harsdorf R. Superoxide induces apoptosis in cardiomyocytes, but proliferation and expression of transforming growth factor-ß1 in cardiac fibroblasts. *FEBS lett.* 1999;448:206-210.
28. Li PF, Dietz R, von Harsdorf R. Reactive oxygen species induce apoptosis of vascular smooth muscle cell. *FEBS Lett.* 1997;404:249-252.
29. Li PF, Dietz R, von Harsdorf R. Differential effect of hydrogen peroxide and superoxide anion on apoptosis and proliferation of vascular smooth muscle cells. *Circulation.* 1997;96:3602-3609.
30. Li PF, Dietz R, von Harsdorf R. Requirement for protein kinases C in reactive oxygen species-induced apoptosis of vascular smooth muscle cells. *Circulation.* 1999;100:in press.

I.2
The mediators of apoptosis

I.2.1
Oncogenes and p53

Franz Kohlhuber, Ph.D., and Dirk Eick, Ph.D.

GSF-Forschungszentrum, München, Germany

INTRODUCTION

The tumor suppressor gene p53 plays a major role in cellular stress response and has been found to be mutated or deleted in more than half of all human tumors. Many signal pathways and factors contribute to control the action of p53. Here we will focus on the control function of p53 after cell cycle activation by oncogenes.

VIRAL ONCOGENES IN CELLULAR TRANSFORMATION

Proliferation, cell cycle arrest, and cell death are central processes in the development and homeostasis of multicellular organisms. Deregulation of these three processes may induce neoplastic diseases e.g. as the result of activation of oncogenes and inactivation of tumor suppressor genes. The large tumor antigen (LT) of simian virus 40 (SV40) has served as paradigm for the study of cell transformation by viral oncogenes. We will use LT to describe how research on viral oncogenes helped during the last two decades to unravel major mechanisms of cell transformation. LT together with the gene products of several other DNA tumor viruses (adenoviruses, papilloma viruses) have been of incredible value for the identification of the cellular factors involved in the process of cell transformation. In fact, p53 has been described first in 1979 as cellular binding factor of LT (1). A decade later it became evident that the gene product of the retinoblastoma tumor suppressor (Rb) gene binds with its pocket motif to LT which thereby inactivates Rb's cell cycle regulatory function (2). Several additional cellular binding factors for LT have been described in the past, e.g. the transcriptional co-activators p300 and CBP, which display acetyltransferases activity. The binding and inactivation of p53 and Rb by LT, however, turned out to be of fundamental importance for LT's oncogenic activity (3).

Growth arrest and differentiation of cells is the basis for the development of multi-cellular organisms. In addition, the development and maintance of multi-cellular organisms also require the programmed elimination of cells. In cancer research, the regulation of cell proliferation has been a central theme from the beginning. Programmed cell death, termed apoptosis, came into focus only in the recent years. Apoptosis occurs through an evolutionarily conserved programme for cell suicide. The characteristic, morphological changes associated with apoptosis include cellular shrinkage, internucleosomal degradation of chromatin, and fragmentation of the cells into apoptotic bodies, which are phagocytosed by macrophages and other surrounding cells without eliciting an inflammatory response (4,5). It is now evident that organisms use apoptosis not only to eliminate cells during development and to maintain homeostasis. Cells also undergo apoptosis after viral infection and after activation of cellular oncogenes. In mammalian cells, p53 turned out to play a central role in the regulation of apoptosis after viral infection and activation of cellular proto-oncogenes (6-11).

ACTIVATION OF THE CELL CYCLE

In adult vertebrates, most cells are kept in a quiescent state. In the few proliferating cells, the cell cycle is driven by the periodic activation of cyclin-dependent kinases (CDKs) which phosphorylate proteins regulating the transition between the different cell cycle phases (Figure 1). Key regulators of the cell cycle are the pocket proteins Rb, and the related proteins P107 and P130, which have an inhibitory effect on G1/S progression. Hyper-phosphorylation of pocket proteins by CDKs dissociates complexes of these pocket proteins with various species of the E2F transcription factor family. Members of the E2F family can drive cell cycle progression by activating a variety of genes required for S phase entry, e.g. the genes encoding dehydrofolate reductase, thymidylate synthetase, and DNA polymerase a (12-14). All these enzymes are not only required for replication of the cellular genome but also of the viral genome in SV40 infected cells. Since propagation of SV40 and other DNA tumor viruses depend on the activity of these enzymes, these viruses encounter a serious problem, if they infect a quiescent cell. In fact, cell cycle arrest is a major barrier for viral multiplication, and some viruses, e.g. retroviruses, are unable to multiply after infecting quiescent cells. In contrast, DNA tumour viruses can multiply after infecting quiescent cells because they have the ablity to activate the cell cycle by specific viral gene products. In the case of SV40, this product is LT. LT binds and inactivates Rb as well as other pocket proteins, thereby liberating and activating E2F (2,15).

In normal cells, phosphorylation of Rb by cyclin dependent kinases leads to inactivation of Rb and defines a particular restriction point of cell cycle control in G1 phase. The finding that LT and other DNA tumour viruses have evolved mechanisms to activate E2F by targeting Rb and other pocket proteins underscores E2F's central role in cell cycle activation.

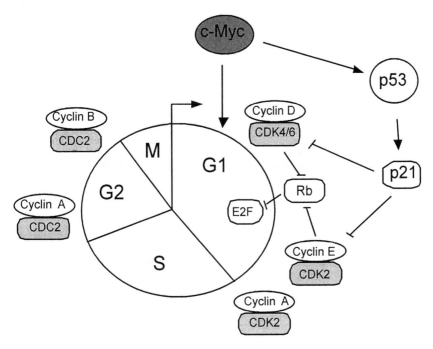

Figure 1 Important players of cell cycle regulation. Complexes of cyclins and cyclin-dependent kinases (CDK) are formed and drive the entry into the different phases of the cell cycle. The activity of these complexes are controlled by CDK phosphorylation and specific inhibitors, e.g. p21. Expression of p21 is inducible by p53. Activation of the cell cycle by Myc in serum-starved fibroblasts leads to expression of cyclins and activation of CDKs. Myc also induces high levels of p53 protein and thereby p21. However, p21 is unable to inhibit CDK activity upon Myc activation. The activation of CDK4/6 and CDK2 leads to phosphorylation and inhibition of Rb thereby liberating and activating E2F from Rb/E2F complexes.

UNSCHEDULED ACTIVATION OF THE CELL CYCLE INDUCES APOPTOSIS

During evolution, activation of the cell cycle by viral infection must have been a continuous problem for multicellular organisms. A major defence mechanism against viral infection, which has been evoved by vertebrates is to recognize the aberrant activation of the cell cycle by viral proteins and to induce apoptosis in infected cells. There is evidence that an infected cell can distinguish between cell cycle activation by growth factors and viral proteins. Activation of the cell cycle by LT and other viral proteins appears to be recognized as foreign and, as a consequence, the cell eliminates itself by apoptosis (Figure 2).

How do cells recognize cell cycle activation by viral proteins, if normal and virally-induced signalling of proliferation involves the same cellular factors? Proliferation signals, as produced by growth factor, are probably complex and split into cell cycle activating and apoptosis inhibiting components. Thus, viruses are faced with two problems after infecting quiescent cells. They must activate the cell cycle and, after activation, must prevent that the infected cells undergo apoptosis, before the virus is multiplied. Among the viral oncoproteins LT appears to be unique. LT combines in a single protein the ability for cell cycle activaton and for inhibition of apoptosis. In quiescent mouse fibroblasts, LT activates the cell cycle by inhibiting the function of Rb, and prevents apoptosis by binding and inactivation of p53 (19,20) (Figure 2).

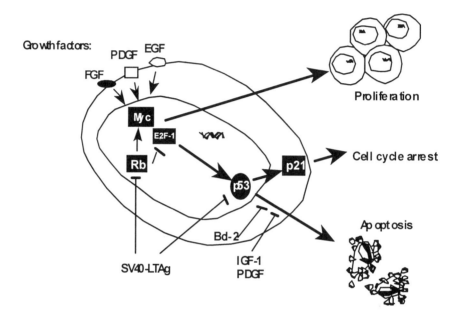

Figure 2 Cell cycle activation by viral oncogenes. Binding to Rb in serum-straved fibroblasts by SV40-LT leads to inactivation of Rb. As consequence, Myc and E2F-1, which are normally under the control of growth factors, activate the cell cycle and induce cell proliferation. Myc and E2F-1 also induce high p53 protein levels. In the absence of survival factors, e.g. IGF-1 and Bcl-2 (16-18), p53 induces apoptosis. Apoptosis is prevented by binding and inactivation of p53 by LT.

The finding that induction of apoptosis in virally infected cells requires the function of p53 suggested that p53 might fulfill a similar task, if the cell cycle is activated in quiescent cells by other mechanisms, e.g. by of activation of cellular proto-oncogenes, or inactivation of tumor-suppressor genes (19). Viruses play also a significant role in heart disease. The extent to which apoptosis contributes to myocyte cell loss during acute carditic viral infection is unknown. First results indicate that despite marked inflammatory activity, myocyte apoptosis is rare in acute coxsackievirus-induced myocarditis in mice (21). There is also no evidence for p53-dependent myocyte apoptosis during acute myocardial infarction in the mouse (22).

p53 MEDIATES MYC INDUCED APOPTOSIS

The linkage of apoptosis to aberrant cell cycle activation is not only a defence mechanism against viral infection. Cells can also undergo apoptosis if the cell cycle is erroneously driven by activated cellular oncogenes. Many of the known proto-oncogenes, e.g. *Ras*, are components of signal transduction pathways which induce proliferation. After conversion to oncogenes, some of these genes are able to activate the cell cycle even in the absence of other growth signals. For example, activation of cellular the proto-oncogene *Myc* in quiescent fibroblasts induces cell cycle re-entry (23). Simultaneously, *Myc* induces apoptosis (24), which is mediated by p53 (25,26). Recent evidence suggests that the Myc protein induces cell cycle progression by antagonizing CDK-inhibitors (28-29), which finally leads to activation of E2F. Consistent with this Myc function, the induction of cell cycle progression after expression of E2F-1 in serum-starved cells is accompanied by p53-mediated apoptosis (14).

p53

p53 is a 393- amino acid protein with major domains characterized as transcriptional activation domain (TAD), proline-rich domain (PRD), DNA-binding domain (DBD), nuclear localization domain (NLS), and carboxy-terminal domain (CTD) (Figure 3). The TAD is also the region where Mdm2 binds. PRD has been described as negative regulatory domain. The DBD is the site where most of the mutations in p53 has been detected. Almost all of these mutations abolishes DNA-binding of p53. DBD is also the domain where large T antigen (LT) binds. The CTD is the region of major allosteric regulation of p53 function and contains sequences necessary for dimerization and tetradimerization. Various serin residues in the TAD are phosphorylated. Serin 15 is phosphorylated by the ATM kinase (the gene mutated in ataxia-telangiectasia patients) upon ionizing radiation. ATM patient are largely deficient in G1-arrest upon ionizing radiation explaining their high radiation sensitivity. Beside the ATM kinase, p53 is phosphorylated by a number of additional kinases including casein kinase I, CDK7, and Pkc. Dephosphorylation of p53 by phosphatases 1 and 2a has also been reported (9,30).

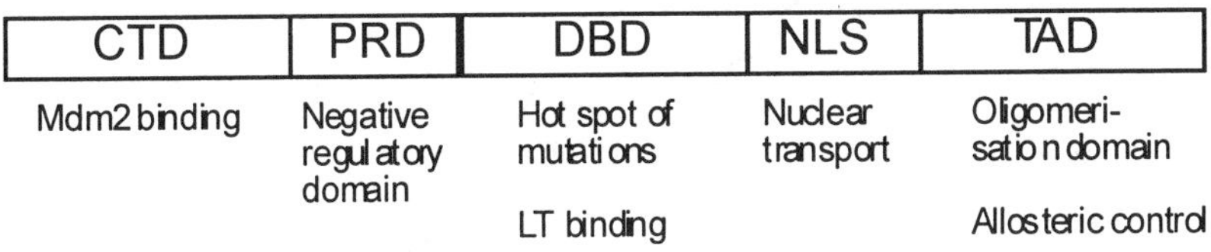

CTD	PRD	DBD	NLS	TAD
Mdm2 binding	Negative regulatory domain	Hot spot of mutations	Nuclear transport	Oligomeri-sation domain
		LT binding		Allosteric control

Figure 3 Structure of the p53 protein. For details see text.

DIFFERENT PATHWAYS ACTIVATE p53

A wide variety of genotoxic and nongenotoxic stimuli induce p53 protein and its activity in cells. Some mechanisms of p53 induction are shared, others are unique. Ionizing and UV radiation, hypoxia, oxidative stress, cell adhesion, nucleotide triphospate depletion and activation of oncogenes, all represent p53 inducing signals (9). Depending on the cellular context these signals can lead to G1 arrest, apoptosis, or differentiation of cells. Here we focus on those signals that induce p53 after activation of oncogenes. Recent evidence indicate that the Ink4a-ARF locus plays an essential role in signalling to p53 (10,11,29-39). The locus encodes p16(Ink4a) and p19(ARF) and is among the most frequently mutated tumor suppressor loci in human cancer. Recent results also showed that the establishment of primary mouse embryo fibroblasts (MEFs) as continuously growing cell lines is normally accompanied by loss of the p53 or p19-ARF, suggesting that both factors may act in a common biochemical pathway (38). Further studies showed that Myc rapidly activates p19-ARF and p53 gene expression in primary MEFs and triggers replicative crisis by inducing apoptosis (11). MEFs that survive Myc overexpression sustain p53 mutation or ARF loss during the process of establishment and become immortal. MEFs lacking p19-ARF or p53 exhibit an attenuated apoptotic response to Myc and rapidly give rise to cell lines that proliferate in chemically defined medium lacking serum. Where can p19-ARF be placed in the signal cascade relatively to Myc and p53? P19-ARF potently suppresses oncogenic transformation in primary cells and this function is abrogated when p53 is neutralized by viral oncoproteins and dominant-negative mutants but not by the p53 antagonist Mdm2. This finding, coupled with the observations that p19-ARF and Mdm2 physically interact (34,36,39) and that p19-ARF blocks Mdm2-induced p53 degradation, suggests that p19-ARF functions mechanistically to prevent Mdm's neutralization of p53 (Figure 4).

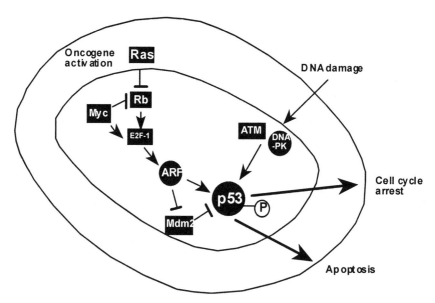

Figure 4 Two important pathways of p53 activation. The Ras and Myc oncogenes can activate the ARF gene expression via E2F-1 activation. ARF controls the stability of p53 by binding and inactivation of Mdm2. Alternatively, p53 is stabilzed after phosphorylation of its amino-terminal domain by the ATM and DNA-PK after irradiation caused DNA damage.

In addition, Mdm2 has a ubiquitin ligase activity for the tumor suppressor p53 protein (33). The binding of Mdm2 to p53 is essential for ubiquitination, but p53's tertiary structure and/or c-terminal region may also be important for this reaction. DNA-dependent protein kinase (DNA-PK) and ATM are known to phosphorylate p53 on Mdm2-binding sites, where DNA damage induces phosphorylation. P53 phosphorylated by these kinases is not a good substrate for Mdm2. This suggests that DNA damage-induced phosphorylation stabilizes p53 by inhibiting its ubiquitination by Mdm2. Similarly, p19-ARF affects the ubiquitin ligase activity of Mdm2 for p53 (33). The ubiquitin ligase activity of p19-ARF-bound Mdm2 was found to be lower than that of free Mdm2, suggesting that p19-ARF promotes the stabilization of p53 by inactivating Mdm2. P19-ARF induction has recently also been shown to be involved in the induction of apoptosis after expression of the oncogene abl (37). How does activation of oncogenes lead to induction of p19-ARF? Recent findings indicate that transcription of the p19-ARF gene is directly activated by E2F-1 (31).

DOWNSTREAM EFFECTORS OF p53

Three different pathways of apoptotic signalling in mammalian cells have been emerged. The best established apoptosis pathway involves signalling by the cell surface death receptors such as TNF and Fas, which through adapter molecules can recruit and activate caspases. A second pathway is initiated by the withdrawal of growth factors and is regulated by the Bcl-2 family of proteins. This pathway results in cytochrom c release from mitochondria and triggering of the caspase cascade. The third and least well characterized pathway is initiated by DNA damage or oncogene activation and involves often p53. How this pathway results in activation of the caspase cascade is not known. In all three cases of these pathways of cell death, caspases and Bcl-2 play a key role in regulation and execution of apoptosis. The disturbances of cellular metabolism imposed by starvation, viral infection, toxins, DNA damage or other signals, results in mitochondrial membran release of cytochrome c and activation of downstream caspases for reviews see (6,7). It appears that many of these signals are first integrated by p53 and then directed to the machinery exicuting apotosis.

References

1. Lane, DP, Crawford, LV. T antigen is bound to a host protein in SV40-transformed cells. Nature 1979; 278:261-3.
2. DeCaprio JA, Ludlow JW, Figge J, Shew JY, Huang CM, Lee WH, Marsilio E, Paucha E, Livingston DM. SV40 large tumor antigen forms a specific complex with the product of the retinoblastoma susceptibility gene. Cell 1988; 54:275-83.
3. Fanning E, Knippers R. Structure and function of simian virus 40 large tumor antigen. Annu Rev Biochem 1992; 61:55-85.
4. Kerr JF, Wyllie AH, Currie AR. Apoptosis: a basic biological phenomenon with wide-ranging implications in tissue kinetics. Br J Cancer 1972; 26:239-57.
5. Wyllie AH. Apoptosis and carcinogenesis. Eur J Cell Biol 1997; 73:189-97.
6. Ding HF, Fisher DE. Mechanisms of p53-mediated apoptosis. Crit Rev Oncog 1998; 9:83-98.

7. Dragovich T, Rudin CM, Thompson CB. Signal transduction pathways that regulate cell survival and cell death. Oncogene 1998; 17:3207-13.
8. Eick D, Hermeking H. Viruses as pacemakers in the evolution of defence mechanisms against cancer. Trends Genet 1996; 12:4-6.
9. Giaccia AJ, Kastan MB. The complexity of p53 modulation: emerging patterns from divergent signals. Genes Dev 1998; 12:2973-83.
10. Sherr CJ. Tumor surveillance via the ARF-p53 pathway. Genes Dev 1998; 12:2984-91.
11. Zindy F, Eischen CM, Randle DH, Kamijo T, Cleveland JL, Sherr CJ, Roussel MF. Myc signaling via the ARF tumor suppressor regulates p53-dependent apoptosis and immortalization. Genes Dev 1998; 12:2424-33.
12. Johnson DG, Schneider-Broussard, R. Role of E2F in cell cycle control and cancer. Front Biosci 1998; 3:d447-8.
13. Weinberg RA. The retinoblastoma protein and cell cycle control. Cell 1995; 81:323-30.
14. Nevins JR. Toward an understanding of the functional complexity of the E2F and retinoblastoma families. Cell Growth Differ 1998; 9:585-93.
15. Wolf DA, Hermeking H, Albert T, Herzinger T, Kind P, Eick D. A complex between E2F and the pRb-related protein p130 is specifically targeted by the simian virus 40 large T antigen during cell transformation. Oncogene 1995; 10:2067-78.
16. Bissonnette RP, Echeverri F, Mahboubi A, Green, DR. Apoptotic cell death induced by c-myc is inhibited by bcl-2. Nature 1992; 359:552-4.
17. Harrington EA, Bennett MR, Fanidi A, Evan GI. c-Myc-induced apoptosis in fibroblasts is inhibited by specific cytokines. Embo J 1994; 13:3286-95.
18. Bennett MR, Evan GI, Schwartz SM. Apoptosis of human vascular smooth muscle cells derived from normal vessels and coronary atherosclerotic plaques. J Clin Invest 1995; 95:2266-74.
19. Hermeking H, Wolf DA, Kohlhuber F, Dickmanns A, Billaud M, Fanning E, Eick D. Role of c-myc in simian virus 40 large tumor antigen-induced DNA synthesis in quiescent 3T3-L1 mouse fibroblasts. Proc Natl Acad Sci U S A 1994; 91:10412-6.
20. Symonds H, Krall L, Remington L, Saenz-Robles M, Lowe S, Jacks T, Van Dyke T. p53-dependent apoptosis suppresses tumor growth and progression in vivo. Cell 1994; 78:703-11.
21. Colston JT, Chandrasekar B, Freeman GL. Expression of apoptosis-related proteins in experimental coxsackievirus myocarditis. Cardiovasc Res 1998; 38:158-68.
22. Bialik S, Geenen DL, Sasson IE, Cheng R, Horner JW, Evans SM, Lord EM, Koch CJ, Kitsis RN. Myocyte apoptosis during acute myocardial infarction in the mouse localizes to hypoxic regions but occurs independently of p53.J Clin Invest 1997; 100:1363-72.
23. Eilers M, Schirm S, Bishop JM. The MYC protein activates transcription of the alpha-prothymosin gene. Embo J 1991; 10:133-41.
24. Evan GI, Wyllie AH, Gilbert CS, Littlewood TD, Land H, Brooks M, Waters CM, Penn LZ, Hancock DC. Induction of apoptosis in fibroblasts by c-myc protein. Cell 1992; 69:119-28.
25. Hermeking H, Eick D. Mediation of c-Myc-induced apoptosis by p53. Science 1994; 265:2091-3.
26. Wagner AJ, Kokontis JM, Hay N. Myc-mediated apoptosis requires wild-type p53 in a manner independent of cell cycle arrest and the ability of p53 to induce p21waf1/cip1. Genes Dev 1994; 8:2817-30.
27. Amati B, Alevizopoulos K, Vlach J. Myc and the cell cycle. Front Biosci 1998;3:250-68.
28. Hermeking H, Funk JO, Reichert M, Ellwart JW, Eick D. Abrogation of p53-induced cell cycle arrest by c-Myc: evidence for an inhibitor of p21WAF1/CIP1/SDI1. Oncogene 1995; 11:1409-15.
29. Vlach J, Hennecke S, Alevizopoulos K, Conti D, Amati B. Growth arrest by the cyclin-dependent kinase inhibitor p27Kip1 is abrogated by c-Myc. Embo J 1996; 15:6595-604.
30. Ko LJ, Prives C. p53: puzzle and paradigm. Genes Dev 1996; 10:1054-72.
31. Bates S, Phillips AC, Clark PA, Stott F, Peters G, Ludwig RL, Vousden KH. p14ARF links the tumour suppressors RB and p53. Nature 1998; 395:124-5.
32. Chin L, Pomerantz J, DePinho RA. The INK4a/ARF tumor suppressor: one gene--two products--two pathways. Trends Biochem Sci 1998; 23:291-6.
33. Honda R, Yasuda H. Association of p19(ARF) with mdm2 inhibits ubiquitin ligase activity of mdm2 for tumor suppressor p53 . Embo J 1999; 18:22-7.
34. Kamijo T, Weber JD, Zambetti G, Zindy F, Roussel MF, Sherr CJ. Functional and physical interactions of the ARF tumor suppressor with p53 and Mdm2. Proc Natl Acad Sci U S A 1998; 95:8292-7.

35. Palmero I, Pantoja C, Serrano M. p19ARF links the tumour suppressor p53 to Ras. Nature 1998; 395:125-6.

36. Pomerantz J, Schreiber-Agus N, Liegeois NJ, Silverman A, Alland L, Chin L, Potes J, Chen K, Orlow I, Lee HW, Cordon-Cardo C, DePinho RA. The Ink4a tumor suppressor gene product, p19Arf, interacts with MDM2 and neutralizes MDM2's inhibition of p53. Cell 1998; 92:713-23.

37. Radfar A, Unnikrishnan I, Lee HW, DePinho RA, Rosenberg N. p19(Arf) induces p53-dependent apoptosis during abelson virus-mediated pre-B cell transformation. Proc Natl Acad Sci U S A 1998; 95:13194-9.

38. de Stanchina E, McCurrach ME, Zindy F, Shieh SY, Ferbeyre G, Samuelson AV, Prives C, Roussel MF, Sherr CJ, Lowe SW. E1A signaling to p53 involves the p19(ARF) tumor suppressor. Genes Dev 1998; 12:2434-42.

39. Stott FJ, Bates S, James MC, McConnell BB, Starborg M, Brookes S, Palmero I, Ryan K, Hara E, Vousden KH, Peters G. The alternative product from the human CDKN2A locus, p14(ARF), participates in a regulatory feedback loop with p53 and MDM2. Embo J 1998; 17:5001-14.

I.2.2
BCL-2 family members and mitochondria

Klaus Schlottmann, M.D., and Jürgen Schölmerich, M.D.
Universität Regensburg, Regensburg, Germany

INTRODUCTION

The process of apoptosis is often subdivided into three phases: the initiation phase which depends on the apoptosis stimulus, the effector phase which underlies regulation of intracellular signaling and the degradation phase which is common to all forms of apoptosis and which is beyond regulation (1). The Bcl-2 family represents one of the most important families of apoptosis relevant proteins acting in the effector phase of apoptosis. In most cases of programmed cell death Bcl-2 proteins influence the decision of a cell to survive or to die. This review will focus on the basic molecular function of Bcl-2 family members in apoptosis as well as the interplay of some of the bcl-2 members with mitochondria in the context of mitochondrial permeability transition and mitochondrial release of apoptogenic factors.

DISCOVERY OF BCL-2

The mammalian homolog of the *Caenorhabditis elegans death* protein CED-9 is the *bcl-2* gene product (2) which was originally cloned from human B cell lymphomas at the interchromosomal breakpoint of the t(14;18) (3-5). The protooncogene Bcl-2 acts by promoting cell survival in contrast to other known oncogenes which induce cell proliferation among which are Src-kinases and Ras. It therefore represented a new class of oncogenes. Other studies indicated that members of the Bcl-2 family may be proapoptotic as well and thus involved in malignant growth (6-8). Subsequent studies revealed that Bcl-2 inhibited apoptosis induced by cytotoxic stimuli in mammalian cells as cytokine withdrawal (9, 10), chemotherapeutic drugs

(11) or ionizing radiation (12) but not by all stimuli of apoptosis as negative selection in the thymus (12) or in some experiments by the proapoptotic surface receptor CD95. Hence, Bcl-2 family members constitute an important checkpoint of apoptosis for intracellular death pathways.

BCL-2 FAMILY MEMBERS

While CED-9 appears to be the only protein of its kind in *C. elegans* a growing number of Bcl-2 homologs have been identified in mammalian cells (Fig.1). Bcl-2 proteins can be devided in pro- and contraapoptotic members (13-15) and they differ in their tissue expression pattern and in structural features.

Contraapoptotic Bcl-2 family members are Bcl-X_L, Mcl-1 and Bfl-1 while proapoptotic homologs are Bcl-X_S, Bak, Bad, DIVA and Bid (Fig.1). Some members of the Bcl-2 family are expressed abundantly in the entire organism (Bcl-2, Bax, Bcl-X_L), while the expression of others is restricted to only one or few tissues (Boo, Bok, DIVA). Knockout models demonstrated functional overlap of Bcl-2 family proteins. Targeted disruption of the *bcl-2* gene resulted in smaller but viable animals, although about half of them die by 6 weeks of age. Organs rich in Bcl-2, like the intestine, develop almost normally while kidneys are polycystic in Bcl-2 null mice (16). Bcl-X deficient mice die at about embryonic day 13. Extensive apoptotic cell death is evident in postmitotic immature neurons of the developing brain, spinal cord, and dorsal root ganglia. Bcl-X functions to support the viability of immature cells during the development of the nervous and hematopoietic systems (17).

Interestingly, Bcl-2 homologs have also been found in the genome of DNA-viruses. Examples are the *E1B-19k* gene which is expressed in Adenovirus or the *BHRF1* gene in Epstein Barr Virus. The functional role of such viral gene products might be the prolongation of cell survival during the period of viral replication.

STRUCTURE AND FUNCTION OF BCL-2 FAMILY PROTEINS

Bcl-2 proteins can form homo- and heterodimers suggesting that at least part of their function is regulated by protein-protein interactions. Bax, a 21-kDa protein is the first proapoptotic Bcl-2 family member which was identified by co-immunoprecipitation experiments with Bcl-2 (18). Besides the heterodimerization with Bcl-2 it can also homodimerize. Overexpression of Bax revealed its proapoptotic capacity resulting in enhanced apoptotic index when cells were exposed to a death stimulus. When cotransfected with Bcl-2 the death inducing effect of Bax was neutralized by heterodimerization with Bcl-2. Accordingly, it was proposed that the death inducing or death inhibiting capacity of these two Bcl-2 family proteins is closely related to their intracellular ratio (18).

Bcl-2 family members share homology in 4 Bcl-2 homology (BH) domains, which have been denoted BH1 through BH4 domains (Fig.1) (19-21). NMR and x-ray crystallography revealed the three-dimensional structure of Bcl-X_L (22). Bcl-X_L consist of two central, primarily hydrophobic alpha-helices, which are surrounded by amphipathic helices. A loop connecting helices α1 and α2 is flexible and non essential for antiapoptotic activity. The three functionally important Bcl-2 homology regions (BH1, BH2 and BH3) are in close spatial proximity and form an elongated hydrophobic cleft that represents the binding site for other Bcl-2 family members. Point mutations in the BH1 or BH2 domains completely abrogate the death inhibiting properties of Bcl-2 and heterodimerization with Bax (19). The BH3 domain of death inducers is required for heterodimerization with Bcl-2 and Bcl-X_L (21, 23). Data generated by NMR suggest that the BH3 domain of Bak forms an α-helix which interacts with the hydrophobic groove formed by the BH1, BH2 and BH3 domains of Bcl-X_L. These interactions depend on highly conserved amino acid residues (24). The death effectors Bid and Bik express only the BH3 domain but no BH1, BH2 and BH4 domains (25, 26). A BH3 mutant from Bid which still heterodimerized with Bcl-2 lost the proapoptotic capacity, but the only BH3 mutant from Bid which had proapoptotic activity heterodimerized with Bax but not with Bcl-2, suggesting that the BH3 domain can be dissected in functional properties (26). A naturally occurring splicing variant of the Bcl-2 related ovarian killer (Bok) which lacks large parts of the BH3 domain retained its proapoptotic function, without binding to death antagonistic Bcl-2 members (27) and Bax BH3-mutants incapable of binding Bcl-2 retained their proapoptotic capacity while the mutation of the IGDE-motif (Residues 66-69) of the BH3 domain resulted in complete lack of the cytotoxic effect of Bax (28). Isolated BH3 domains from the proapoptotic proteins Bax and Bak, but not the BH3 domain of the contraapoptotic protein Bcl-2, induced apoptosis in a cell-free system based on extracts of *Xenopus* eggs, as determined by the rapid activation of caspases, cytochrome c release and by DNA fragmentation. The BH3 domains of pro-apoptotic proteins are sufficient to inactivate the normal capacity of Bcl-2 to suppress apoptosis (29) underlining the central role of this domain for the apoptotic process. It has also been suggested that heterodimerization between the death repressor Bcl-X_L and the proapoptotic Bax is essential for the anti-death activity of Bcl-X_L. However, specific mutations that disrupt the ability of Bcl-X_L to interact with Bax or Bak still preserve most of the contraapoptotic activity of Bcl-X_L. Hence, the interaction with Bax is not necessarily required for Bcl-X_L to exert death repressing activity (30) and other members of the Bcl-2 protein family exhibit proapoptotic function without interaction with cytoprotective members via heterodimerization (31).

Another site of sequence homology, the BH4 domain which is located at the N-terminus is shared by various death inhibiting as well as death promoting Bcl-2 family members (32-34). This domain is not required for protein dimerization *in vivo*, but its deletion imparted a dominant negative phenotype, yielding mutants that promoted rather than inhibited apoptotic death (33). BH4 is also important for the interaction of Bcl-2 and Bcl-X_L with apoptosis regulating proteins which are not structurally related to Bcl-2 as Raf-1 (35, 36), calcineurin (37), and Ced-4 (38). A unique feature of the Bcl-2 family protein Bfl-1 is the presence of a glycine-rich N-terminal region that overlaps with the BH4 domain. This domain has been functionally related to proliferation permission of Bfl-1. Unlike other BCL-2 family proteins, expression of Bfl-1 permits limited cell proliferation over an extended period of time when cells are induced to undergo apoptosis (39-41).

Pro-survival

Bcl-2-subfamily: Bcl-2, Bcl-X

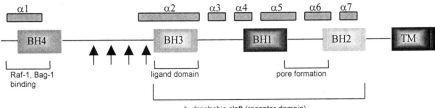

Pro-apoptosis

Bax-subfamily: Bax, Bak, Bok

BH3-subfamily: Bik, Blk, Bad, Bid

BH4-subfamily: DIVA, Mtd

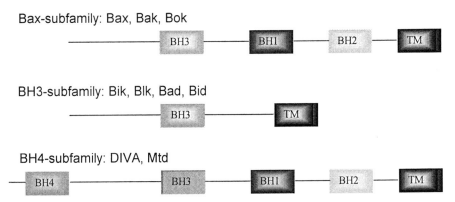

Figure 1 The Bcl-2 protein family. Bcl-2 proteins can be distinguished by functional properties (pro-survival and pro-apoptosis). Both functional classes contain subclasses. Members of the subclasses can be structurally distinguished. The function of Bcl-2 proteins is closely related to structural features. Not all Bcl-2 family members are shown. The BH3 domain of DIVA is not functionally active. Some of the BH3-subfamily members do not express a transmembrane domain. The arrows indicate phosphorylation sites. For the explanation of structural features (α-domains) and functional properties see also Text.

A carboxy-terminal hydrophobic region functions as a transmembrane domain. The transmembrane domain often decides about the localization of Bcl-2 members. It is also believed to be involved in channel formation by Bcl-2 family proteins.

Thus, some but not all Bcl-2 family members interact by homo- or heterodimerization. This death/life rheostat is mediated, at least in part, by competitive dimerization between selective pairs of Bcl-2 family death antagonists and agonists. Therefore, the expression level of these proteins is part of the tight regulation of cellular homeostasis and the disposition of a cell to undergo apoptosis upon a death stimulus.

CELLULAR DISTRIBUTION OF BCL-2 FAMILY MEMBERS

Bcl-2 and Bcl-XL localize to the outer mitochondrial membrane, to the outer nuclear envelope and to the endoplasmic reticulum (42-44). Bcl-2 is found predominantly in close vicinity to contact sites between the outer and inner mitochondrial membrane, generating a patchy pattern in electron microscopy. Bcl-2 and other members contain a single predicted transmembrane segment located at its carboxy-terminus. The transmembrane domain of human Bcl-2 functions as a mitochondrial signal anchor sequence that targets and inserts the protein into the outer membrane leaving the polypeptide facing the cytosole. Insertion of Bcl-2 into the mitochondrial outer membrane is mechanistically different to its association with microsomes (45). The localization of Bcl-2 to the mitochondrial membrane is sufficient to inhibit apoptosis. Elimination of the C-terminus of Bcl-2 abrogates or diminishes the contraapoptotic function of Bcl-2 and Bcl-X$_L$ in some studies (14, 46) but not in others (47, 48). At present it is not clear whether experimentally truncated Bcl-2 and Bcl-Xβ protein in the latter investigations interact with their homologs still residing in the mitochondrial membrane or whether death-inducing Bcl-2 family members are sequestered from the mitochondria by the overexpressed mutants.

Some death agonists as Bax and Bak also contain a transmembrane domain which targets them to mitochondrial, nuclear and ER membranes (49). However, in the normal state of a cell Bax is rather located in the cytosole. After an apoptotic stimulus Bax translocates to the mitochondrion and inserts into the mitochondrial membrane (50). These data have been confimed in vitro with isolated mitochondria, showing that both, Bax and Bak influence basic mitochondrial mechanisms required for the induction of apoptosis (51). The incapability of Bax to insert into the mitochondrial membrane in the absence of a death signal correlates with repression of the transmembrane signal-anchor function of Bax by the NH$_2$-terminal domain. Caspase inhibitors partially blocked the ability to insert into mitochondria which suggests a caspase-dependent processing of Bax causing attenuation of the repressor effect of the NH2-terminal domain (52). Other Bcl-2 proteins as the BH3-only members Bid and Bad completely lack a transmembrane domain but still exert proapoptotic function. After a death-inducing stimulus from the CD95/Fas or TNFα death receptors Bid is cleaved by caspase-8 into a 15 kDa COOH-terminal and a 13 kDa NH2-terminal part. The 15 kDa cleavage product translocates to mitochondria and induces apoptosis (53, 54). Indeed, the p15 Bid cleavage product became an integral mitochondrial membrane protein after stimulating cells with TNF-α, indicating other mechanisms for membrane integration than a transmembrane domain in these transmembrane domain lacking members (55). Hence, molecular interactions within the Bid molecule itself are most likely responsible for the repression of the Bid carboxy-terminal domain, leading to Bid translocation and mitochondrial membrane integration.

In conclusion, transmembrane domains seem to play an important role for the localization and function of Bcl-2 proteins. Translocation to and insertion into the outer mitochondrial membrane of death-inducing as well as death inhibitory members are strongly involved in the decision about the fate of a cell.

RECRUITMENT OF NON BCL-2 FAMILY SIGNAL TRANSDUCTION MODULES BY BCL-2 PROTEINS

As mentioned above, Bcl-2 proteins do not regulate cell death exclusively by the relative expression level of Bcl-2 related death agonists and antagonists. Homo- and heterodimers of Bcl-2 homologs mainly locate to the mitochondrial outer membrane facing the cytosole, where they can interact with cytosolic effectors such as signal transduction molecules (Fig. 2). The small GTP-binding protein p21-Ras is a main signaling molecule in growth factor- and antigen-mediated cellular activation and proliferation. Ras directly activates the serine threonine kinase Raf-1 which in turn activates the ERK pathway. In most investigations the Ras/Raf-1 pathway functions as a cell survival pathway. Interestingly, Ras and Raf-1 can be coimmunoprecipitated with Bcl-2 which functionally reflects a cross talk between the Ras/Raf-1 pathway and Bcl-2 family proteins. Bcl-2 can target Raf-1 to the mitochondrial membrane (35) and mitochondria associated Raf-1 can induce serine phosphorylation of the proapoptotic Bcl-2 family protein Bad (56, 57). Phosphorylation of Bad is observed under growth factor receptor ligation (e.g. IL-3). Upon phosphorylation Bad is distributed to the cytosole and here it binds phosphorylation dependently to the 14-3-3 protein (57). Under growth factor deprivation, a strong proapoptotic stimulus, Bad is dephosphorylated, released from 14-3-3, translocated to the mitochondrial membrane and here, interacting with Bcl-2 family proteins, it finally triggers apoptosis. Another Bcl-2 interacting protein is Bag-1 which enhances the cytoprotective effect of Bcl-2 (58). Upon growth factor withdrawal Bag-1 is recruited to growth factor receptors as hepatocyte growth factor or platelet-derived growth factor and thereby is not available for the cytoprotective cooperation with mitochondrial Bcl-2 (59). Furthermore, Bag-1 can bind to and activate Raf-1, another possible contraapoptotic function of this molecule (36).

Besides interactions of Bcl-2 with cytoplasmic signaling molecules Bcl-2 family proteins underlie posttranslational modifications. Bcl-2 can be phosphorylated on serine and threonine residues reverting the contraapoptotic capacity. The kinase responsible for Bcl-2 phosphorylation remains elusive. Bcl-X_L is cleaved into two 18 kDa fragments by Caspase-3 in the interleukin-2 dependent T cell clone CTLL-2 upon deprivation of IL-2 from culture medium. Transfection of the COOH-terminal fragment resulted in enhanced apoptosis, suggesting that fragments from cytoprotective Bcl-2 family proteins can reverse the initial function (60). Moreover, cell lines infected with alpha virus revealed that BH4 can be removed from Bcl-2 by caspases indicating that alphaviruses can trigger a caspase-mediated inactivation of Bcl-2 in order to evade the death protection imposed by this survival factor (61). Furthermore, the loop domain of Bcl-2 was shown to be cleaved at Asp34 by caspase-3 in vitro, in cells overexpressing caspase-3, and after induction of apoptosis by CD95 ligation and interleukin-3 withdrawal. The COOH-terminal Bcl-2 cleavage product triggered cell death and accelerated Sindbis virus-induced apoptosis, which was dependent on the BH3 homology and transmembrane domains of Bcl-2. Inhibitor studies indicated that cleavage of Bcl-2 may further activate downstream caspases and contribute to amplification of the caspase cascade.

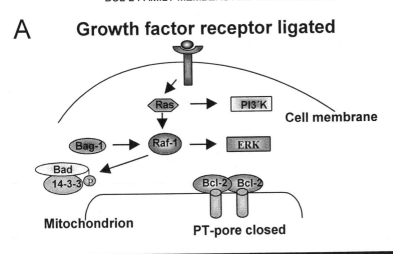

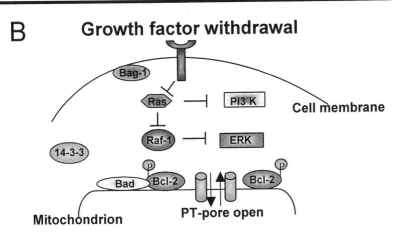

Figure 2 Growth factor receptor ligation (A) and growth factor withdrawal (B) influence cellular susceptibility to apoptosis by serine-phosporylation of Bcl-2 and Bad. (A): Ligation of e.g. the IL-3 receptor induces phosphorylation of Bad leading to sequestration and binding of Bad to 14-3-3. The growth inhibitory protein Bag-1 can probably activate Raf-1 kinase upon occupancy of e.g. hepatocyte growth factor receptor. (B) Upon growth factor withdrawal no Raf-1 phosphorylating kinases are active resulting in dephosphorylation of Bad and release from 14-3-3. Bad heterodimerizes with Bcl-2 and thereby triggers apoptosis. Additionally, the contraapoptotic protein Bag-1 is sequestered to the plasma membrane. Bcl-2 is phosphorylated on serine and thereby inactivated by a yet unidentified kinase.

These data indicate that Bcl-2 family proteins underlie posttranslational modifications and degradation, which control the function of this apoptosis regulating protein family.

MITOCHONDRIAL PERMEABILITY TRANSITION

The apoptotic process is oxygen independent and does neither require oxidative phosphorylation nor mitochondrial DNA. However, there is strong evidence that mitochondria and mitochondrial products play a central role in the programmed signaling events finally leading to cell death.

The mitochondrial permeability transition, initially described by Hunter and Haworth (62-66), is a process representing a rapid increase in the permeability of the inner mitochondrial membrane involved in apoptosis and necrosis of mammalian cells (67, 68). With the recognition that cyclosporin A mediates a saturable inhibitory effect on mitochondrial permeability transition, the theory of a protein pore regulating the PT was strongly supported (69, 70). Applying the patch clamp technique, Szabo and Zoratti identified a cyclosporin inhibitable pore in mitochondrial membranes (71) the opening of which today is believed to be responsible for the permeability transition.

Although the exact molecular composition of the mitochondrial permeability transition-pore has not yet been elucidated, it is proposed that the pore is a dynamic multiprotein complex located at contact sites between the inner and outer mitochondrial membranes (Fig. 3). The PT-pore involves cytosolic proteins such as hexokinase, outer mitochondrial membrane proteins as the voltage dependent anion channel and the mitochondrial benzodiazepine receptor (72, 73) as well as inner mitochondrial membrane proteins like the adenine nucleotide transporter (74) and mitochondrial matrix proteins as cyclophilin D.

It should be emphasized that the mitochondrial permeability transition-pore is regulated by multiple factors (reviewed in (67)) and that it has physiological functions besides the critical role in apoptosis. The permeability transition-pore is by no means a cellular tool designed solely for the execution of programmed cell death. Ca^{2+} induced release of Ca^{2+} from mitochondria dependent on transitory opening of the mitochondrial permeability transition-pore operating in a low conductance mode is one physiological role of the pore not associated with programmed cell death. The Ca^{2+} fluxes taking place during Ca^{2+} induced release of Ca^{2+} from mitochondria are a direct consequence of the mitochondrial depolarization spike caused by pore opening. Both mitochondrial depolarization spike and Ca^{2+} induced release of Ca^{2+} from mitochondria can propagate from one mitochondrion to another in vitro, generating traveling depolarization and Ca^{2+} waves. Mitochondria thus appear to be excitable organelles capable of generating and conveying electrical and Ca^{2+} signals. In living cells, mitochondrial depolarization spike and Ca^{2+} induced release of Ca^{2+} from mitochondria are triggered during IP3- induced Ca^{2+} mobilization and results in the amplification of the Ca^{2+} signals primarily emitted from the endoplasmic reticulum (64, 65, 75, 76). This way a significant amount of the intracellular calcium transits through mitochondria by entering the cell via the Ca^{2+} uniporter and leaving this organelle via the mitochondrial permeability transition-pore. The molecular cutoff of the mitochondrial permeability transition-pore in the low conductance state is <300 Da, and therefore permeable only to small ions like Ca^{2+} or K^+.

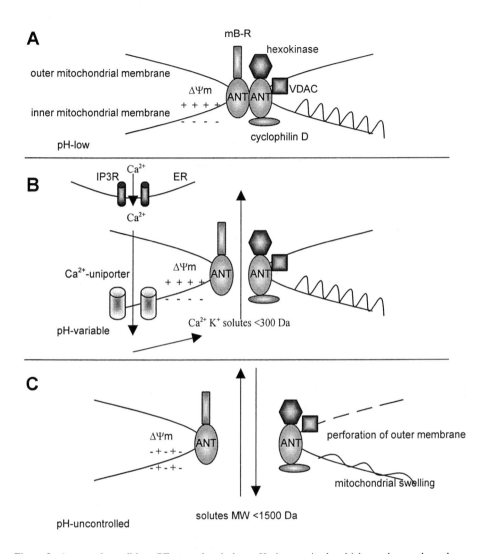

Figure 3 **A** normal condition: PT-pore closed, low pH, inner mitochondrial membrane charged negatively on the inner surface, cristae folded. **B** subconductance state during calcium induced calcium release: uptake of Ca^{2+} from endoplasmic reticulum via uniporter causes charge compensation by respiratory chain, increased matrix pH, PT-pore opening collapses proton gradient, Ca^{2+} is released. **C** high conductance state during MPT: stimuli causing high conductance state lead to dissipation of $\Delta\Psi$m, free leakage of solutes and mitochondrial swelling with consecutive disruption of the outer mitochondrial membrane and release of factors involved in apoptosis. ANT: adenine nucleotide transporter; mB-R: mitochondrial benzodiazepine receptor; VDAC: voltage dependent anionic channel; CICR: calcium induced calcium release; MPT: mitochondrial permeability transition, ER: endoplasmic reticulum; IP3: inositol-3-phosphate.

In the low conductance state the mitochondrial permeability transition-pore is mainly regulated by the matrix pH, inasfar as a low pH closes the pore and a high pH triggers pore opening. Hence, in the low conductance state the PT-pore does not impair mitochondrial functions like volume homeostasis, it is operated by changes in matrix pH accompanying mitochondrial Ca^{2+} uptake and it is involved in the regulation of cellular Ca^{2+} homeostasis as a calcium release channel. In contrast to the high conductance state, the low conductance state does not seem to be involved in programmed cell death (76).

Mitochondrial changes occur early in the process of cell death. Induction of the mitochondrial permeability transition in the high conductance state causes dissipation of the inner mitochondrial transmembrane potential $\Delta\Psi m$ rendering the inner mitochondrial membrane unselectively permeable to solutes with a molecular mass <1500 Da (62-65). Due to the extremely high conductance with single channel currents of >1 nanoSiemens the permeability transition-pore was also termed "mitochondrial megachannel" or "multiple conductance channel" (67). Under normal conditions there is a strong negative charge in the mitochondrion building up a proton (pH) and chemical gradient which is essential for mitochondrial function. Inducers of apoptosis like ionizing radiation, ceramide or anti-CD95 have shown to result in disruption of the electron transport chain at the cytochrome b-c1/cytochrome c step In this scenario the mitochondrion cannot sustain electron transport, oxidative phosphorylation, and adenosine trisphosphate production. However, the maintenance of a permissive ATP concentration seems to be important for the apoptotic process while low ATP concentrations are usually found in necrotic cell death (77-81). The volume dysregulation which takes place during mitochondrial permeability transition-pore opening leads to entry of water into the protein-rich matrix of mitochondria causing the matrix space to expand finally resulting in the rupture of the outer mitochondrial membrane. This observation allowed the assumption that permeability transition-pore opening in situ with subsequent arrest of aerobic ATP-synthesis and electron transport could participate in toxic cell death. The high conductance state is regulated by Ca^{2+}, voltage and pH as well as cyclophiln D, by the reactive oxygen species leaking from the respiratory chain and by the rate of electron transfer across the respiratory chain complex I (67, 68, 76, 82).

First data indicating that cellular apoptosis involves mitochondria were generated by using cationic lipophilic fluorochromes (e.g. $DiOC_6(3)$, JC-1 or CMXRos) which enter the mitochondrial matrix due to the negative charge inside the mitochondrion. The authors realized that flow cytometric signs of apoptosis were preceded by a collaps in $\Delta\Psi m$ resulting in reduced incorporation of the $\Delta\Psi m$-sensitive dyes and in structural changes in mitochondria as well as release of reactive oxygen species (83-85). These events were observed at early stages of the apoptotic process, when most of the cells were not irreversibly committed to death. No DNA-degradation or exposure of phosphatidylserine were detectable by the point of dissipation of the $\Delta\Psi m$, showing that the mitochondrial permeability transition is an early process in programmed cell death (85-87). In subsequent studies a plenitude of receptor and non-receptor apoptotic stimuli applied in different *ex vivo* and tumor cell lines reproduced these results (68).

Interestingly, Cyclosporin A a known inhibitor of the PT (via cyclophilin D) and a non immunosuppressant derivative of Cyclosporin A which does not interfere with the calcineurin pathway, inhibited the PT and apoptosis under a variety of stimuli, again suggesting, that $\Delta\Psi$m plays a causative role in apoptosis. Many other substances like bongkrekate, a ligand of the adenine nucleotide transporter or oligomycin can inhibit the permeability transition (extensively reviewed in (67))

Together, these data point to mitochondria as a crucial component of apoptosis. One key regulator is opening of the permeability transition-pore in the high conductance state with subsequent $\Delta\Psi$m, the inhibition of which is a powerful tool to abrogate apoptosis in cells.

BCL-2 FAMILY PROTEINS AND MITOCHONDRIA

The $\Delta\Psi$m is not the only mitochondrial factor to participate in the orchestration of cell death components. Upon an apoptotic stimulus mitochondria can release at least two proteins which are capable of triggering apoptosis: apoptosis inducing factor, a flavoprotein of relative molecular mass 57 kDa which shares homology with the bacterial oxidoreductases and cytochrome-c, an essential component of the mitochondrial respiratory chain. (88-91). Apoptosis inducing factor is normally confined to mitochondria but translocates to the nucleus when apoptosis is induced. Recombinant apoptosis inducing factor causes chromatin condensation in isolated nuclei and large-scale fragmentation of DNA. It induces purified mitochondria to release the apoptogenic proteins cytochrome c and caspase-9. Microinjection of apoptosis inducing factor into the cytoplasm of intact cells induces condensation of chromatin, dissipation of the mitochondrial transmembrane potential, and exposure of phosphatidylserine on the plasma membrane. None of these effects is prevented by the caspase inhibitor Z-VAD.fmk. Overexpression of Bcl-2, which controls the opening of mitochondrial permeability transition pores, prevents the release of apoptosis inducing factor from the mitochondrion but does not affect its apoptogenic activity indicating that apoptosis inducing factor is a mitochondrial effector of apoptotic cell death (91).

Cytochrome-c is a soluble heme containing protein that is located in the mitochondrial intermembrane space loosely attached to the inner membrane. Cytochrome-c accepts an electron from cytochrome-c reductase and passes it on to to cytochrome-c oxidase. Translocation of cytochrome-c from mitochondria to the cytosole has been shown to be a crucial step in rpogrammed cell death in various death models including anti-CD95, staurosporine or etoposide in a cell-free system using *Xenopus* egg extract or dATP-primed cytosol and UV-light (88-90, 92). Cytochrome-c (Apaf-2) activates caspases through binding to the cytosolic protein apoptosis protease activating factor-1 (Apaf-1) a mammalian homolog of CED-4 (93) thereby likely changing the molecular conformation of Apaf-1. Another member of this complex required for induction of apoptosis is dATP (94). Subsequently the Apaf-1/cytochrome-c/dATP complex can bind to the zymogen of the proapoptotic caspase-9 (Apaf-3) via the amino-terminal CARD-domains of Apaf-1 and Caspase-9 resulting in activation of caspase-9 probably by autoproteolysis (94). Oligomerization of caspase-9 by Apaf-1 has been proposed further explaining the caspase-9 proteolytic activation by the Apaf-1/cytochrome-c complex (95). Caspase-9 in turn can activate procaspase-3 leading to activation of the caspase cascade and cleavage of fodrin, PARP and laminB$_1$. However, Apaf-1 is not required for all apoptosis stimuli, since the CD95 pathway is preserved in Apaf-1 knockout mice suggesting distinct pathways for mitochondrial apoptosis among apoptosis inducers (79, 96). Bcl-X$_L$, an antiapoptotic member of the Bcl-2 family, was shown to physically interact with Apaf-1 and caspase-9 in mammalian cells. The association of Apaf-1 with Bcl-X$_L$ was mediated through both, its CED-4-like domain and the C-terminal domain containing WD-40 repeats. Expression of Bcl-X$_L$ inhibited the association of Apaf-1 with caspase-9 in mammalian cells. Significantly, recombinant Bcl-X$_L$ inhibited Apaf-1-dependent processing of caspase-9. Furthermore, Bcl-X$_L$ failed to inhibit caspase-9 processing mediated by a constitutively active Apaf-1 mutant, suggesting that Bcl-X$_L$ regulates caspase-9 through Apaf-1 (Fig. 4). These experiments demonstrate that Bcl-X$_L$ associates with caspase-9 and Apaf-1, and Bcl-X$_L$ inhibits the maturation of caspase-9 mediated by Apaf-1 (97, 98). However, despite the large body of evidence which implements cytochrome-c in the signaling of programmed cell death other authors have described cytochrome-c independent apoptosis (99, 100).

Several theories exist explaining the mechanism of cytochrome-c release from mitochondria: As mentioned above disruption of the outer mitochondrial membrane by mitochondrial matrix swelling with subsequent release of cytochrome-c and other proapoptotic factors from the intermembrane space would be one possibility. However, morphological changes are no typical aspect of mitochondria during early apoptosis and cytochrome-c is also part of the respiratory chain which generates ATP needed for the apoptotic process.

This is where Bcl-2 family members come into the play. Overexpression of the cytoprotective Bcl-2 and Bcl-X$_L$ inhibit apoptosis, PT-pore opening, release of apoptosis inducing factor and cytochrome-c. Bcl-2 but not Bcl-2 mutants which fail to suppress apoptosis blocked PT-pore opening *in vitro* (88-90, 101). On the other hand, the proapoptotic protein Bax has been shown to bind to the PT-pore constituent ANT, to induce $\Delta\Psi$m and to release cytochrome-c (74, 102, 103).

Other studies suggest, that besides PT-pore regulation Bcl-2 exerts functions which might not be closely related to PT-pore opening. Comparison of the time course of cytochrome-c release and $\Delta\Psi$m in growth factor deprived or cancer drug treated cells indicated that cytochrome-c release can precede the $\Delta\Psi$m (88, 89, 104). This could lead to caspase activation with only a portion of the available cytochrome-c being released and a sufficient amount of cytochrome-c remaining in the mitochondria in order to preserve the electron transport in the respiratory chain (105, 106). If cytochrome-c can be released while leaving the inner mitochondrial membrane intact the question arises how cytochrome-c can enter the cytoplasm from the mitochondrial intermembrane space. Jürgensmeier et al. showed that recombinant Bax can induce cytochrome-c release from mitochondria without mitochondrial swelling proposing that mitochondrial permeability transition-pore opening is not necessarily required for cytochrome-c release (105). Eskes et al. suggest the existence of two distinct mechanisms leading to cytochrome-c release: one stimulated by calcium and inhibited by cyclosporin A, the other Bax dependent,

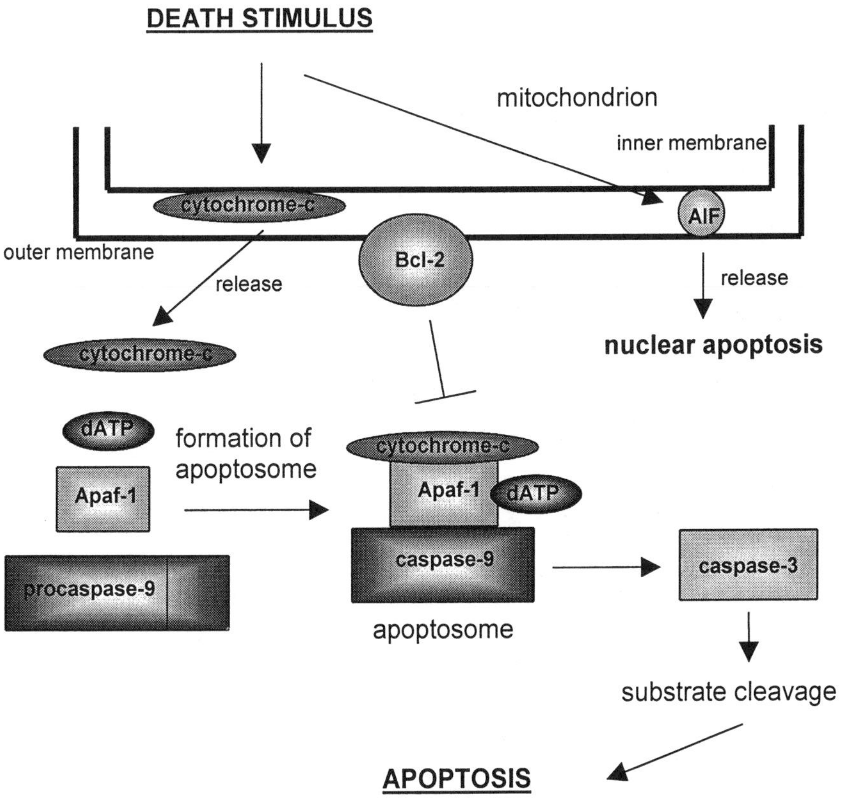

Figure 4 A death stimulus induces mitochondrial cytochrome-c release which triggers assembly of cytochrome-c (Apaf-2), apoptosis protease activating factor-1 (Apaf-1), dATP and caspase-9 (Apaf-3). The complex of these molecules is also called the apoptosome. Apaf-1 most likely oligomerizes caspase-9 which allows for autoproteolysis and activation of caspase-9. In a cascade caspase-9 activates the distal effector caspase-3 which can cleave multiple specific intracellular substrates. Apoptosis inducing factor is the second factor released from mitochondria in cells targeted by an apoptotic stimulus. Apoptosis inducing factor induces nuclear changes of apoptosis. Note that caspase-2, caspase-3 and caspase-9 been shown to be located in mitochondria and can be released from mitochondria upon induction of cellular apoptosis.

Mg2+ sensitive but cyclosporin insensitive (107). In this scenario it is important to realize that certain caspases can induce permeability transition-pore opening when added to isolated mitochondria (108, 109) and caspase inhibition has no effect on release of cytochrome-c (110). Recent data also suggest that procaspase-2 and procaspase-9 are released from purified mitochondria upon induction of apoptosis and pore opening. Both procaspases redistribute from the mitochondrion to the cytosole and are processed to generate enzymatically active caspases. This redistribution is inhibited by Bcl-2 (111).

Together, these data allow to generate a model in which cytochrome-c released in small amounts targets procaspase-9 with consecutive opening of the permeability transition-pore and release of more cytochrome-c, apoptosis inducing factor and procaspases-2/3/9 (112). Small amounts of extramitochondrial caspase-9 would be required to induce this feed forward mechanism. However, at present it is not clear whether other caspases besides caspase-9 can be targeted by the Apaf-1/cytochrome-c complex, since apoptosis is not completely blocked in caspase-9 knockout mice (113).

PORE FORMATION – ION CHANNELS

The elucidation of the three-dimensional structure of Bcl-X_L and the structural similarity of Bcl-X_L to pore forming bacterial toxins such as diphtheria toxin A and colicins A and E1 (22) prompted further investigation on pore-forming capacity of Bcl-2 family members. Bcl-X_L, Bcl-2 and Bax form cation selective channels in the lipid bilayer reconstitution system *in vitro* (114-118). Channel formation has been linked to the cytoprotective effect in the case of Bcl-2 and Bcl-X_L or to the cytotoxic function of Bax. The channel forming fifth and sixth α-helices of Bcl-2 are essential for the contraapoptotic function in this context (119). In contrast, deletion or substitution of alpha5-alpha6 in Bax reduced but did not abrogate apoptosis induction in human cells, whereas it did completely abrogate cytotoxic activity in yeast, implying that the pore-forming segments of Bax are critical for confering a lethal phenotype in yeast but not necessarily in human cells (119).

Characterisation of the ion channels formed by the proapoptotic Bcl-2 and the contraapoptotic Bax showed that Bax and Bcl-2 each form channels in artificial membranes but have distinct characteristics including ion selectivity, conductance, voltage dependence, and rectification (117, 118).

Thus, one role of these molecules may include pore activity at selected membrane sites. However, the exact regulatory properties of these channels are currently unknown.

CONCLUSION

Mitochondria are crucially involved in the cell death machinery. Bcl-2 and mitochondria may both prevent and initiate the apoptotic cell death. Cellular homeostasis and the integrity of the entire organism require tight regulation of these processes. At present it is believed that the final outcome of cell death, necrosis or apoptosis depends on the energy state of a cell. This is underlined in studies where one and the same death stimulus can cause both modes of death, a fact which has led to the introduction of the term „necrapoptosis" (80). This might explain why mitochondria which constitute the power plant of a cell play a central role in apoptosis. The mitochondrial permeability transition and mitochondrial release of apoptosis influencing factors are regulated and modulated by Bcl-2 family proteins. Albeit rapidly growing knowledge on the molecular regulation of processes involved in programmed cell death and although we are aware of the crucial role programmed cell death plays in many diseases it is only to begin that we consciously exploit the resources which emerge from the theoretical background. The introduction of powerful agents to selectively influence defined steps of the apoptotic machinery into clinical medicine is a matter of time.

References

1.   Kroemer G, Petit P, Zamzami N, Vayssiere JL, Mignotte B: The biochemistry of programmed cell death. Faseb J 1995; 9:1277-87.
2.   Hengartner MO, Horvitz HR: C. elegans cell survival gene ced-9 encodes a functional homolog of the mammalian proto-oncogene bcl-2. Cell 1994; 76:665-76.
3.   Bakhshi A, Minowada J, Arnold A, Cossman J, Jensen JP, Whang-Peng J, Waldmann TA, Korsmeyer SJ: Lymphoid blast crises of chronic myelogenous leukemia represent stages in the development of B-cell precursors. N Engl J Med 1983; 309:826-31.
4.   Tsujimoto Y, Yunis J, Onorato-Showe L, Erikson J, Nowell PC, Croce CM: Molecular cloning of the chromosomal breakpoint of B-cell lymphomas and leukemias with the t(11;14) chromosome translocation. Science 1984; 224:1403-6.
5.   Cleary ML, Smith SD, Sklar J: Cloning and structural analysis of cDNAs for bcl-2 and a hybrid bcl- 2/immunoglobulin transcript resulting from the t(14;18) translocation. Cell 1986; 47:19-28.
6.   Rampino N, Yamamoto H, Ionov Y, Li Y, Sawai H, Reed JC, Perucho M: Somatic frameshift mutations in the BAX gene in colon cancers of the microsatellite mutator phenotype. Science 1997; 275:967-9.
7.   Brimmell M, Mendiola R, Mangion J, Packham G: BAX frameshift mutations in cell lines derived from human haemopoietic malignancies are associated with resistance to apoptosis and microsatellite instability. Oncogene 1998; 16:1803-12.
8.   Ouyang H, Furukawa T, Abe T, Kato Y, Horii A: The BAX gene, the promoter of apoptosis, is mutated in genetically unstable cancers of the colorectum, stomach, and endometrium. Clin Cancer Res 1998; 4:1071-84.
9.   Vaux DL, Cory S, Adams JM: Bcl-2 gene promotes haemopoietic cell survival and cooperates with c- myc to immortalize pre-B cells. Nature 1988; 335:440-2.
10.   Nunez G, London L, Hockenbery D, Alexander M, McKearn JP, Korsmeyer SJ: Deregulated Bcl-2 gene expression selectively prolongs survival of growth factor-deprived hemopoietic cell lines. J Immunol 1990; 144:3602-10.
11.   Kamesaki S, Kamesaki H, Jorgensen TJ, Tanizawa A, Pommier Y, Cossman J: bcl-2 protein inhibits etoposide-induced apoptosis through its effects on events subsequent to topoisomerase II-induced DNA strand breaks and their repair. Cancer Res 1993; 53:4251-6.
12.   Sentman CL, Shutter JR, Hockenbery D, Kanagawa O, Korsmeyer SJ: bcl-2 inhibits multiple forms of apoptosis but not negative selection in thymocytes. Cell 1991; 67:879-88.
13.   Chao DT, Korsmeyer SJ: BCL-2 family: regulators of cell death. Annu Rev Immunol 1998; 16:395-419.
14.   Minn AJ, Swain RE, Ma A, Thompson CB: Recent progress on the regulation of apoptosis by Bcl-2 family members. Adv Immunol 1998; 70:245-79.
15.   Adams JM, Cory S: The Bcl-2 protein family: arbiters of cell survival. Science 1998; 281:1322-6.
16.   Nakayama K, Negishi I, Kuida K, Sawa H, Loh DY: Targeted disruption of Bcl-2 alpha beta in mice: occurrence of gray hair, polycystic kidney disease, and lymphocytopenia. Proc Natl Acad Sci U S A 1994; 91:3700-4.
17.   Motoyama N, Wang F, Roth KA, Sawa H, Nakayama K, Negishi I, Senju S, Zhang Q, Fujii S, et al.: Massive cell death of immature hematopoietic cells and neurons in Bcl-x- deficient mice. Science 1995; 267:1506-10.
18.   Oltvai ZN, Milliman CL, Korsmeyer SJ: Bcl-2 heterodimerizes in vivo with a conserved homolog, Bax, that accelerates programmed cell death. Cell 1993; 74:609-19.
19.   Yin XM, Oltvai ZN, Korsmeyer SJ: BH1 and BH2 domains of Bcl-2 are required for inhibition of apoptosis and heterodimerization with Bax. Nature 1994; 369:321-3.

20. Chittenden T, Flemington C, Houghton AB, Ebb RG, Gallo GJ, Elangovan B, Chinnadurai G, Lutz RJ: A conserved domain in Bak, distinct from BH1 and BH2, mediates cell death and protein binding functions. Embo J 1995; 14:5589-96.

21. Zha H, Aime-Sempe C, Sato T, Reed JC: Proapoptotic protein Bax heterodimerizes with Bcl-2 and homodimerizes with Bax via a novel domain (BH3) distinct from BH1 and BH2. J Biol Chem 1996; 271:7440-54.

22. Muchmore SW, Sattler M, Liang H, Meadows RP, Harlan JE, Yoon HS, Nettesheim D, Chang BS, Thompson CB, Wong SL, Ng SL, Fesik SW: X-ray and NMR structure of human Bcl-xL, an inhibitor of programmed cell death. Nature 1996; 381:335-41.

23. Hunter JJ, Parslow TG: A peptide sequence from Bax that converts Bcl-2 into an activator of apoptosis. J Biol Chem 1996; 271:8521-34.

24. Sattler M, Liang H, Nettesheim D, Meadows RP, Harlan JE, Eberstadt M, Yoon HS, Shuker SB, Chang BS, Minn AJ, Thompson CB, Fesik SW: Structure of Bcl-xL-Bak peptide complex: recognition between regulators of apoptosis. Science 1997; 275:983-6.

25. Boyd JM, Gallo GJ, Elangovan B, Houghton AB, Malstrom S, Avery BJ, Ebb RG, Subramanian T, Chittenden T, Lutz RJ, et al.: Bik, a novel death-inducing protein shares a distinct sequence motif with Bcl-2 family proteins and interacts with viral and cellular survival-promoting proteins. Oncogene 1995; 11:1921-8.

26. Wang K, Yin XM, Chao DT, Milliman CL, Korsmeyer SJ: BID: a novel BH3 domain-only death agonist. Genes Dev 1996; 10:2859-69.

27. Hsu SY, Hsueh AJ: A splicing variant of the Bcl-2 member Bok with a truncated BH3 domain induces apoptosis but does not dimerize with antiapoptotic Bcl-2 proteins in vitro. J Biol Chem 1998; 273:30139-46.

28. Zha H, Reed JC: Heterodimerization-independent functions of cell death regulatory proteins Bax and Bcl-2 in yeast and mammalian cells. J Biol Chem 1997; 272:31482-8.

29. Cosulich SC, Worrall V, Hedge PJ, Green S, Clarke PR: Regulation of apoptosis by BH3 domains in a cell-free system. Curr Biol 1997; 7:913-20.

30. Cheng EH, Levine B, Boise LH, Thompson CB, Hardwick JM: Bax-independent inhibition of apoptosis by Bcl-XL. Nature 1996; 379:554-6.

31. Inohara N, Ekhterae D, Garcia I, Carrio R, Merino J, Merry A, Chen S, Nunez G: Mtd, a novel Bcl-2 family member activates apoptosis in the absence of heterodimerization with Bcl-2 and Bcl-XL. J Biol Chem 1998; 273:8705-10.

32. Hanada M, Aime-Sempe C, Sato T, Reed JC: Structure-function analysis of Bcl-2 protein. Identification of conserved domains important for homodimerization with Bcl-2 and heterodimerization with Bax. J Biol Chem 1995; 270:11962-9.

33. Hunter JJ, Bond BL, Parslow TG: Functional dissection of the human Bcl2 protein: sequence requirements for inhibition of apoptosis. Mol Cell Biol 1996; 16:877-83.

34. Inohara N, Gourley TS, Carrio R, Muniz M, Merino J, Garcia I, Koseki T, Hu Y, Chen S, Nunez G: Diva, a Bcl-2 homologue that binds directly to Apaf-1 and induces BH3- independent cell death. J Biol Chem 1998; 273:32479-86.

35. Wang HG, Rapp UR, Reed JC: Bcl-2 targets the protein kinase Raf-1 to mitochondria [see comments]. Cell 1996; 87:629-38.

36. Wang HG, Takayama S, Rapp UR, Reed JC: Bcl-2 interacting protein, BAG-1, binds to and activates the kinase Raf- 1. Proc Natl Acad Sci U S A 1996; 93:7063-8.

37. Shibasaki F, Kondo E, Akagi T, McKeon F: Suppression of signalling through transcription factor NF-AT by interactions between calcineurin and Bcl-2. Nature 1997; 386:728-31.

38. Chinnaiyan AM, K OR, Lane BR, Dixit VM: Interaction of CED-4 with CED-3 and CED-9: a molecular framework for cell death. Science 1997; 275:1122-6.

39. Choi SS, Park IC, Yun JW, Sung YC, Hong SI, Shin HS: A novel Bcl-2 related gene, Bfl-1, is overexpressed in stomach cancer and preferentially expressed in bone marrow. Oncogene 1995; 11:1693-8.

40. D'Sa-Eipper C, Subramanian T, Chinnadurai G: bfl-1, a bcl-2 homologue, suppresses p53-induced apoptosis and exhibits potent cooperative transforming activity. Cancer Res 1996; 56:3879-82.

41. D'Sa-Eipper C, Chinnadurai G: Functional dissection of Bfl-1, a Bcl-2 homolog: anti-apoptosis, oncogene-cooperation and cell proliferation activities. Oncogene 1998; 16:3105-14.

42. Nakai M, Takeda A, Cleary ML, Endo T: The bcl-2 protein is inserted into the outer membrane but not into the inner membrane of rat liver mitochondria in vitro. Biochem Biophys Res Commun 1993; 196:233-9.

43. Krajewski S, Tanaka S, Takayama S, Schibler MJ, Fenton W, Reed JC: Investigation of the subcellular distribution of the bcl-2 oncoprotein: residence in the nuclear envelope, endoplasmic reticulum, and outer mitochondrial membranes. Cancer Res 1993; 53:4701-14.
44. Akao Y, Otsuki Y, Kataoka S, Ito Y, Tsujimoto Y: Multiple subcellular localization of bcl-2: detection in nuclear outer membrane, endoplasmic reticulum membrane, and mitochondrial membranes. Cancer Res 1994; 54:2468-71.
45. Nguyen M, Millar DG, Yong VW, Korsmeyer SJ, Shore GC: Targeting of Bcl-2 to the mitochondrial outer membrane by a COOH- terminal signal anchor sequence. J Biol Chem 1993; 268:25265-78.
46. Nguyen M, Branton PE, Walton PA, Oltvai ZN, Korsmeyer SJ, Shore GC: Role of membrane anchor domain of Bcl-2 in suppression of apoptosis caused by E1B-defective adenovirus. J Biol Chem 1994; 269:16521-34.
47. Gonzalez-Garcia M, Garcia I, Ding L, O'Shea S, Boise LH, Thompson CB, Nunez G: bcl-x is expressed in embryonic and postnatal neural tissues and functions to prevent neuronal cell death. Proc Natl Acad Sci U S A 1995; 92:4304-8.
48. Zhu W, Cowie A, Wasfy GW, Penn LZ, Leber B, Andrews DW: Bcl-2 mutants with restricted subcellular location reveal spatially distinct pathways for apoptosis in different cell types. Embo J 1996; 15:4130-41.
49. Krajewski S, Krajewska M, Reed JC: Immunohistochemical analysis of in vivo patterns of Bak expression, a proapoptotic member of the Bcl-2 protein family. Cancer Res 1996; 56:2849-55.
50. Hsu YT, Wolter KG, Youle RJ: Cytosol-to-membrane redistribution of Bax and Bcl-X(L) during apoptosis. Proc Natl Acad Sci U S A 1997; 94:3668-72.
51. Narita M, Shimizu S, Ito T, Chittenden T, Lutz RJ, Matsuda H, Tsujimoto Y: Bax interacts with the permeability transition pore to induce permeability transition and cytochrome c release in isolated mitochondria. Proc Natl Acad Sci U S A 1998; 95:14681-6.
52. Goping IS, Gross A, Lavoie JN, Nguyen M, Jemmerson R, Roth K, Korsmeyer SJ, Shore GC: Regulated targeting of BAX to mitochondria. J Cell Biol 1998; 143:207-15.
53. Luo X, Budihardjo I, Zou H, Slaughter C, Wang X: Bid, a Bcl2 interacting protein, mediates cytochrome c release from mitochondria in response to activation of cell surface death receptors. Cell 1998; 94:481-90.
54. Li H, Zhu H, Xu CJ, Yuan J: Cleavage of BID by caspase 8 mediates the mitochondrial damage in the Fas pathway of apoptosis. Cell 1998; 94:491-501.
55. Gross A, Yin XM, Wang K, Wei MC, Jockel J, Milliman C, Erdjument-Bromage H, Tempst P, Korsmeyer SJ: Caspase cleaved BID targets mitochondria and is required for cytochrome c release, while BCL-XL prevents this release but not tumor necrosis factor-R1/Fas death. J Biol Chem 1999; 274:1156-63.
56. Yang E, Zha J, Jockel J, Boise LH, Thompson CB, Korsmeyer SJ: Bad, a heterodimeric partner for Bcl-XL and Bcl-2, displaces Bax and promotes cell death. Cell 1995; 80:285-91.
57. Zha J, Harada H, Yang E, Jockel J, Korsmeyer SJ: Serine phosphorylation of death agonist BAD in response to survival factor results in binding to 14-3-3 not BCL-X(L). Cell 1996; 87:619-28.
58. Takayama S, Sato T, Krajewski S, Kochel K, Irie S, Millan JA, Reed JC: Cloning and functional analysis of BAG-1: a novel Bcl-2-binding protein with anti-cell death activity. Cell 1995; 80:279-84.
59. Bardelli A, Longati P, Albero D, Goruppi S, Schneider C, Ponzetto C, Comoglio PM: HGF receptor associates with the anti-apoptotic protein BAG-1 and prevents cell death. Embo J 1996; 15:6205-12.
60. Fujita N, Nagahashi A, Nagashima K, Rokudai S, Tsuruo T: Acceleration of apoptotic cell death after the cleavage of Bcl-XL protein by caspase-3-like proteases. Oncogene 1998; 17:1295-304.
61. Grandgirard D, Studer E, Monney L, Belser T, Fellay I, Borner C, Michel MR: Alphaviruses induce apoptosis in Bcl-2-overexpressing cells: evidence for a caspase-mediated, proteolytic inactivation of Bcl-2. Embo J 1998; 17:1268-78.
62. Hunter DR, Haworth RA, Southard JH: Relationship between configuration, function, and permeability in calcium-treated mitochondria. J Biol Chem 1976; 251:5069-77.
63. Hunter DR, Haworth RA: The Ca2+-induced membrane transition in mitochondria. I. The protective mechanisms. Arch Biochem Biophys 1979; 195:453-59.
64. Haworth RA, Hunter DR: The Ca2+-induced membrane transition in mitochondria. II. Nature of the Ca2+ trigger site. Arch Biochem Biophys 1979; 195:460-7.

65.   Hunter DR, Haworth RA: The Ca2+-induced membrane transition in mitochondria. III. Transitional Ca2+ release. Arch Biochem Biophys 1979; 195:468-77.

66.   Haworth RA, Hunter DR: Allosteric inhibition of the Ca2+-activated hydrophilic channel of the mitochondrial inner membrane by nucleotides. J Membr Biol 1980; 54:231-6.

67.   Zoratti M, Szabo I: The mitochondrial permeability transition. Biochim Biophys Acta 1995; 1241:139-76.

68.   Kroemer G, Dallaporta B, Resche-Rigon M: The mitochondrial death/life regulator in apoptosis and necrosis. Annu Rev Physiol 1998; 60:619-42.

69.   Fournier N, Ducet G, Crevat A: Action of cyclosporine on mitochondrial calcium fluxes. J Bioenerg Biomembr 1987; 19:297-303.

70.   Crompton M, Ellinger H, Costi A: Inhibition by cyclosporin A of a Ca2+-dependent pore in heart mitochondria activated by inorganic phosphate and oxidative stress. Biochem J 1988; 255:357-60.

71.   Szabo I, Zoratti M: The giant channel of the inner mitochondrial membrane is inhibited by cyclosporin A. J Biol Chem 1991; 266:3376-9.

72.   Pastorino JG, Simbula G, Gilfor E, Hoek JB, Farber JL: Protoporphyrin IX, an endogenous ligand of the peripheral benzodiazepine receptor, potentiates induction of the mitochondrial permeability transition and the killing of cultured hepatocytes by rotenone. J Biol Chem 1994; 269:31041-6.

73.   Hirsch T, Decaudin D, Susin SA, Marchetti P, Larochette N, Resche-Rigon M, Kroemer G: PK11195, a ligand of the mitochondrial benzodiazepine receptor, facilitates the induction of apoptosis and reverses Bcl-2-mediated cytoprotection. Exp Cell Res 1998; 241:426-34.

74.   Marzo I, Brenner C, Zamzami N, Jurgensmeier JM, Susin SA, Vieira HL, Prevost MC, Xie Z, Matsuyama S, Reed JC, Kroemer G: Bax and adenine nucleotide translocator cooperate in the mitochondrial control of apoptosis. Science 1998; 281:2027-31.

75.   Ichas F, Jouaville LS, Mazat JP: Mitochondria are excitable organelles capable of generating and conveying electrical and calcium signals. Cell 1997; 89:1145-53.

76.   Ichas F, Mazat JP: From calcium signaling to cell death: two conformations for the mitochondrial permeability transition pore. Switching from low- to high- conductance state. Biochim Biophys Acta 1998; 1366:33-50.

77.   Eguchi Y, Shimizu S, Tsujimoto Y: Intracellular ATP levels determine cell death fate by apoptosis or necrosis. Cancer Res 1997; 57:1835-40.

78.   Leist M, Single B, Castoldi AF, Kuhnle S, Nicotera P: Intracellular adenosine triphosphate (ATP) concentration: a switch in the decision between apoptosis and necrosis. J Exp Med 1997; 185:1481-6.

79.   Ferrari D, Stepczynska A, Los M, Wesselborg S, Schulze-Osthoff K: Differential regulation and ATP requirement for caspase-8 and caspase-3 activation during CD95- and anticancer drug-induced apoptosis. J Exp Med 1998; 188:979-84.

80.   Lemasters JJ: V. Necrapoptosis and the mitochondrial permeability transition: shared pathways to necrosis and apoptosis. Am J Physiol 1999; 276:G1-G6.

81.   Qian T, Herman B, Lemasters JJ: The Mitochondrial Permeability Transition Mediates Both Necrotic and Apoptotic Death of Hepatocytes Exposed to Br-A23187. Toxicol Appl Pharmacol 1999; 154:117-25.

82.   Kroemer G, Zamzami N, Susin SA: Mitochondrial control of apoptosis. Immunol Today 1997; 18:44-51.

83.   Vayssiere JL, Petit PX, Risler Y, Mignotte B: Commitment to apoptosis is associated with changes in mitochondrial biogenesis and activity in cell lines conditionally immortalized with simian virus 40. Proc Natl Acad Sci U S A 1994; 91:11752-6.

84.   Petit PX, Lecoeur H, Zorn E, Dauguet C, Mignotte B, Gougeon ML: Alterations in mitochondrial structure and function are early events of dexamethasone-induced thymocyte apoptosis. J Cell Biol 1995; 130:157-67.

85.   Zamzami N, Marchetti P, Castedo M, Decaudin D, Macho A, Hirsch T, Susin SA, Petit PX, Mignotte B, Kroemer G: Sequential reduction of mitochondrial transmembrane potential and generation of reactive oxygen species in early programmed cell death. J Exp Med 1995; 182:367-77.

86.   Zamzami N, Marchetti P, Castedo M, Zanin C, Vayssiere JL, Petit PX, Kroemer G: Reduction in mitochondrial potential constitutes an early irreversible step of programmed lymphocyte death in vivo. J Exp Med 1995; 181:1661-72.

87. Castedo M, Hirsch T, Susin SA, Zamzami N, Marchetti P, Macho A, Kroemer G: Sequential acquisition of mitochondrial and plasma membrane alterations during early lymphocyte apoptosis. J Immunol 1996; 157:512-21.
88. Kluck RM, Bossy Wetzel E, Green DR, Newmeyer DD: The release of cytochrome c from mitochondria: a primary site for Bcl-2 regulation of apoptosis [see comments]. Science 1997; 275:1132-6.
89. Yang J, Liu X, Bhalla K, Kim CN, Ibrado AM, Cai J, Peng TI, Jones DP, Wang X: Prevention of apoptosis by Bcl-2: release of cytochrome c from mitochondria blocked. Science 1997; 275:1129-32.
90. Susin SA, Zamzami N, Castedo M, Hirsch T, Marchetti P, Macho A, Daugas E, Geuskens M, Kroemer G: Bcl-2 inhibits the mitochondrial release of an apoptogenic protease. J Exp Med 1996; 184:1331-41.
91. Susin SA, Lorenzo HK, Zamzami N, Marzo I, Snow BE, Brothers GM, Mangion J, Jacotot E, Costantini P, Loeffler M, Larochette N, Goodlett DR, Aebersold R, Siderovski DP, Penninger JM, Kroemer G: Molecular characterization of mitochondrial apoptosis-inducing factor. Nature 1999; 397:441-6.
92. Krippner A, Matsuno-Yagi A, Gottlieb RA, Babior BM: Loss of function of cytochrome c in Jurkat cells undergoing fas- mediated apoptosis. J Biol Chem 1996; 271:21629-36.
93. Zou H, Henzel WJ, Liu X, Lutschg A, Wang X: Apaf-1, a human protein homologous to C. elegans CED-4, participates in cytochrome c-dependent activation of caspase-3. Cell 1997; 90:405-13.
94. Li P, Nijhawan D, Budihardjo I, Srinivasula SM, Ahmad M, Alnemri ES, Wang X: Cytochrome c and dATP-dependent formation of Apaf-1/caspase-9 complex initiates an apoptotic protease cascade. Cell 1997; 91:479-89.
95. Srinivasula SM, Ahmad M, Fernandes-Alnemri T, Alnemri ES: Autoactivation of procaspase-9 by Apaf-1-mediated oligomerization. Mol Cell 1998; 1:949-57.
96. Yoshida H, Kong YY, Yoshida R, Elia AJ, Hakem A, Hakem R, Penninger JM, Mak TW: Apaf1 is required for mitochondrial pathways of apoptosis and brain development. Cell 1998; 94:739-50.
97. Hu Y, Benedict MA, Wu D, Inohara N, Nunez G: Bcl-XL interacts with Apaf-1 and inhibits Apaf-1-dependent caspase-9 activation. Proc Natl Acad Sci U S A 1998; 95:4386-91.
98. Pan G, O'Rourke K, Dixit VM: Caspase-9, Bcl-XL, and Apaf-1 form a ternary complex. J Biol Chem 1998; 273:5841-5.
99. Tang DG, Li L, Zhu Z, Joshi B: Apoptosis in the absence of cytochrome c accumulation in the cytosol. Biochem Biophys Res Commun 1998; 242:380-4.
100. Chauhan D, Pandey P, Ogata A, Teoh G, Krett N, Halgren R, Rosen S, Kufe D, Kharbanda S, Anderson K: Cytochrome c-dependent and -independent induction of apoptosis in multiple myeloma cells. J Biol Chem 1997; 272:29995-7.
101. Kluck RM, Martin SJ, Hoffman BM, Zhou JS, Green DR, Newmeyer DD: Cytochrome c activation of CPP32-like proteolysis plays a critical role in a Xenopus cell-free apoptosis system. Embo J 1997; 16:4639-49.
102. Marzo I, Brenner C, Zamzami N, Susin SA, Beutner G, Brdiczka D, Remy R, Xie ZH, Reed JC, Kroemer G: The permeability transition pore complex: a target for apoptosis regulation by caspases and bcl-2-related proteins. J Exp Med 1998; 187:1261-71.
103. Marzo I, Brenner C, Kroemer G: The central role of the mitochondrial megachannel in apoptosis: evidence obtained with intact cells, isolated mitochondria, and purified protein complexes. Biomed Pharmacother 1998; 52:248-51.
104. Bossy-Wetzel E, Newmeyer DD, Green DR: Mitochondrial cytochrome c release in apoptosis occurs upstream of DEVD- specific caspase activation and independently of mitochondrial transmembrane depolarization. Embo J 1998; 17:37-49.
105. Jurgensmeier JM, Xie Z, Deveraux Q, Ellerby L, Bredesen D, Reed JC: Bax directly induces release of cytochrome c from isolated mitochondria. Proc Natl Acad Sci U S A 1998; 95:4997-5002.
106. Vander Heiden MG, Chandel NS, Williamson EK, Schumacker PT, Thompson CB: Bcl-xL regulates the membrane potential and volume homeostasis of mitochondria [see comments]. Cell 1997; 91:627-37.
107. Eskes R, Antonsson B, Osen-Sand A, Montessuit S, Richter C, Sadoul R, Mazzei G, Nichols A, Martinou JC: Bax-induced cytochrome C release from mitochondria is independent of the permeability transition pore but highly dependent on Mg2+ ions. J Cell Biol 1998; 143:217-24.

108. Susin SA, Zamzami N, Castedo M, Daugas E, Wang HG, Geley S, Fassy F, Reed JC, Kroemer G: The central executioner of apoptosis: multiple connections between protease activation and mitochondria in Fas/APO-1/CD95- and ceramide- induced apoptosis. J Exp Med 1997; 186:25-37.
109. Marzo I, Susin SA, Petit PX, Ravagnan L, Brenner C, Larochette N, Zamzami N, Kroemer G: Caspases disrupt mitochondrial membrane barrier function. FEBS Lett 1998; 427:198-202.
110. Finucane DM, Bossy-Wetzel E, Waterhouse NJ, Cotter TG, Green DR: Bax-induced Caspase Activation and Apoptosis via Cytochrome c Release from Mitochondria Is Inhibitable by Bcl-xL. J Biol Chem 1999; 274:2225-2233.
111. Susin SA, Lorenzo HK, Zamzami N, Marzo I, Brenner C, Larochette N, Prvost MC, Alzari PM, Kroemer G: Mitochondrial Release of Caspase-2 and -9 during the Apoptotic Process. J Exp Med 1999; 189:381-394.
112. Reed JC, Jurgensmeier JM, Matsuyama S: Bcl-2 family proteins and mitochondria. Biochim Biophys Acta 1998; 1366:127-37.
113. Kuida K, Haydar TF, Kuan CY, Gu Y, Taya C, Karasuyama H, Su MS, Rakic P, Flavell RA: Reduced apoptosis and cytochrome c-mediated caspase activation in mice lacking caspase 9. Cell 1998; 94:325-37.
114. Minn AJ, Velez P, Schendel SL, Liang H, Muchmore SW, Fesik SW, Fill M, Thompson CB: Bcl-x(L) forms an ion channel in synthetic lipid membranes. Nature 1997; 385:353-7.
115. Antonsson B, Conti F, Ciavatta A, Montessuit S, Lewis S, Martinou I, Bernasconi L, Bernard A, Mermod JJ, Mazzei G, Maundrell K, Gambale F, Sadoul R, Martinou JC: Inhibition of Bax channel-forming activity by Bcl-2. Science 1997; 277:370-2.
116. Schendel SL, Xie Z, Montal MO, Matsuyama S, Montal M, Reed JC: Channel formation by antiapoptotic protein Bcl-2. Proc Natl Acad Sci U S A 1997; 94:5113-8.
117. Schlesinger PH, Gross A, Yin XM, Yamamoto K, Saito M, Waksman G, Korsmeyer SJ: Comparison of the ion channel characteristics of proapoptotic BAX and antiapoptotic BCL-2. Proc Natl Acad Sci U S A 1997; 94:11357-62.
118. Lam M, Bhat MB, Nunez G, Ma J, Distelhorst CW: Regulation of Bcl-xl channel activity by calcium. J Biol Chem 1998; 273:17307-10.
119. Matsuyama S, Schendel SL, Xie Z, Reed JC: Cytoprotection by Bcl-2 requires the pore-forming alpha5 and alpha6 helices. J Biol Chem 1998; 273:30995-1001.

I.2.3
Inhibition of cardiac myocyte apoptosis by gp130-dependent cytokines

Kai C. Wollert, M.D.
Medizinische Hochschule Hannover, Hannover, Germany

INTRODUCTION

In animal models and in patients with end-stage heart failure, a small fraction of cardiac myocytes undergoes programmed cell death (apoptosis) (1-4). In general, cardiac failure is preceded by a hypertrophic response of the myocardium, that allows the heart to maintain cardiac output despite a chronic increase in hemodynamic load. However, sustained hemodynamic overloading eventually causes a transition from hypertrophy to heart failure, characterized by chamber dilatation, progressive contractile dysfunction and impaired survival. The observation that the prevalence of apoptotic cardiomyocytes is increased in the failing heart but not during the initial stage of compensatory hypertrophy has given rise to the hypothesis that cardiac myocyte dropout by apoptosis may be one mechanism contributing to the progression of cardiac hypertrophy to heart failure (5,6).

Considerable research efforts have focussed on the elucidation of the molecular mechanisms that regulate cardiac myocyte hypertrophy and apoptosis. In this regard, growth factors and cytokines acting in an autocrine and/or paracrine manner are thought to play a key role in the activation of cardiac myocyte hypertrophy (7-13). Moreover, growth factors and cytokines are emerging as potent regulators of cardiac myocyte apoptosis (14-18). In this context, TNF-α and IL-1β have been shown to *promote* apoptosis in cultured cardiac myocytes (15,18). In contrast to these observations, recent data indicate that cytokines belonging to the interleukin

(IL)-6 cytokine family *inhibit* cardiac myocyte apoptosis and stimulate cardiac myocyte hypertrophy, via the signal-transducing receptor component gp130.

INTERLEUKIN-6 CYTOKINE FAMILY - SIGNALING PATHWAYS

IL-6 related cytokines regulate growth, differentiation and apoptosis of various tissues and cells, including hematopoietic and lymphoid cells, neuronal cells, hepatocytes and osteoclasts (reviewed in 19). The members of the IL-6 cytokine family are distantly related with regard to their primary amino acid sequence and share a common four α-helix bundle topology. Besides IL-6, this cytokine family encompasses IL-11, leukemia inhibitory factor (LIF), oncostatin M (OSM), ciliary neurotrophic factor (CNTF) and cardiotrophin-1 (CT-1) (20-25). A characteristic feature of the IL-6 related cytokines is their functional redundancy, i.e. the fact that different cytokines can mediate the same biological activities in a given cell or tissue system. This functional redundancy can be explained on a molecular level by the use of common receptor subunits by different members of the IL-6 cytokine family (Figure 1).

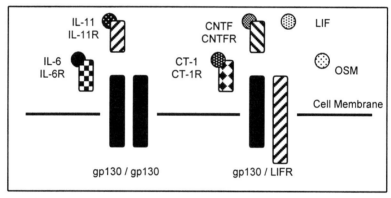

Figure 1 Receptor complexes of the IL-6 cytokine family. Downstream signaling events are triggered by the homodimerization of gp130 or the heterodimerisation of gp130 with the LIF receptor (LIFR). In the case of IL-6, IL-11, CNTF and, probably, CT-1, dimerization of gp130 requires cytokine-specific receptor α-subunits.

The IL-6 related cytokines signal through multisubunit cell surface receptors that share the transmembrane signal transducer gp130. In the case of the IL-6 and IL-11 receptor systems, intracellular signaling is triggered through a homodimerization of gp130 (26). By contrast, LIF, OSM, CNTF and CT-1 signaling requires the heterodimerization of gp130 with a structurally related transmembrane signal transducer, the low-affinity LIF receptor (LIFR) (27). LIF and OSM trigger intercellular signaling through a direct interaction with gp130 and the LIFR. By contrast, IL-6, IL-11, CNTF and, at least in some cell types, CT-1 cannot bind to gp130 and the LIFR directly, but must first associate with receptor α-subunits, the IL-6R, IL-11R, CNTFR, and CT-1R respectively (28-31). Subsequently, the IL-6/IL-6R and IL-11/IL-11R complexes induce gp130 homodimerization, whereas the

CNTF/CNTFR and CT-1/CT-1R complexes induce gp130/LIFR heterodimerization (reviewed in 19).

Following ligand-induced gp130 dimerization, intracellular signaling proceedes through several cascades, including the Janus kinase (JAK) - signal transducer and activator of transcription (STAT) pathway and the p21ras-mitogen-activated protein kinase (MAPK) pathway (Figure 2).

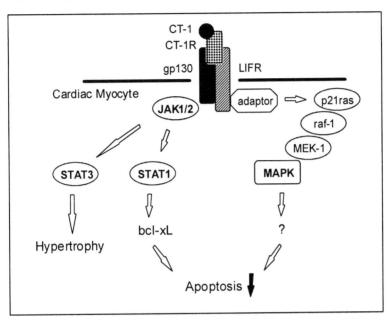

Figure 2 Activation of the JAK-STAT and p21ras-MAPK signal transduction pathways in cardiac myocytes by gp130-stimulatory cytokines. The inhibition of apoptosis and the induction of hypertrophy are mediated by divergent signaling pathways.

Homo- or heterodimerization of gp130 results in the activation and auto/trans-phosphorylation of the gp130-associated Janus kinases (32). The pattern of JAK activation has been shown to be cell type specific (33). Upon activation, Janus kinases phosphorylate gp130 at cytoplasmic tyrosine residues, thereby creating docking sites for the SH2 domain containing transcription factors of the STAT family. Recruited STATs become tyrosine phosphorylated and form homo- or heterodimers which then translocate into the nucleus to bind to cognate DNA response elements and activate target gene transcription (reviewed in 34). Activation of the MAPK's ERK1 and ERK2 by the IL-6 related cytokines proceeds through a signaling cascade involving the stepwise activation of p21ras, raf-1 and MAPK kinase 1 (MEK-1) (35,36). It has been suggested that the activation of p21ras through gp130 depends on the prior tyrosine phosphorylation of the adaptor protein Shc followed by complex formation with Grb2 and SOS (36). However, the precise mechanism(s) linking gp130 to the MAPK cascade remain to be established.

In cardiomyocytes, dimerization of gp130 induces a rapid tyrosine phosphorylation of JAK1 and JAK2, but not Tyk2 (37,38). Janus kinase activation is quickly followed by STAT1α/β and STAT3 tyrosine phosphorylation and nuclear translocation (37,38). In addition, stimulation of gp130 induces MAPK activity in cardiac myocytes (37). Co-immunoprecipitation of MAPK with STAT1 and STAT3 suggests a cross-talk between the MAPK and JAK-STAT signaling pathways (38).

GP130-DEPENDENT SIGNALING PATHWAYS PROMOTE CARDIAC MYOCYTE HYPERTROPHY AND INHIBIT APOPTOSIS

In recent years, IL-6 related cytokines have been shown to activate a hypertrophic growth response in cardiac myocytes, and to enhance cardiac myocyte survival by inhibiting apoptotic cell death (reviewed in 39). Moreover, several groups have begun to dissect the signaling pathways that mediate these biological responses (Figure 2). Stimulation of cultured neonatal cardiac myocytes with IL-6 related cytokines activates several morphological and molecular markers that define a hypertrophic response, including cell growth, sarcomere organisation and increased gene transcription (40). CT-1, LIF, and a complex of IL-6 and the IL-6R promote cardiomyocyte hypertrophy in vitro, indicating that similar signaling cascades are activated in cardiomyocytes by gp130/LIFR heterodimers and gp130 homodimers, respectively (40). Double transgenic mice overexpressing IL-6 and the IL-6R provide evidence that an activation of gp130 dependent pathways induces cardiac hypertrophy in vivo as well: IL-6/IL-6R transgenic mice display tyrosine phosphorylation, i.e. activation, of gp130 and STAT3 in the myocardium and develop dramatic increases in cardiac weights and cardiomyocyte size (41).

To investigate whether IL-6 related cytokines can promote the survival of postnatal cardiac myocytes, Sheng et. al. developed an assay system in which cell death is induced in neonatal cardiac myocytes by serum deprivation (42). As evidenced by DNA agarose gel-electrophoresis and by in situ nick end-labeling, cardiac myocyte death following serum deprivation is primarily due to apoptosis. In this assay system, IL-6 related cytokines enhance cardiac myocyte survival by blocking apoptosis (42). In a similar study, Stephanou et al. demonstrated that CT-1 can protect cultured cardiac myocytes from ischemia-induced apoptosis (43). Transfection of a MEK-1 dominant negative mutant cDNA and cotreatment with a MEK-1 inhibitor abolished the survival effects of the IL-6 related cytokines in serum-deprived cardiac myocytes, indicating a requirement for MAPK(s) (42). Inhibition of MEK-1 does not alter cardiac myocyte hypertrophy in response to stimulation with IL-6 related cytokines, suggesting that divergent signaling pathways promote hypertrophy and survival in cardiac myocytes (42). By contrast, transfection of a dominant negative STAT3 cDNA inhibits cardiac myocyte hypertrophy in response to IL-6 related cytokines, indicating that the JAK-STAT signal transduction pathway is required for the induction of hypertrophy (44). Little is known regarding the molecular mechanisms that mediate the cytoprotective effect of IL-6 related cytokines in cardiac myocytes. In this regard, IL-6 related cytokines have been shown to upregulate the anti-apoptotic regulator bcl-xL in cardiac myocytes via a STAT1 dependent transcriptional mechanism (45). Moreover, the cytoprotective effect of CT-1 in ischemic cardiac myocytes is associated with the induction of heat shock proteins (43). In conclusion, inhibition of cardiac myocyte apoptosis by IL-6 related cytokines appears to be mediated by MAPK and, presumably, JAK-STAT1-dependent signaling pathways.

TARGETED DISRUPTION OF GP130 REVEALS A CRITICAL ROLE FOR GP130-DEPENDENT CYTOKINES IN VIVO

Using a Cre-lox technology, Hirota et al. have recently generated mice with a cardiac myocyte-specific knockout of the gp130 receptor component (46). These mice display normal embryonic viability and show no evidence of congenital heart defects. This is in striking contrast to the cardiac morphogenic defects observed in conventional gp130 knockout animals (47). Therefore, during normal embryonic development, there is no cardiomyocyte cell-autonomous requirement for the gp130 signaling pathway. The cardiac defects reported previously for the conventional gp130 knockout mice may rather arise as a consequence of severe associated hematopoietic defects resulting in oxygen deprivation and/or may be secondary to the deletion of gp130 in non-cardiac myocyte cell types in the heart. Cardiac-specific gp130 knockout mice survive to adulthood, display no apparent histological abnormalities of the heart and exhibit normal cardiac function as assessed by echocardiography (46). Strikingly, however, in the setting of chronic pressure overload, cardiac-specific gp130 knockout mice rapidly develop cardiac dilatation associated with a depression of cardiac contractility and a dramatic increase in mortality (46). In contrast, control mice develop concentric hypertrophy consistent with an adaptive physiological response. As evidenced by the normal expression of embryonic genes in response to pressure overload, the rapid chamber dilatation in cardiac-specific gp130 knockout mice may not be due to an inability to activate a hypertrophic response. Instead, in cardiac-specific gp130 knockout mice, cardiac deterioration is associated with a dramatic increase in cardiac myocyte apoptosis (46). It appears therefore, that gp130-dependent signaling pathways are critical for myocyte survival and the prevention of heart failure during pressure overload. Moreover, these studies provide direct evidence that myocyte apoptosis is a pivotal event in the transition from compensatory hypertrophy to overt heart failure.

EXPRESSION OF IL-6 RELATED CYTOKINES IN THE HEART

Considering the potent hypertrophic and anti-apoptotic effects of IL-6 related cytokines, is has become critical to determine which of the IL-6 cytokine family members activate gp130-dependent signaling cascades in cardiomyocytes *in vivo*. In this regard, none of the IL-6 related cytokines appears to be expressed abundantly in the normal adult myocardium. However, recent studies indicate that the expression of IL-6 related cytokines may be upregulated in the myocardium and in cardiac myocytes under pathophysiological conditions. Cardiac myocytes have been shown to synthesize and release IL-6 in response to hypoxic stress *in vitro* (48). Moreover, the expression of IL-6 and CT-1 is upregulated in the infarcted myocardium early after experimental coronary artery ligation (49,50). Considering that IL-6 related cytokines can protect cultured cardiac myocytes from ischemia-induced apoptosis (43), one may speculate that the increased levels of IL-6 and CT-1 promote cardiac myocyte survival in the ischemic heart. Hemodynamic overload has been shown to be associated with increased expression levels of IL-6 and LIF in the myocardium, suggesting that IL-6 related cytokines may play a role in the development of cardiac hypertrophy in response to pressure overload *in vivo* (51,52). Little is known regarding the mechanisms that promote the expression of IL-6 related cytokines in the myocardium. However, it has been shown that tumor necrosis factor (TNF)-α can induce the expression of IL-6 and LIF in cultured cardiac myocytes, suggesting that IL-6 related cytokines may be part of a cytokine cascade (51,53). In agreement with this hypothesis, the expression levels of TNF-α, IL-6 and CT-1 are increased in the failing left ventricular myocardium late after experimental myocardial infarction (49,50). With regard to the human situation, clinical studies have indicated that circulating levels of IL-6 are increased in patients with unstable angina, acute myocardial infarction or heart failure (54-56). In heart failure patients, the peripheral circulation appears to be an important site of IL-6 generation (57). The expression of IL-6 related cytokines in the human heart remains to be determined.

CONCLUSIONS

Cytokines from the IL-6 cytokine family are emerging as potent regulators of cardiomyocyte hypertrophy and programmed cell death. IL-6 related cytokines signal through the common receptor component gp130 and activate the MAPK and JAK-STAT signal transduction pathways in cardiac myocytes. The recent generation of mice with a cardiac-specific knockout of gp130 has provided strong evidence that gp130-dependent cytokines mediate a myocyte survival pathway that blocks the onset of apoptosis and prevents the progression to heart failure in pressure overload hypertrophy *in vivo*.

ACKNOWLEDGEMENT

The author would like to thank Kenneth R. Chien, M.D., Ph.D. for his critical discussion of the manuscript.

References

1. Cheng W, Kajstura J, Nitahara JA, Li B, Reiss K, Liu Y, Clark WA, Krajewski S, Reed JC, Olivetti G, Anversa P. Programmed myocyte cell death affects the viable myocardium after infarction in rats. Exp Cell Res 1996;226:316-327.
2. Li Z, Bing OHL, Long X, Robinson KG, Lakatta EG. Increased cardiomyocyte apoptosis during the transition to heart failure in the spontaneously hypertensive rat. Am J Physiol 1997;272:H2313-H2319.
3. Narula J, Haider N, Virmani R, di Salvo TG, Kolodgie FD, Hajjar RJ, Schmidt U, Semigran MJ, Dec GW, Khaw BA. Apoptosis in myocytes in end-stage heart failure. N Engl J Med 1996;335:1182-1189.

4.   Olivetti G, Abbi R, Quaini F, Kajstura J, Cheng W, Nitahara JA, Quaini E, di Loreto C, Beltrami CA, Krajewski S, Reed JC, Anversa P. Apoptosis in the failing human heart. N Engl J Med 1997;336:1131-1141.
5.   Bing OHL. Hypothesis: apoptosis may be a mechanism for the transition to heart failure with chronic pressure overload. J Mol Cell Cardiol 1994;26:943-948.
6.   Colucci WS. Apoptosis in the heart. N Engl J Med 1996;335:1224-1226.
7.   Knowlton KU, Michel MC, Itani M, Shubeita HE, Ishihara K, Brown JH, Chien KR. The α_{1A}-adrenergic receptor subtype mediates biochemical, molecular, and morphologic features of cultured myocardial cell hypertrophy. J Biol Chem 1993;268:15374-15380.
8.   Shubeita HE, McDonough PM, Harris AN, Knowlton KU, Glembotski CC, Brown JH, Chien KR. Endothelin induction of inositol phospholipid hydrolysis, sarcomere assembly, and cardiac gene expression in ventricular myocytes. A paracrine mechanism for myocardial cell hypertrophy. J Biol Chem 1990;265:20555-20562.
9.   Sadoshima J, Izumo S. Molecular characterization of angiotensin II-induced hypertrophy of cardiac myocytes and hyperplasia of cardiac fibroblasts. Critical role of the AT_1 receptor subtype. Circ Res 1993;73:413-423.
10.   Parker TG, Packer SE, Schneider MD. Peptide growth factors can provoke fetal contractile protein gene expression in rat cardiac myocytes. J Clin Invest 1990;85:507-514.
11.   Ito H, Hiroe M, Hirata Y, Tsujino M, Adachi S, Schichiri M, Koike A, Nogami A, Marumo F. Insulin-like growth factor-I induces hypertrophy with enhanced expression of muscle specific genes in cultured rat cardiomyocytes. Circulation 1993;87:1715-1721.
12.   Thaik CM, Calderone A, Takahashi N, Colucci WS. Interleukin-1β modulates the growth and phenotype of neonatal rat cardiac myocytes. J Clin Invest 1995;96:1093-1099.
13.   Yokoyama T, Nakano M, Bednarczyk JL, McIntyre BW, Entmann ML, Mann DL. Tumor necrosis factor-α provokes a hypertrophic growth response in adult cardiac myocytes. Circulation 1997;95:1247-1252.
14.   Kajstura J, Cigola E, Malhotra A, Li P, Cheng W, Meggs LG, Anversa P. Angiotensin II induces apoptosis of adult ventricular myocytes in vitro. J Mol Cell Cardiol 1997;29:859-870.
15.   Krown KA, Page MT, Nguyen C, Zechner D, Gutierrez V, Comstock KL, Glembotski CC, Quintana PJE, Sabbadini RA. Tumor necrosis factor alpha-induced apoptosis in cardiac myocytes. Involvement of the sphingolipid signaling cascade in cardiac cell dearth. J Clin Invest 1996;98:2854-2865.
16.   Wang L, Ma W, Markovich R, Chen JW, Wang PH. Regulation of cardiomyocyte apoptotic signaling by insulin-like growth factor I. Circ Res 1998;83:516-522.
17.   Nakano M, Knowlton AA, Dibbs Z, Mann DL. Tumor necrosis factor-α confers resistance to hypoxic injury in the adult mammalian cardiac myocyte. Circulation 1998;97:1392-1400.
18.   Ing DJ, Zang J, Dzau VJ, Webster KA, Bishopric NH. Modulation of cytokine-induced cardiac myocyte apoptosis by nitric oxide, bak, and bcl-x. Circ Res 1999;84:21-33.
19.   Kishimoto T, Akira S, Narazaki M, Taga T. Interleukin-6 family of cytokines and gp130. Blood 1995;86:1243-1254.
20.   Hirano T, Yasukawa K, Harada H, Taga T, Watanabe Y, Matsuda T, Kashiwamura SI, Nakajima K, Koyama K, Iwamatsu A, Tsunasawa S, Sakiyama F, Matsui H, Takahara Y, Taniguchi T, Kishimoto T. Complementary DNA for a novel human interleukin (BSF-2) that induces B lymphocytes to produce immunoglobulin. Nature 1986;324:73-76.
21.   Paul SR, Bennett F, Calvetti JA, Kelleher K, Wood CR, O'Hara RM, Leary AC, Sibley B, Clark SC, Williams DA, Yang YC. Molecular cloning of a cDNA encoding interleukin 11, a stromal cell-derived lymphopoietic and hematopoietic cytokine. Proc Natl Acad Sci USA 1990;87:7512-7516.
22.   Gearing DP, Gough NM, King JA, Hilton DJ, Nicola NA, Simpson RJ, Nice EC, Kelso A, Metcalf D. Molecular cloning and expression of cDNA encoding a murine myeloid leukaemia inhibitory factor (LIF). EMBO J 1987;6:3995-4002.
23.   Malik N, Kallestad JC, Gunderson NL, Austin SD, Neubauer MG, Ochs V, Marquardt H, Zarling JM, Shoyab M, Wei CM, Linsley PS, Rose TM. Molecular cloning, sequence analysis, and functional expression of a novel growth regulator, oncostatin M. Mol Cell Biol 1989;9:2847-2853.
24.   Stöckli KA, Lottspeich F, Sendtner M, Masiakowski P, Carroll P, Götz R, Lindholm D, Thoenen H. Molecular cloning, expression and regional distribution of rat ciliary neurotrophic factor. Nature 1989;342:920-923.

25. Pennica D, King KL, Shaw KJ, Luis E, Rullamas J, Luoh SM, Darbonne WC, Knutzon DS, Yen R, Chien KR, Baker JB, Wood WI. Expression cloning of cardiotrophin 1, a cytokine that induces cardiac myocyte hypertrophy. Proc Natl Acad Sci USA 1995;92:1142-1146.
26. Hibi M, Murakami M, Saito M, Hirano T, Taga T, Kishimoto T. Molecular cloning and expression of an IL-6 signal transducer, gp130. Cell 1990;63:1149-1157.
27. Gearing DP, Thut CJ, VandenBos T, Gimpel SD, Delaney PB, King J, Price V, Cosman D, Beckmann MP. Leukemia inhibitory factor receptor is structurally related to the IL-6 signal transducer, gp130. EMBO J 1991;10:2839-2848.
28. Yamasaki K, Taga T, Hirata Y, Yawata H, Kawanishi Y, Seed B, Taniguchi T, Hirano T, Kishimoto T. Cloning and expression of the human interleukin-6 (BSF-2/IFNβ 2) receptor. Science 1988;241:825-828.
29. Hilton DJ, Hilton AA, Raicevic A, Rakar S, Harrison-Smith M, Gough NM, Begley CG, Metcalf D, Nicola NA, Willson TA. Cloning of a murine IL-11 receptor a-chain; requirement for gp130 for high affinity binding and signal transduction. EMBO J 1994;13:4765-4775.
30. Davis S, Aldrich TH, Valenzuela DM, Wong V, Furth ME, Squinto SP, Yancopoulos GD. The receptor for ciliary neurotrophic factor. Science 1991;253:59-63.
31. Robledo O, Fourcin M, Chevalier S, Guillet C, Auguste P, Pouplard-Barthelaix A, Pennica D, Gascan H. Signaling of the cardiotrophin-1 receptor. Evidence for a third receptor component. J Biol Chem 1997;272:4855-4863.
32. Narazaki M, Witthuhn BA, Yoshida K, Silvennoinen O, Yasukawa K, Ihle JN, Kishimoto T, Taga T. Activation of JAK2 kinase mediated by the interleukin 6 signal transducer gp130. Proc Natl Acad Sci USA 1994;91:2285-2289.
33. Stahl N, Boulton TG, Farruggella T, Ip NY, Davis S, Witthuhn BA, Quelle FW, Silvennoinen O, Barbieri G, Pellegrini S, Ihle JN, Yancopoulos GD. Association and activation of Jak-Tyk kinases by CNTF-LIF-OSM-IL-6 β receptor components. Science 1994;263:92-95.
34. Ihle JN. STATs: signal transducers and activators of transcription. Cell 1996;84:331-334.
35. Daeipour M, Kumar G, Amaral MC, Nel AE. Recombinant IL-6 activates p42 and p44 mitogen-activated protein kinases in the IL-6 responsive B cell line, AF10. J Immunol 1993;150:4743-4753.
36. Kumar G, Gupta S, Wang S, Nel AE. Involvement of janus kinases, p52shc, Raf-1, and MEK-1 in the IL-6-induced mitogen-activated protein kinase cascade of a growth-responsive B cell line. J Immunol 1994;153:4436-4447.
37. Kunisada K, Hirota H, Fujio Y, Matsui H, Tani Y, Yamauchi-Takihara K, Kishimoto T. Activation of JAK-STAT and MAP kinases by leukemia inhibitory factor through gp130 in cardiac myocytes. Circulation 1996;94:2626-2632.
38. Kodama H, Fukuda K, Pan J, Makino S, Baba A, Hori S, Ogawa S. Leukemia inhibitory factor, a potent cardiac hypertrophic cytokine, activates the JAK/STAT pathway in rat cardiomyocytes. Circ Res 1997;81:656-663.
39. Wollert KC, Chien KR. Cardiotrophin-1 and the role of gp130-dependent signaling pathways in cardiac growth and development. J Mol Med 1997;75:492-501.
40. Wollert KC, Taga T, Saito M, Narazaki M, Kishimoto T, Glembotski CC, Vernallis AB, Heath JK, Pennica D, Wood WI, Chien KR. Cardiotrophin-1 activates a distinct form of cardiac muscle cell hypertrophy. Assembly of sarcomeric units in series via gp130/leukemia inhibitory factor receptor-dependent pathways. J Biol Chem 1996;271:9535-9545.
41. Hirota H, Yoshida K, Kishimoto T, Taga T. Continuous activation of gp130, a signal-transducing receptor component for interleukin 6-related cytokines, causes myocardial hypertrophy in mice. Proc Natl Acad Sci USA 1995;92:4862-4866.
42. Sheng Z, Knowlton K, Chen J, Hoshijima M, Brown JH, Chien KR. Cardiotrophin-1 inhibition of cardiac myocyte apoptosis via a mitogen-activated protein kinase-dependent pathway. Divergence from downstream CT-1 signals for myocardial cell hypertrophy. J Biol Chem 1997;272:5783-5791.
43. Stephanou A, Brar B, Heads R, Knight RD, Marber MS, Pennica D, Latchman DS. Cardiotrophin-1 induces heat shock protein accumulation in cultured cardic myocytes and protects them from stressful stimuli. J Mol Cell Cardiol 1998;30:849-855.
44. Kunisada K, Tone E, Fujio Y, Matsui H, Yamauchi-Takihara K, Kishimoto T. Activation of gp130 transduces hypertrophic signals via STAT3 in cardiac myocytes. Circulation 1998;98:346-352.

45. Fujio Y, Kunisada K, Hirota H, Yamauchi-Takihara K, Kishimoto T. Signals through gp130 upregulate *bcl-x* gene expression via STAT1-binding *cis*-element in cardiac myocytes. J Clin Invest 1997;99:2898-2905.

46. Hirota H, Chen J, Betz UAK, Rajewsky K, Gu Y, Ross J, Müller W, Chien KR. Loss of a gp130 cardiac muscle cell survival pathway is a critical event in the onset of heart failure during biomechanical stress. Cell 1999; 97:189-198.

47. Yoshida K, Taga T, Saito M, Suematsu S, Kumanogoh A, Tanaka T, Fujiwara H, Hirata M, Yamagami T, Nakahata T, Hirabayashi T, Yoneda Y, Tanaka K, Wang WZ, Mori C, Shiota K, Yoshida N, Kishimoto T. Targeted disruption of gp130, a common signal transducer for the interleukin 6 family of cytokines, leads to myocardial and hematological disorders. Proc Natl Acad Sci USA 1996;93:407-411.

48. Yamauchi-Takihara K, Ihara Y, Ogata A, Yoshizaki K, Azuma J, Kishimoto T. Hypoxic stress induces cardiac myocyte-derived interleukin-6. Circulation 1995;91:1520-1524.

49. Ono K, Matsumori A, Shioi T, Furukawa Y, Sasayama S. Cytokine gene expression after myocardial infarction in rat hearts. Possible implication in left ventricular remodeling. Circulation 1998;98:149-156.

50. TakimotoY, Aoyama T, Pennica D, Shinoda E, Keyamura R, Hattori R, Yui Y, Sasayama S. Augmented gene expression of cardiotrophin-1 and its receptor component, gp130, in both ventricles after myocardial infarction in the rat. Circulation 1998 (suppl);98:I-839.

51. Wang F, Seta Y, Baumgarten G, Mann DL. Expression of leukemia inhibitory factor in the adult mammalian heart. Dynamic regulation and functional significance. Circulation 1998 (suppl);98:I-247.

52. Sakai S, Miyauchi T, Kobayashi T, Yamaguchi I, Sugishita Y. Involvement of endogenous interleukin-6 (IL-6) and leukemia inhibitory factor (LIF) in the development of cardiac hypertrophy induced by pressure-overload in vivo in rats. Circulation 1998 (suppl);98:I-421.

53. Gwechenberger M, Mendoza LH, Youker KA, Frangogiannis NG, Smith W, Michael LH, Entmann ML. Cardiac myocytes produce interleukin-6 in culture and in viable border zone of reperfused infarctions. Circulation 1999;99:546-551.

54. Biasucci LM, Vitelli A, Liuzzo G, Altamura S, Caligiuri G, Monaco C, Rebuzzi AG, Ciliberto G, Maseri A.. Elevated levels of interleukin-6 in unstable angina. Circulation 1996;94:874-877.

55. Ikeda U, Ohkawa F, Seino Y, Yamamoto K, Hidaka Y, Kasahara T, Kawai T, Shimada K. Serum interleukin 6 levels become elevated in acute myocardial infarction. J Mol Cell Cardiol 1992;24:579-584.

56. Torre-Amione G, Kapadia S, Benedict C, Oral H, Young JB, Mann DL. Proinflammatory cytokine levels in patients with depressed left ventricular ejection fraction. A report from the studies of left ventricular dysfunction (SOLVD). J Am Coll Cardiol 1996;27:1201-1206.

57. Tsutamoto T, Hisanaga T, Wada A, Maeda K, Ohnishi M, Fukai D, Mabuchi N, Sawaki M, Kinoshita M. Interleukin-6 spillover in the peripheral circulation increases with the severity of heart failure, and the high plasma level of interleukin-6 is an important prognostic predictor in patients with congestive heart failure. J Am Coll Cardiol 1998;31:391-398.

I.2.4
Cell cycle regulation and apoptotic cell death

Lothar Jahn, M.D., and Harald Bär, M.D.
Ruprecht-Karls-Universität Heidelberg, Heidelberg, Germany

INTRODUCTION

The number of cells in any cellular biological system is determined by the balance of cell proliferation and cell death. Changes result in tissue growth or atrophy. The control of this equilibrium is crucial for the developing and the fully differentiated organism. Morphogenesis, gain and maintenance of organ function and response to various types of cell stress require mechanisms tightly controlling this equilibrium. The development of digits and the reorganisation and loss of thymic cells during mammalian development, the remodelling of bones in response to various forces are examples for processes depending on major shifts of this equilibrium that must be regulated extraordinarily accurate. An imbalance of cell proliferation and cell death may be the primary cause of diseases. Moreover, the seize of organs, animals and human beings eventually are determined by this balance.

Thus far cell proliferation and cell death have been studied predominantly as two separated processes. While cell proliferation was investigated extensively already over the last decades cell death, particularly apoptosis, only more recently became a central issue in cell biology. Most studies focused either only on cell proliferation or on cell death. However, cell proliferation and cell death are not only intimately connected to each other due to their counteracting effects, but even more because of the composition of players regulating both processes. Recent studies demonstrate that molecules regulating cell proliferation, i.e. cell cycle control, also are directly involved in the regulation of cell cycle exit, differentiation and apoptosis.

CELL CYCLE CONTROL

Proliferation of eukaryotic cells is regulated by highly complex and specific mechanisms. Proliferating cells must pass a certain sequence of control points during the cell cycle. After having doubled the DNA content during S phase cells go through G2 phase before entering mitosis or M phase. Between mitosis and S-phase cells are in G1 and have two options, either to enter a new round of the cell cycle or to go into a resting state, G0. Major control points of the cell cycle are the G1/S and the G2/M transition. Over the last several years studies using yeast mutants defective in specific points of the cell cycle have provided the basis of biochemical events regulating the cell cycle in eukaryotic cells. Important components in cell cycle control are three classes of proteins the cyclins, the cyclin-dependent kinases and the recently discovered cyclin-dependent kinase inhibitors.

COMPONENTS OF THE CELL CYCLE REGULATORY MACHINERY: CYCLINS, CYCLIN-DEPENDENT KINASES AND CYCLIN-DEPENDENT KINASE INHIBITORS

Cyclins

Cyclins are proteins that have been named according to their oscillating levels during the cell cycle. They were initially found in marine invertebrates (1), but later also described in yeast, vertebrates (2) and plants (3). Cyclins associate with cyclin-dependent kinases regulating the cyclin-dependent kinase activity. They are regulated by the activity of kinases, phosphatases and ubiquitin dependent proteases. In proliferating cells different combinations of cyclin/cyclin dependent kinase are necessary to pass the checkpoints of the cell cycle. In most cells the transition from G1 to S phase and the G2/M phase transition are crucial checkpoints that are tightly controlled. Differential association of the various cyclins with different cyclin dependent kinases and cyclin dependent kinase inhibitors provide an almost unlimited variability of complexes and consecutively of cell cycle regulation. The members of these families reveal specific affinities to their counterparts.

Cyclin dependent kinases

The cyclin dependent kinases (cdk) are proteins closely related to the cdc2+ gene product of *Schizosaccharomyces pombe*, $p34^{cdc2}$, a serine/threonine kinase (4,5,6; for review, see 7). The first hints about their function were obtained using inactivating antibodies. Depletion of CDK2 from Xenopus egg extracts blocked DNA synthesis (8) indicating that CDK2 is involved in G1/S transition. On the other hand, depletion of $p34^{cdc2}$ did not affect DNA replication, but delayed mitosis (8) confirming observations suggesting a crucial role of $p34^{cdc2}$ in concert with cyclin B for G2/M transition (9). Accumulation and association of certain cyclins with the various CDKs at specific points of the cell cycle was also studied to gain insight into the function of these proteins. At the G1/S transition an association of D-type cyclins with CDK4 and CDK6 and of cyclin E with CDK2 was observed. At

G2/M complexes consisting of cyclin A and CDK 2 or CDC 2 and cyclin B and CDC 2 were found. The activity of these complexes is regulated by phosphorylation of threonine and tyrosine residues of CDKs (10, 11, 12).

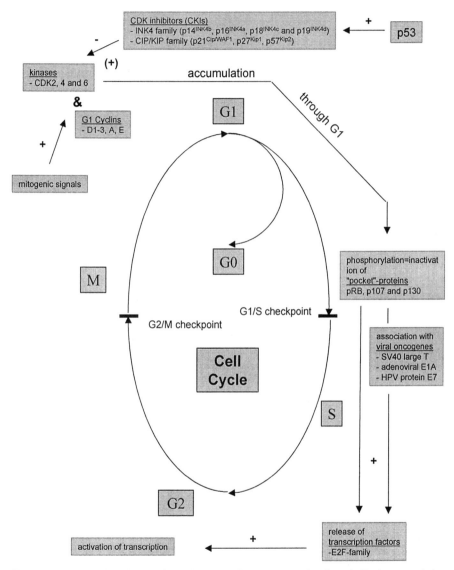

Figure 1   Representation of cell cycle regulating proteins. For progression through G1 phase association of CDKs and G1 cyclins is necessary, while p53 via CDK inhibitors mainly retards progression. At the G1/S transition pRB is inactivated inducing the release of transcription factors and, through largely unknown mechanisms, triggering DNA replication. The transcriptional activation by pRB inactivation is mimicked by viral oncogenes. (+) activation; (-) inhibition. See text for details.

Cyclin dependent kinase inhibitors

More recently a new class of regulators of cdk activity, the so called CDK inhibitors (CKIs) has been described (13,14). One class of CKIs is the INK4 family consisting of $p14^{INK4b}$, $p16^{INK4a}$, $p18^{INK4c}$ and $p19^{INK4d}$. CKIs of the INK4 family specifically inhibit CDK4 and CDK6 at the G1 checkpoint (13) and depend on the tumour suppressor protein pRB (15). A second class of CKIs, the Cip/Kip family acts non-specifically and targets various cyclin/CDK complexes. Three members of this family of negative regulators of cell cycle control are characterised thus far, $p21^{Cip1/WAF1}$, $p27^{kip1}$ and $p57^{Kip2}$ (16, 17, 18).

Very recently this concept of inhibition of CDKs by CDK inhibitors was challenged by the observation that the assembly of the cyclin D/CDK4 complex depends on $p21^{Cip1/WAF1}$ and $p27^{kip1}$ (19), thought to be negative regulators of CDKs. Moreover, the nuclear accumulation of this complex depends on CDK inhibitors. These results suggest, that CDK inhibitors not only specifically interact with different CDKs, but also differentially regulate CDKs, by inhibiting CDK2 and activating CDK4. This complex regulation targets the action of CDK inhibitors to specific checkpoint of cell cycle regulation. The same molecule may positively regulate mitogenic signals via its effect on CDK4 and negatively regulate G1/S transition through the inactivation of CDK2.

REGULATION OF APOPTOSIS BY THE CYCLIN DEPENDENT KINASE INHIBITOR $p21^{CIP1/WAF1}$

The differential effect of CDK inhibitors does not only depend on the target CDK, but also on its cellular localisation. While the well known inhibitory effect on G1/S transition correlates with a nuclear localisation, in certain cells $p21^{Cip1/WAF1}$ remains cytoplasmic and inhibits apoptosis (20). In accordance, a negative regulation of $p21^{Cip1/WAF1}$ on apoptosis by interaction with p53 was described in malignomas such as colorectal cancer (21) and in melanomas (22). In vitro studies using a carcinoma cell line also suggested an inhibition of stress-induced apoptosis by $p21^{Cip1/WAF1}$ (23). The mechanism by which $p21^{Cip1/WAF1}$ inhibits apoptosis seems to be based on an interaction of $p21^{Cip1/WAF1}$ with the apoptosis signal-regulating kinase 1 (ASK1) and results in an upstream inhibition of stress-activated MAP-kinases (20). To make this complex regulation even more complicated the „anti-apoptotic" cytoplasmic localisation of $p21^{Cip1/WAF1}$ depends on a certain level of the cellular differentiation program. This observation is of particular interest regarding the interplay between cell proliferation, differentiation and cell death. $p21^{Cip1/WAF1}$ may be a multifunctional key player of signal transduction of these different cellular pathways. The pivotal role of CDK inhibitors during development is documented by the phenotype of $p27^{kip1}$-deficient mice, which are about 30% larger than control animals (24).

It is well established that the induction of apoptosis by DNA damaging agents such as UV- or γ-radiation is mediated by the tumour suppressor p53 (25, 26) which in turn activates a whole set of genes (27) including the cyclin dependent kinase inhibitor $p21^{Cip1/WAF1}$ in its "typical" nuclear localisation (28). In p53 deficient/mutated cells $p21^{Cip1/WAF1}$ expression and apoptosis did not occur, suggesting that functional p53 is necessary to induce the activity of $p21^{Cip1/WAF1}$ at the G1/S transition and eventually apoptosis. (29). On the other hand, experiments using p53 deficient cells derived from p53 deficient mice clearly demonstrate that there must be alternative p53 independent pathways to induce apoptosis mediated by activation of $p21^{Cip1/WAF1}$ (30). In normal hepatocytes IFN-gamma induces p53 as well as $p21^{Cip1/WAF1}$ mRNA expression, but cell death is also induced in p53-deficient hepatocytes (apoptotic bodies were not detectable, however; 31). Other inducers of p53 independent apoptosis that act through activation of $p21^{Cip1/WAF1}$ are 12-0-tetradecanoyl phorbol-13-acetate (TPA), 1,25-dihydroxyvitamin D3, retinoic acid, dimethylsulfoxid (32), serum or individual growth factors such as platelet-derived growth factor, fibroblast growth factor and epidermal growth factor (30). Interestingly, these are all compounds known to be involved in cellular proliferation and/or induction of differentiation, the latter being a process that normally depends on the exit of cells from the cell cycle. These results indicate that the "classic" p53-dependent pathway of apoptosis induction through $p21^{Cip1/WAF1}$ may be bypassed by the direct activation of downstream $p21^{Cip1/WAF1}$. In addition, p21Cip1/WAF1 may be directly down regulated in a p53-independent way by the tumour repressor retinoblastoma protein pRB (33).

THE TUMOUR REPRESSOR RETINOBLASTOMA PROTEIN (PRB)

A large body of evidence indicates that pRB is involved in proliferation and cell cycle control. The initial observation, that mutation of the retinoblastoma gene is the cause of retinoblastoma tumours is the basis of its classification as a tumour repressor (34). pRB is a nuclear protein that shows changing levels of phosphorylation while the cell proceeds through the cell cycle. It is a member of the "pocket" protein family consisting of pRB, pRB2/p130, and p107. pRB is un- or hypophosphorylated during the G1 phase of the cell cycle and becomes phosphorylated by cyclin/CDK complexes at the G1/S transition (35). The first links between specific function of pRB and its state of phosphorylation came from experiments looking for binding partners of viral oncoproteins. SV40 T antigen, human papilloma virus protein E7 and adenoviral protein E1A are able to bind hypophosphorylated pRB. This binding displaces an ubiquitous cellular transcription factor (E2F) from the so called "pocket" region of pRB, enabling the cell to enter and pass the G1/S checkpoint of the cell cycle (35, 36). According to this model of cell cycle regulation hypophosphorylated pRB is the active protein that binds and inactivates common transcription factors of the E2F family. Strong support for this hypothesis comes from binding studies monitoring the transcriptional activity of free E2F as compared to E2F bound to pRB (37). Very recent studies suggest that pRB also plays a regulatory role in apoptotic cell death. During the onset of apoptosis pRB becomes hypophosphorylated by a specific protein-serine/ threonine phosphatase and is cleaved by a caspase-like protease. According to these results unphosphorylated pRB seems to be an inhibitor of apoptosis (38), although the cleavage of a 5 kDa fragment from the C-terminus of pRB seems to mimic this effect, indicating that proteolytic cleavage of pRB also may be responsible for the demonstrated inhibition of apoptosis (39).

CONCLUDING REMARKS

Tissue homeostasis must be balanced by a tight regulation of cell proliferation and cell death. This regulation is crucial during early embryogenesis for developing tissues and organogenesis as well as for maintenance of specific organ function. It must be extraordinarily dynamic requiring numerous negative and positive regulating elements. Thus far our understanding of this complex regulation is limited. Research is dissecting different pathways or single steps of cell proliferation and apoptosis neglecting the intimate interaction of both processes. Moreover, the level of differentiation of the cell or the intracellular localisation of the molecule determines the mode of action of cell cycle regulating proteins. The fact that "classic" negative regulators of cell cycle control the CDK inhibitors are also activators of cyclin dependent kinases demonstrates not only the complexity of cell cycle regulation but also illustrates the difficulty and future challenge to understand the interplay of cell proliferation and cell death.

References

1. Evans T, Rosenthal E, Youngblom J, Distel D Hunt T. Cyclin: a protein specified by maternal mRNA in sea urchin eggs that is destroyed at each cleavage division. *Cell*. 1983; 33,389-396.
2. Pines J. Cell proliferation and control. *Curr Opin Cell Biol*. 1992; 4, 144-148.
3. Hata S, Kouchi H, Suzuka K Ishii T. Isolation and characterization of cDNA clones for plant cyclins. *EMBO J*. 1991; 10, 2681-2688.
4. Dunphy W, Brizuela L, Bech D, Newport J. The Xenopus cdc2 protein is a component of MPF, a cytoplasmic regulator of mitosis. *Cell*. 1988; 54,423-431.
5. Gautier J, Norbury C, Lohka M, Nurse P, Maller J. Purified maturation-promoting factor contains the product of a Xenopus homolog of the fission yeast cell cycle control gene cdc2+. *Cell*. 1988; 54,433-439.
6. Meyerson M, Enders GH, Wu CL, Su LK, Gorka C, Nelson C, Harlow E Tsai LH. A family of human cdc2-related protein kinases. *EMBO J*. 1992; 11, 2909-2917.
7. Lewin B. Driving the cell cycle: M phase kinase, its partners, and substrates. *Cell*. 1990; 61,743-52.
8. Fang F Newport J. Evidence that the G1-S and G2-M transitions are controlled by different cdc2 proteins in higher eukaryotes. *Cell*. 1991; 66,731-742.
9. Draetta G, Luca F, Westendorf J, Brizuela L, Ruderman J, Beach D. Cdc2 protein kinase is complexed with both cyclin A and B: evidence for proteolytic inactivation of MPF. *Cell*. 1989; 56,829-838.
10. Gu Y, Rosenblatt J, Morgan D. Cell cycle regulation of CDK2 activity by phosphorylation of Thr160 and Tyr15. *EMBO J*. 1992; 11,3995-4005.
11. Lorca T, Labbe J, Devault A, Fesquet D, Capony J, Cavadore J, Le Bouffant F Doree M. Dephosphorylation of cdc2 on threonine 161 is required for cdc2 kinase inactivation and normal anaphase. *EMBO J*. 1992; 11, 2381-2390.
12. Solomon M, Lee T Kirschner M. Role of phosphorylation in p34cdc2 activation: identification of an activating kinase. *Mol Biol Cell*. 1992; 3, 13-27.
13. Sherr CJ, Roberts JM. Inhibitors of mammalian G1 cyclin-dependent kinases. *Genes Dev*. 1995; 9,1149-63.
14. Elledge SJ, Harper JW. Cdk inhibitors: on the threshold of checkpoints and development. *Curr Opin Cell Biol*. 1994; 6,847-52.

15. Guan KL, Jenkins CW, Li Y, Nichols MA, Wu X, O'Keefe CL, Matera AG, Xiong Y. Growth suppression by p18, a p16INK4/MTS1- and p14INK4B/MTS2-related CDK6 inhibitor, correlates with wild-type pRB function. *Genes Dev.* 1994; 8, 2939-52.

16. Harper JW, Adami GR, Wei N, Keyomarsi K, Elledge SJ. The p21 Cdk-interacting protein Cip1 is a potent inhibitor of G1 cyclin-dependent kinases. *Cell.* 1993; 75, 805-16.

17. Polyak K, Lee MH, Erdjument-Bromage H, Koff A, Roberts JM, Tempst P, Massague J. Cloning of p27Kip1, a cyclin-dependent kinase inhibitor and a potential mediator of extracellular antimitogenic signals. *Cell.* 1994; 78, 59-66.

18. Toyoshima H Hunter T. p27, a novel inhibitor of G1 cyclin-Cdk protein kinase activity, is related to p21. *Cell.* 1994; 78, 67-74.

19. Cheng M, Olivier P, Diehl JA, Fero M, Roussel MF, Roberts JM, Sherr CJ. The p21(Cip1) and p27(Kip1) CDK 'inhibitors' are essential activators of cyclin D-dependent kinases in murine fibroblasts. *EMBO J.* 1999; 18:1571-1583.

20. Asada M, Yamada T, Ichijo H, Delia D, Miyazono K, Fukumuro K, Mizutani S. Apoptosis inhibitory activity of cytoplasmic p21(Cip1/WAF1) in monocytic differentiation. *EMBO J.* 1999; 18:1223-1234.

21. Polyak K, Waldman T, He TC, Kinzler KW, Vogelstein B. (1996). Genetic determinants of p53-induced apoptosis and growth arrest. *Genes Dev.* 1996; 10:1945-1952.

22. Gorospe M, Cirielli C, Wang X, Seth P, Capogrossi MC, Holbrook NJ. p21(Waf1/Cip1) protects against p53-mediated apoptosis of human melanoma cells. *Oncogene* 1997; 27:929-935.

23. Guadagno TM, Newport JW. Cdk2 kinase is required for entry into mitosis as a positive regulator of Cdc2-cyclin B kinase activity. *Cell.* 1996; 84:73-82.

24. Kiyokawa H, Kineman RD, Manova-Todorova KO, Soares VC, Hoffman ES, Ono M, Khanam D, Hayday AC, Frohman LA, Koff A. Enhanced growth of mice lacking the cyclin-dependent kinase inhibitorfunction of p27(Kip1). *Cell.* 1996; 85:721-732.

25. Clarke AR, Purdie CA, Harrison DJ, Morris RG, Bird CC, Hooper ML, Wyllie AH. Thymocyte apoptosis induced by p53-dependent and independent pathways. *Nature.* 1993; 362:849-852.

26. Lowe SW, Schmitt EM, Smith SW, Osborne BA, Jacks T. p53 is required for radiation-induced apoptosis in mouse thymocytes. *Nature.* 1993; 362:847-849.

27. Polyak K, Xia Y, Zweier JL, Kinzler KW, Vogelstein B. A model for p53-induced apoptosis. *Nature.* 1997; 389:300-305.

28. El-Deiry WS, Tokino T, Velculescu VE, Levy DB, Parsons R, Trent JM, Lin D, Mercer WE, Kinzler KW, Vogelstein B. WAF1, a potential mediator of p53 tumor suppression. *Cell.* 1993; 75:817-825.

29. El-Deiry WS, Harper JW, O'Connor PM, Velculescu VE, Canman CE, Jackman J, Pietenpol JA, Burrell M, Hill, DE, Wang Y, et al. WAF1/CIP1 is induced in p53-mediated G1 arrest and apoptosis. *Cancer Res.* 1994; 54:1169-1174.

30. Michieli P, Chedid M, Lin D, Pierce JH, Mercer WE, Givol D. Induction of WAF1/CIP1 by a p53-independent pathway. *Cancer Res.* 1994; 54:3391-3395.

31. Kano A, Watanabe Y, Takeda N, Aizawa S, Akaike T. Analysis of IFN-gamma-induced cell cycle arrest and cell death in hepatocytes. *J Biochem (Tokyo).* 1997; 121:677-683.

32. Jiang H, Lin J, Su ZZ, Collart FR, Huberman E, Fisher PB. Induction of differentiation in human promyelocytic HL-60 leukemia cells activates p21, WAF1/CIP1, expression in the absence of p53. *Oncogene.* 1994; 9:3397-3406.

33. Yin Y, Solomon G, Deng C, Barrett JC. Differential regulation of p21 by p53 and Rb in cellular response to oxidative stress. *Mol Carcinog.* 1999; 24:15-24.

34. Knudson AG Jr. Mutation and cancer: statistical study of retinoblastoma. *Proc Natl Acad Sci U S A.* 1971; 68:820-823.

35. Hollingsworth RE Jr, Chen PL, Lee WH. Integration of cell cycle control with transcriptional regulation by the retinoblastoma protein. *Curr Opin Cell Biol.* 1993; 5:194-200.

36. Nevins JR. E2F: a link between the Rb tumor suppressor protein and viral oncoproteins. *Science.* 1992; 258:424-429.

37. Hiebert SW, Chellappan SP, Horowitz JM, Nevins JR. The interaction of RB with E2F coincides with an inhibition of the transcriptional activity of E2F. *Genes Dev.* 1992; 6:177-85.

38. Morana SJ, Wolf CM, Li J, Reynolds JE, Brown MK, Eastman A. The involvement of protein phosphatases in the activation of ICE/CED-3 protease, intracellular acidification, DNA digestion, and apoptosis. *J Biol Chem.* 1996; 271:18263-1871.

39. Chen WD, Otterson GA, Lipkowitz S, Khleif SN, Coxon AB, Kaye FJ. Apoptosis is associated with cleavage of a 5 kDa fragment from RB which mimics dephosphorylation and modulates E2F binding. *Oncogene*. 1997; 14:1243-1248.

I.3
The execution of apoptosis

I.3.1
Caspase cascades and caspase targets

Thomas Rudel, Ph.D.

Max-Planck Institut Berlin, Berlin

INTRODUCTION

Apoptosis is an evolutionarily conserved form of cell suicide. Cells that die by apoptosis are disassembled in a stereotypical manner resulting in a characteristic 'apoptotic morphology'. It was this characteristic, uniform morphology displayed by cells during apoptosis which led to the assumption that cells contain a similar execution machinery running according to a program present in all cells. The apoptosis-inducing stimuli are extremely diverse, engage sometimes totally different signalling pathways but are finally translated into the same response of a co-ordinated cell death. Furthermore, induction of apoptosis is sometimes very rapid, in the range of minutes to hours from receiving the signal until the first apoptotic signs appear. For such a fast event, time is too short to start the synthesis of new proteins executing the apoptotic program. Thus, all the components of the death machinery are present in a dormant form and are rapidly converted if necessary. In recent years many of the molecules involved in apoptotic death have been identified and functionally assigned to different stages of apoptosis. The final stage, also called execution, is initiated and co-ordinated by a recently identified class of cysteine proteases termed caspases.

CASPASES, THE CENTRAL EXECUTIONERS OF PROGRAMMED CELL DEATH

Caspases have been recognised as the mammalian homologues of the nematode *Caenorhabditis elegans* CED-3, an essential gene product required for apoptotic cell death (1,2). To date, a large family of 14 different caspases has been identified which play a role in inflammation (Casp-1, -4,-5,-11,-13) and apoptosis; the best characterised members are depicted in table 1. Caspases share similarities in sequence, structure and substrate specificity (3). They are all produced as inactive precursors (zymogens) which contain a N-terminal prodomain, a large (~20 kDa) and a small subunit (~10 kDa). The N-terminal domain is highly variable between

Table 1 Caspase Family.

Proteases	Other names	Ideal cleavage sequence	Substrates
caspase-1	ICE	WEHD	pro-IL1β, pro-caspase-3,-4
caspase-4	ICErel-II, TX, ICH-2	W/LEHD	pro-caspase-1
caspase-5	ICErelII, TY	W/LHD	not pro-IL1β
caspase-2	ICH-1	DEHD	not PARP
caspase-3	CPP32, YAMA, apopain	DEVD	PARP, DNA-PK, SRE/BP, rho-GDI, PAK2, pro-caspase-6,-9
caspase-6	Mch2	VEHD	Lamin
caspase-7	Mch3, ICE-LAP3, CMH-1	DEVD	PARP, pro-caspase-6
caspase-8	FLICE, MACH, Mch5	LETD	pro-caspase-3,-4,-7,-9
caspase-9	ICE-LAP6, Mch6	LEHD	pro-caspase-3,-7
caspase-10	Mch4	LEAD	pro-caspase-3,-7

the different members and is important for the subcellular localisation and activation (see below). Activation requires processing of the precursor into the large and small subunit, in some cases the prodomain is removed as well. The individual subunits dimerise and associate to form a α2β2 hetero-tetramer with two, independent active sites (Figure 1)(4-6). A special feature of caspases is their high specificity with an absolute requirement for cleavage after aspartic acid. The cleavage recognition site includes a stretch of 4 amino acids N-terminal to the cleavage site. Individual caspases prefer different tetrapeptide motifs, a feature, that might explain the substrate specificity (Table 1)(7).

It is of special interest that all pro-forms of caspases contain perfect caspase recognition and cleavage sites at junctions of their functional domains implying that activation occurs either autocatalytically or by other caspases. Two major apoptotic pathways of caspase activation exist, either mediated by death receptors or by mitochondria.

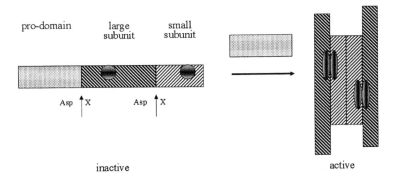

Figure 1 Molecular structure of caspases and mechanism of activation.
Subunits of caspases are separated by caspase-recognition sequences (Asp – X). Upon cleavage, small and large subunits dimerise to form the active site (double oval).

ACTIVATION OF CASPASES BY DEATH RECEPTORS

In recent years, several death receptors have been identified all of which belong to the tumor necrosis factor (TNF)-receptor family (8). Activation of these receptors, e.g. CD95 (Fas/Apo-1) or TNF-receptor 1, results in induction of programmed cell death within hours. This extremely rapid mode of cell death reflects the fact that all components of apoptotic execution are pre-formed in the cell and time-consuming synthesis of new proteins is not required to run the death program. Immediately after activation a number of adaptor and effector molecules are recruited in an highly ordered manner to the cytoplasmic domain of the receptor. The assembly of this multi-protein complex involves interaction modules present in the cytoplasmic domain of the receptor, the adaptors and the effectors (Fig. 2). Three types of protein-protein interaction domains are present in apoptotic molecules: death domains (DDs), death effector domains (DEDs) and caspase interaction and recruitment domains (CARDs). DDs are common in death receptors and molecules that are recruited to these receptors, whereas DEDs and CARDs are responsible for recruiting initiator caspases to death complexes through adaptor molecules some of which are depicted in table 2.

Table 2 Caspase – adaptor pairs and their interaction domains.

Caspase	Adaptor	Type of interaction	Reference
CED-3	CED-4	CARD-CARD	(9)
Caspase-1	CARDIAK	CARD-CARD	(10)
Caspase-2	RAIDD	CARD-CARD	(11)
Caspase-8	FADD	DED-DED	(12,13)
Caspase-9	APAF-1	CARD-CARD	(14)
Caspase-10	FADD	DED-DED	(12,13)

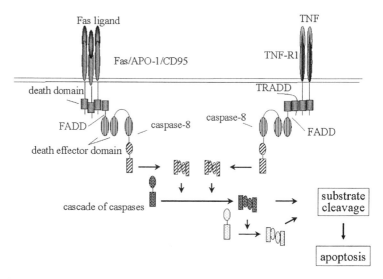

Figure 2 Receptor-mediated activation of caspases.
Ligation of death receptors results in the formation of protein complexes which recruit and activate initiator caspases. Following initiator caspase activation second level caspases are processed which cleave cellular substrates and co-ordinate apoptosis.

The cytoplasmic domain of CD95 (Fas/Apo-1) contains a DD which interacts with the DD present in the adaptor molecule FADD (Fas-associated protein with death domain) (15). FADD also contains a death effector domain (DED) which associates with the DED present in the large N-terminal prodomain of caspase-8 (12,13). The key to the activation of the first level caspase-8 (initiator caspase) is the very low intrinsic activity of the pro-caspase which is, however, sufficient for cleavage and activation when the molecules are in close proximity in the complex (16,17). This 'induced proximity' auto- or trans-activation of initiator caspases (16) results in their release from the receptor complex and the subsequent cleavage and activation of downstream effector caspases. Following effector caspase activation a set of substrates is cleaved and the cell is disassembled in a co-ordinate manner.

MITOCHONDRIAL CONTROL OF CASPASES ACTIVATION

Unlike the ligands of death receptors which induce apoptosis in a well defined way, numerous substances, cytotoxic stress or toxic cell metabolites initiate apoptotic cell death by a less well understood pathway. It is remarkable, however, that although the inducers of apoptosis can be so diverse, the phenotype of apoptotic cells is very uniform. Thus, the major pathways of the effector phase in apoptotic execution are probably conserved. This assumption is substantiated by the fact that, independent of the nature of the inducers, apoptotic cell death can be prevented or delayed by inhibiting caspase function (3,18). But how can such diverse stimuli as oxygen stress, γ-irradiation or staurosporine treatment be translated into a co-ordinate response of the cell leading to apoptotic death? Central to this question are mitochondria which appear to be the integrators of many different apoptotic stimuli (19). Mitochondria respond to apoptotic stimuli with the release of caspase-activating proteins like cytochrome c. Cytochrome c is required as co-factor in a complex with the adaptor molecule Apaf-1 and dATP for caspase-9 activation (14). Active caspase-9 cleaves and activates effector caspases which co-ordinate the execution phase of the death program (Figure 3).

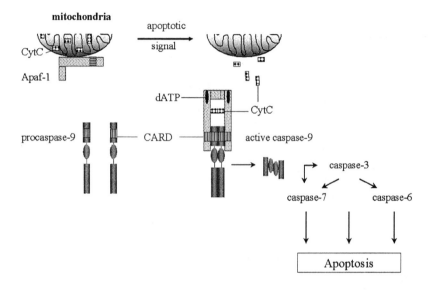

Figure 3 Mitochondria controlled induction of apoptosis.
A complex consisting of Apaf-1, cytochrome C, dATP and pro-caspase-9 is formed upon induction of apoptosis. Pro-caspase-9 is converted to the active caspase-9, the first level caspase in caspase cleavage and activation cascade.

Thus, the common theme of caspase activation either by death receptors or by mitochondria involves initiator caspases which are bound by their specific adaptor molecules (Table 2). Apoptotic stimuli modify the adaptor in a way that it is able to bind and activate the first level caspases of a complex caspase cascade. As a consequence, a similar set of effector caspases is activated during the later phases of apoptosis. This model explains, how different signals induce the same biochemical and morphological changes in apoptotic cells.

Although the receptor-mediated and the mitochondria-mediated pathways of apoptosis are distinct in terms of their activation mechanisms and the molecules involved, there are multiple examples of cross-talk. Several inducers of apoptosis have been shown to up-regulate the expression of Fas-receptor or Fas- ligand (20-23), leading to activation of the Fas-pathway by an auto- or paracrine mechanism. Also, direct engagement of the Fas-receptor pathway results in activation of and apoptosis-signalling by mitochondria in many cell types (24). This explains why mitochondrial inhibitors of apoptosis are able to prevent apoptosis in certain cells stimulated to apoptosis by the Fas-pathway (25). One example how the apoptotic receptor pathways talk to the mitochondria is given by the caspase-mediated cleavage of the Bcl-2 like molecule Bid. Cleavage of Bid results in the recruitment of the Bid-cleavage product to mitochondria where it induces the release of cytochrome C and subsequently the activation of caspase-9 (26,27).

CASPASE CASCADES

Independent of the pathways by which caspases are activated, it is now clear, that the initial signal is amplified by a chain-reaction-like activation of the second level caspases (executioner caspases). The precise molecular hierarchy of caspases below the initiator caspases is, however, still unclear. Using purified caspases *in vitro*, several investigators demonstrated the cleavage and activation of second level caspases by first level caspases and also by active second level caspases. It has, however, been extremely difficult to demonstrate the relevance of the *in vitro* findings also *in vivo*. The generation and analysis of caspase knock outs (see below) were helpful to elucidate some of the caspase activation pathways. From the phenotype of caspase-9 knock out mice it appears that different cascades of caspase activation are engaged depending on the stimulus used to induce apoptosis and on the cell type (28,29). It is, however, clear from these results that caspase-9 and caspase-3 form a linear and obligate proteolytic cascade under certain conditions (29). Whether caspase-9 is also able to directly activate caspases-6 and -7 *in vivo* is not known. Although caspase activation cascades have not been described for caspase-8 knock outs so far, some *in vitro* results and time course experiments suggest caspase-8 directly upstream of caspase-3. Other caspases processed and activated by caspase-8 *in vitro* include caspases-4, -7 and –9.

CASPASE KNOCK OUT MICE

Knock out mice are extremely valuable in order to discriminate the *in vivo* function of individual caspases. The analysis of knock outs unravelled unexpected roles of caspases. It was a surprise, that little or no effect on apoptosis was observed upon disruption of caspases-1, -2 (30) or caspase-11 (31), although over-expression of these caspases induces apoptosis in different cell types. Knock out of caspases-1 and -11 did, however, affect cytokine processing. In contrast, knock outs of caspase-3 and –9 (28,29) had profound developmental defects, especially in the brain. Interestingly, the requirement for caspase-3 and –9 depends on the inducers of apoptosis and in addition differs from cell type to cell type. Thus, one or both caspases are required for apoptosis in a given setting but not in others (28).

Also, caspase-8 knock outs die early during development due to a defect in heart development (32). In contrast to the development of the brain, where cell death regulates the pool of progenitor cells, heart development has no component of cell death. Thus, the caspase-8 phenotype was also unexpected since it suggests that caspase-8 has other functions than inducing cell death.

Table 3 Phenotypes in knock-out mice.

Caspase-1 $^{-/-}$	normal , no IL-1α, IL-1β, reduced TNFα and IL-6
Caspase-2 $^{-/-}$	normal, accelerated neuronal apoptosis during development
Caspase-3 $^{-/-}$	die at week 1-3, abnormal brain development, no role in thymocyte apoptosis
Caspase-8 $^{-/-}$	die prenatally, abnormal heart development, absolute defect in Fas- and TNF-receptor initiated apoptosis
Caspase-9 $^{-/-}$	die perinatally, abnormal brain development, no caspase-3 activation, thymocytes resist apoptosis

HOW CASPASES CO-ORDINATE APOPTOSIS

Central to the understanding of the molecular mechanism of cell death is the identification of caspase targets and the elucidation of the consequences of proteolytic cleavage. Most substrates are cleaved only once and therefore activation of caspases results not in a proteolytic degradation of cellular proteins but rather in an highly ordered 'clipping' of substrates at functionally relevant sites. While some substrates are functionally inactivated upon caspase-mediated cleavage, other proteins and enzymes can be activated, particularly by proteolytic removal of regulatory domains.

Although about 60 different substrates for caspases have been identified so far, only in a few cases their proteolysis can be linked to a discrete apoptotic phenotype. In general one can distinguish three major mechanisms by which caspases modify the function of substrates in order to control the apoptotic program: (i) Destruction or inactivation of substrates, (ii) direct activation of substrates sometimes leading to a gain of function and (iii) inactivation of apoptosis inhibitors. Cleavage of nuclear lamins by caspase-6 is a good example for the first mechanism. Lamin cleavage very likely facilitates the disassembly of the nuclear envelope and disintegration of the nucleus (33). Gain of function is given in the case of Bcl-2 cleavage by caspases which converts an inhibitor to an inducer or promoter of apoptosis (34). Cleavage of gelsolin, an actin-severing protein, results in a constitutive active fragment which depolymerises actin and may contribute to membrane blebbing (35). Different kinases are activated by caspases one example of which is the caspase-mediated formation of apoptotic bodies induced by the p21-activated kinase 2 (PAK2). Tightly regulated by GTPases in living cells, processing of PAK2 by caspase-3 generates an permanently active kinase fragment (36). Blocking of PAK2 by a dominant-negative mutant prevented apoptotic body formation while DNA degradation and exposure of phosphtidylserine remained unaffected (36). Another interesting example of selective functions of caspase substrates is also given by the recently identified caspase-activated DNAse (CAD; (37)). CAD is sequestered in the cytosol in its inactive form by binding to a protein called inhibitor of CAD (ICAD), whose human homologue has been previously identified as DNA fragmentation factor (DFF) (38). Upon induction of apoptosis, caspase-3 cleaves ICAD/DFF which allows the DNAse to enter the nucleus and degrade DNA.

Disassembly of cell structures

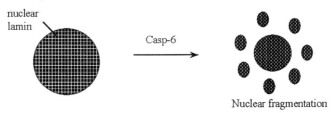

Modification of apoptotic regulators

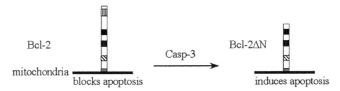

Inactivation of apoptotic inhibitors

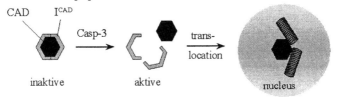

Figure 4 Co-ordination of apoptosis by caspases.

Interestingly, overexpression of ICAD blocks chromatin changes in apoptotic cells but does not affect other phenotypes, e.g. apoptotic body formation (37). Therefore, the cleavage of PAK2 and ICAD are examples of how different features of apoptosis might be discriminated at the level of caspase substrates.

Still the question remains if there is a single caspase substrate whose cleavage is critical for cell death. So far, none of the cleavage events have been shown to be absolutely required to kill cells. It is more likely that apoptosis requires 'a thousand cuts' (39) each contributing to a part of the apoptotic phenotype. The cleavage of multiple substrates with key functions may then collectively culminate in the systematic and orderly disassembly of the apoptotic cell.

CASPASES IN MYOCYTE APOPTOSIS

Apoptosis has been recognised in recent years as important principle in numerous disorders including cardiac diseases. Apoptotic cardiomyocytes have been identified in animal models of cardiac injury and in patients with congestive heart failure or acute myocardial infarction. Since caspases are such important general regulators and effectors of apoptosis, they very likely play also a major role in apoptosis of cardiomyocytes. Support for this assumption comes from *in vitro* experiments with cultured cardiomyocytes which where shown to require caspases to undergo apoptosis induced by staurosporine (40). Yue and colleges (41) tested for activity of caspase-1, -3, -4, -7 and -8 in staurosporine-treated myocytes. The only significant caspase activity present in myocytes after staurosporine treament was caspase-3, whereas activity of caspases-1, -4 and -8 was absent. In addition, there is evidence from *in vivo* studies for up-regulation of caspase-3 upon cardiac injury in an ischemia-reperfusion model (41). Interestingly, elevated caspase-3 levels were detected in the ischemic-reperfused region of the heart only in those regions, where significantly more apoptotic myocytes were found. These results taken together are a first hint of a prominent role of caspase-3 in myocyte apoptosis but they do not exclude a function of other caspases in myocyte apoptosis *in vivo*.

Although the role of caspases in myocyte apoptosis is still elusive, the current reports suggest, that caspases might be potential targets in the treatment of heart disease that are caused by apoptosis. First promising results were reported from *in vivo* studies with caspase inhibitors in ischemia-reperfusion models. In a rat brain model of transient ischemia, a non-selective irreversible inhibitor of caspases significantly reduced brain infarct size after the onset of reperfusion (42). Likewise, caspase inhibitors reduced the ischemia/reperfusion-induced damage of cardiomyocytes in rats, probably by preventing apoptosis (43).

Thus, there is some evidence the caspases play a role in cardiac disease. But, as in the case of other diseases that have a component of apoptosis, it still has to be shown that these powerful molecules can be targeted in a highly specific and selective way for therapeutic intervention.

References

1. Yuan J, Shaham S, Ledoux S, Ellis HM, Horvitz HR: The C. elegans cell death gene ced-3 encodes a protein similar to mammalian interleukin-1 beta-converting enzyme. *Cell* 1993;75:641-652.
2. Thornberry NA, Bull HG, Calaycay JR, Chapman KT, Howard AD, Kostura MJ, Miller DK, Molineaux SM, Weidner JR, Et A: A novel heterodimeric cysteine protease is required for Interleukin-1-beta processing in monocytes. *Nature* 1992;356:768-776.
3. Nicholson DW, Thornberry NA: Caspases: killer proteases. *Trends in Biochemical Sciences* 1997;22:299-306.
4. Walker NP, Talanian RV, Brady KD, Dang LC, Bump NJ, Ferenz CR, Franklin S, Ghayur T, Hackett MC, Hammill LD: Crystal structure of the cysteine protease interleukin-1 beta-converting enzyme: a (p20/p10)2 homodimer. *Cell* 1994;78:343-352.
5. Wilson KP, Black JA, Thomson JA, Kim EE, Griffith JP, Navia MA, Murcko MA, Chambers SP, Aldape RA, Raybuck SA: Structure and mechanism of interleukin-1 beta converting enzyme. *Nature* 1994;370:270-275.

6.   Rotonda J, Nicholson DW, Fazil KM, Gallant M, Gareau Y, Labelle M, Peterson EP, Rasper DM, Ruel R, Vaillancourt JP, Thornberry NA, Becker JW: The three-dimensional structure of apopain/CPP32, a key mediator of apoptosis. *Nature Structural Biology* 1996;3:619-625.
7.   Thornberry NA, Rano TA, Peterson EP, Rasper DM, Timkey T, Garcia-Calvo M, Houtzager VM, Nordstrom PA, Roy S, Vaillancourt JP, Chapman KT, Nicholson DW: A combinatorial approach defines specificities of members of the caspase family and granzyme B. Functional relationships established for key mediators of apoptosis. *Journal of Biological Chemistry* 1997;272:17907-17911.
8.   Ashkenazi A, Dixit VM: Death receptors: signaling and modulation. *Science* 1998;281:1305-1308
9.   Chou JJ, Matsuo H, Duan H, Wagner G: Solution structure of the raidd card and model for card/card interaction in caspase-2 and caspase-9 recruitment. *Cell* 1998;94:171-180.
10. Thome M, Hofmann K, Burns K, Martinon F, Bodmer JL, Mattmann C, Tschopp J: Identification of cardiak, a rip-like kinase that associates with caspase-1. *Current Biology* 1998;8:885-888.
11. Duan H, Dixit VM: RAIDD is a new 'death' adaptor molecule. *Nature* 1997;385:86-89.
12. Boldin MP, Goncharov TM, Goltsev YV, Wallach D: Involvement of MACH, a novel MORT1/FADD-interacting protease, in Fas/APO-1- and TNF receptor-induced cell death. *Cell* 1996;85:803-815.
13. Muzio M, Chinnaiyan AM, Kischkel FC, Orourke K, Shevchenko A, Ni J, Scaffidi C, Bretz JD, Zhang M, Gentz R, Mann M, Krammer PH, Peter ME, Dixit VM: FLICE, a novel FADD-homologous ICE/CED-3-like protease, is recruited to the CD95 (Fas/Apo-1) death-inducing signaling complex. *Cell* 1996;85:817-827.
14. Zou H, Henzel WJ, Liu X, Lutschg A, Wang X: Apaf-1, a human protein homologous to C. elegans CED-4, participates in cytochrome c-dependent activation of caspase-3. *Cell* 1997;90:405-413.
15. Chinnaiyan AM, O'Rourke K, Tewari M, Dixit VM: FADD, a novel death domain-containing protein, interacts with the death domain of Fas and initiates apoptosis. *Cell* 1995;81:505-512.
16. Muzio M, Stockwell BR, Stennicke HR, Salvesen GS, Dixit VM: An induced proximity model for caspase-8 activation. *Journal of Biological Chemistry* 1998;273:2926-2930.
17. Yang X, Chang HY, Baltimore D: Autoproteolytic activation of pro-caspases by oligomerization. *Molecular Cell* 1998;1:319-325.
18. Salvesen GS, Dixit VM: Caspases: intracellular signaling by proteolysis. *Cell* 1997;91:443-446
19. Green DR, Reed JC: Mitochondria and apoptosis. *Science* 1998;281:1309-1312.
20. Krammer PH: Drug-induced cd95 (apo-1/fas)-mediated apoptosis. *Annals of Oncology* 1998;9:39-39.
21. Dhein J, Walczak H, Baumler C, Debatin KM, Krammer PH: Autocrine T-cell suicide mediated by APO-1/(Fas/CD95). *Nature* 1995;373:438-441.
22. Faris M, Kokot N, Latinis K, Kasibhatla S, Green DR, Koretzky GA, Nel A: The c-jun n-terminal kinase cascade plays a role in stress- induced apoptosis in jurkat cells by up-regulating fas ligand expression. *Journal of Immunology* 1998;160:134-144.
23. Kasibhatla S, Brunner T, Genestier L, Echeverri F, Mahboubi A, Green DR: Dna-damaging agents induce expression of fas ligand and subsequent apoptosis in t-lymphocytes via the activation of nf-kb and ap-1. *Molecular Cell* 1998;1:543-551.
24. Peter ME, Krammer PH: Mechanisms of CD95 (APO-1/Fas)-mediated apoptosis. *Current Opinion in Immunology* 1998;10:545-551.
25. Scaffidi C, Fulda S, Srinivasan A, Friesen C, Li F, Tomaselli KJ, Debatin KM, Krammer PH, Peter ME: Two CD95 (APO-1/Fas) signaling pathways. *EMBO Journal* 1998;17:1675-1687
26. Li HL, Zhu H, Xu CJ, Yuan JY: Cleavage of bid by caspase-8 mediates the mitochondrial damage in the fas pathway of apoptosis. *Cell* 1998;94:491-501.
27. Luo X, Budihardjo I, Zou H, Slaughter C, Wang XD: Bid, a bcl2 interacting protein, mediates cytochrome-c release from mitochondria in response to activation of cell- surface death receptors. *Cell* 1998;94:481-490.
28. Hakem R, Hakem A, Duncan GS, Henderson JT, Woo M, Soengas MS, Elia A, Delapompa JL, Kagi D, Khoo W, Potter J, Yoshida R, et al.: Differential requirement for caspase-9 in apoptotic pathways in- vivo. *Cell* 1998;94:339-352.
29. Kuida K, Haydar TF, Kuan CY, Gu Y, Taya C, Karasuyama H, Su MSS, Rakic P, Flavell RA: Reduced apoptosis and cytochrome-c-mediated caspase activation in mice lacking caspase-9. *Cell* 1998;94:325-337.

30. Bergeron L, Perez GI, Macdonald G, Shi LF, Sun Y, Jurisicova A, Varmuza S, Latham KE, Flaws JA, Salter JCM, Hara H, Moskowitz MA, et al.: Defects in regulation of apoptosis in caspase-2-deficient mice. *Genes & Development* 1998;12:1304-1314.

31. Wang SY, Miura M, Jung YK, Zhu H, Li E, Yuan JY: Murine caspase-11, an ice-interacting protease, is essential for the activation of ice. *Cell* 1998;92:501-509.

32. Varfolomeev EE, Schuchmann M, Luria V, Chiannilkulchai N, Beckmann JS, Mett IL, Rebrikov D, Brodianski VM, Kemper OC, Kollet O, Lapidot T, Soffer D, Sobe T, Avraham KB, Goncharov T, Holtmann H, Lonai P, Wallach D: Targeted disruption of the mouse Caspase 8 gene ablates cell death induction by the TNF receptors, Fas/Apo1, and DR3 and is lethal prenatally. *Immunity* 1998;9:267-276.

33. Rao L, Perez D, White E: Lamin proteolysis facilitates nuclear events during apoptosis. *Journal of Cell Biology* 1996;135:1441-1455.

34. Cheng EHY, Kirsch DG, Clem RJ, Ravi R, Kastan MB, Bedi A, Ueno K, Hardwick JM: Conversion of bcl-2 to a bax-like death effector by caspases. *Science* 1997;278:1966-1968.

35. Kothakota S, Azuma T, Reinhard C, Klippel A, Tang J, Chu KT, Mcgarry TJ, Kirschner MW, Koths K, Kwiatkowski DJ, Williams LT: Caspase-3-generated fragment of gelsolin - effector of morphological change in apoptosis. *Science* 1997;278:294-298.

36. Rudel T, Bokoch GM: Membrane and morphological changes in apoptotic cells regulated by caspase-mediated activation of PAK2. *Science* 1997;276:1571-1574.

37. Enari M, Sakahira H, Yokoyama H, Okawa K, Iwamatsu A, Nagata S: A caspase-activated DNase that degrades DNA during apoptosis, and its inhibitor ICAD. *Nature* 1998;393:396-396.

38. Liu X, Zou H, Slaughter C, Wang X: DFF, a heterodimeric protein that functions downstream of caspase-3 to trigger DNA fragmentation during apoptosis. *Cell* 1997;89:175-184.

39. Martin SJ, Green DR: Protease activation during apoptosis: death by a thousand cuts? *Cell* 1995;82:349-352.

40. Yue TL, Wang C, Romanic AM, Kikly K, Keller P, DeWolf WEJ, Hart, TK, Thomas HC, Storer B, Gu JL, Wang X, Feuerstein GZ: Staurosporine-induced apoptosis in cardiomyocytes: A potential role of caspase-3. *Journal of Molecular & Cellular Cardiology* 1998;30:495-507.

41. Black SC, Huang JQ, Rezaiefar P, Radinovic S, Eberhart A, Nicholson, DW, Rodger IW: Co-localization of the cysteine protease caspase-3 with apoptotic myocytes after in vivo myocardial ischemia and reperfusion in the rat. *Journal of Molecular & Cellular Cardiology* 1998;30:733-742.

42. Hara H, Friedlander RM, Gagliardini V, Ayata C, Fink K, Huang Z, Shimizu-Sasamata M, Yuan J, Moskowitz MA: Inhibition of interleukin 1beta converting enzyme family proteases reduces ischemic and excitotoxic neuronal damage. *Proceedings of the National Academy of Sciences of the United States of America* 1997;94:2007-2012.

43. Yaoita H, Ogawa K, Maehara K, Maruyama Y: Attenuation of ischemia/reperfusion injury in rats by a caspase inhibitor. *Circulation* 1998;97:276-281.

I.3.2
Apoptosis: a distinctive form of cell death

L.B. Jordan, M.D., and D.J. Harrison, M.D.
University of Edinburgh, Edinburgh, United Kingdom

INTRODUCTION

As we have seen in the previous chapters, apoptosis is an evolutionary conserved process that is ubiquitous within the living multicellular organism, essential for function and development. In this chapter we aim to introduce the concept of necrosis to highlight the unique process of apoptosis, discuss the features of apoptosis and importantly discuss the difficulties in identifying programmed cell death.

Furthermore, to interpret the significance of 'numbers' of apoptotic cells within a tissue and the vital importance of appropriate resolution of apoptosis, that may have profound implications for Cardiac pathology.

APOPTOSIS VS. NECROSIS

'Apoptosis', a term derived from the classical Greek referring to the falling of leaves from a tree in autumn or the loss of petals from a flower, was proposed by Kerr *et al* (1) after the morphological identification of unique cellular events, now synonymous with this process. This is continually contrasted with necrosis, as an active versus passive form of death. However attitudes may be changing.

Recently several authors (2, 3), have proposed a revised terminology, claiming that necrosis is an all encompassing ancient term to describe post mortem changes in any cell, regardless of the pre-lethal changes or events that lead to death. They have proposed the term 'oncosis', derived from the Greek word for swelling, be resurrected from the original use by Von Recklinghausen in 1910 (2, 4). Dividing pre-lethal morphological changes into apoptosis and oncosis, with necrosis possible sequelae to both. However tempting this revision is, it adds to a field dominated by confused and conflicting terminology and as this has not been widely accepted, we will refrain from its use and compare apoptosis with 'necrosis'.

The next misinterpretation must be addressed; the concept of accidental versus programmed death. As Trump *et al* (2) suggest, apoptosis has gradually become interchangeable with programmed cell death over time, as the apoptotic process has been associated with physiological timed deletion of cells in processes such as development.

NECROSIS	APOPTOSIS
Plasma membrane alterations	Cell and Cytosol Shrinkage
- Blebbing, blunting, distortion of microvilli, failed integrity causing cellular oedema, loss of intercellular attachments. (Functional - loss of ion flux control, Ca^{2+} build up). - Cytoplasmic protein denaturation and clumping.	- (Functional alteration of ion flux and build up of intracellular calcium).
Variable mitochondrial changes	Nuclear Changes.
- Swelling, rarefaction, formation of phospholipid rich amorphous densities. (Functional loss of ATP production, impairing Na^+K^+ ATPase pump contributing to cellular swelling).	- Chromatin condensation and clumping - Site specific cleavage of DNA by a cation dependent endonuclease. - Nuclear fragmentation (karryohexis)
Dilatation of endoplasmic reticulum	Cytoplasmic blebbing.
- Detachment of ribosomes.	
Nuclear changes	Variable endoplasmic reticulum changes.
- Disaggregation of nuclear skeleton and chromatin clumping. - Karyolysis or karryohexis. - Random dissociation and cleavage of DNA.	
Cellular dissociation.	Condensation or no alteration of mitochondria.
	Cytoplasmic Budding.
Clearance.	- Production of vesicles or apoptotic bodies containing chromatin /organelles. (Packaging).
- Probable activation of inflammatory pathways.	Clearance. - Phagocytosis by surrounding cells without inducing an inflammatory response (ideal situation).
NO ENERGY REQUIREMENT.	ENERGY REQUIRED.

Not all death under such circumstances is apoptotic and it is crucial to realise that every cell is 'programmed' for death under the appropriate stimulus (2). However, the activation of that program may produce varied morphology, although the biomechanics involved may be similar.

Tabulated below is a classic morphological comparison of necrosis and apoptosis arranged in approximate chronological observation, derived from many sources (1, 2, 5, 6, 7).

APOPTOTIC STIMULI

Apoptosis can be initiated by numerous stimuli in a wide variety of settings. For simplification, physiological and pathological division can be used.

Physiologic stimuli include those encountered during development, where apoptosis is the most common pre-lethal morphology associated with programmed deletion on a schedule set by external and internal environment factors, e.g. hormones, body mass and nutrition (2, 5, 8, 9). This is also applicable to adult life, with regression of hyperplastic tissues no longer required or deletion of excess cell produced by mitosis. A further example would be the deletion of self reactive T cell clones within the thymus.

Pathological stimuli are those that are injurious to the cell outwith physiological expectation, such as chemical, microbiological, radiological or genetic factors, inducing an apoptotic response often with a self protective motive. Such a response may be appropriate, preventing the spread of a genetic lesion that may lead to neoplasia. Alternatively these may be inappropriate, for example after an occlusion of blood supply to the myocardium; both apoptosis and necrosis are initiated. In this case the program for death is activated by the ischaemic injury. If the blood supply is not reinstated, apoptotic cells die from necrosis as the energy to continue an active process is unavailable. If the blood supply returns rapidly, many cells may be lost by completing their suicide programs as part of reperfusion injury. This can be viewed as inappropriate as the injurious agent has fled and such losses may be detrimental to tissue, organ and organism function. This is the subject of intense research for the medical implications alone (5). Obviously, anti-apoptotic pathways exist to curb some of this loss, but it appears the overall dangers of not responding to an apoptotic stimulus, far outweighs any inappropriate loss of cells.

FEATURES OF APOPTOSIS

The apoptotic process can be subdivided into three distinct stages: commitment, execution and clearance (5). Commitment is the initial stage where an injurious stimulus such as anoxia/hypoxia causes an irreversible commitment to death. Execution is the main subject of this section and includes the majority of the typical morphological changes of apoptosis. Clearance is the final stage, when cellular remnants are removed. This will be dealt with exclusively in a later section.

Kerr *et al* (1) were the first to describe the morphological changes synonymous with the execution phase in 1972. The changes are co-ordinated structural and biochemical events experienced throughout the cell. The easiest events to visualise via microscopy are the nuclear changes (Figure 1).

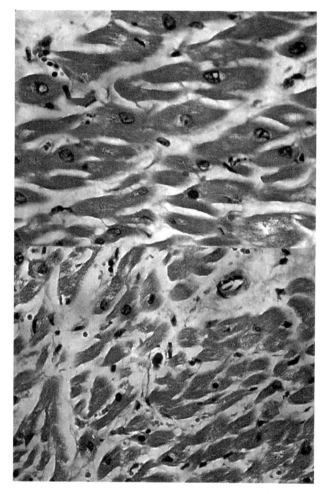

Figure 1 Two photomicrographs of human left ventricular myocardium, retrieved from autopsy material of a 72-year-old female. Note the characteristic nuclear features of two apoptotic cardiomyocytes (top) and the cytoplasmic shrinkage and budding during apoptosis (bottom).

Chromatin condenses and aggregates in a crescent distribution within the nucleus. Examination of this chromatin reveals cleaved DNA fragments in multiples of 180-200 base pairs (7), cleavage being performed by a cation dependent endonuclease initially into 30-50 kilobase pairs. This is not essential and does not occur in some cell types, as its inhibition does not halt the process or ultimate outcome (10, 11). Simultaneously with the condensation, nuclear integrity is altered. The nuclear lamina (intermediate fibre skeleton) responsible for membrane and nuclear pore stability is cleaved, allowing fragmentation of nuclear contents into membrane bound vesicles (12, 13, 14, 15). Remaining intracellular organelles remain structurally intact, although mitochondrial dysfunction occurs with altered transmembrane potential and uncoupling the electron transport pathway from ATP generation with production of more reactive oxygen species (16). Within the cytoplasm, transaglutaminase cross-links various proteins (17) and cytoskeletal filaments aggregate in parallel arrays. The endoplasmic reticulum may dilate and fuse with the plasma membrane; this combined with the loss of membrane phospholipid asymmetry, microvilli and cell-cell contacts destabilises the plasma membrane. The net result is the dissociation from neighbouring cells, continued shrinking and budding of apoptotic bodies into the surrounding tissue. The apoptotic bodies are recognised by surrounding cells or professional phagocytes (such as macrophages) and are phagocytosed rapidly; otherwise these bodies will undergo dissolution, like necrosis and initiate an inflammatory response.

The time to perform the execution phase, once initiated is rapid and conserved, possibly indicating a final common pathway (18). However, the time from exposure to the noxious stimulus to resolution of apoptosis is highly variable and appears dependent on the type of stimulus, cell type (phenotype, genotype and gene expression) and the internal/external environmental milieu. This appears to be related to the variability of reception and transduction of the apoptotic stimulus, followed by the initiation of the response. Perhaps unsurprisingly, many of the pathways involved play a role in carcinogenesis (5).

IDENTIFICATION OF APOPTOSIS

Originally, apoptosis was only identifiable by morphological criteria via microscopy. Subsequent developments have led to an expanding variety of detection methods, each with particular drawbacks that often resort to morphological criteria for confirmation or corroboration of those results. Morphology remains the gold standard at present.

Features of apoptotic cells significantly vary depending on the nature of the apoptotic stimulus, cell type, stage of apoptosis (19), and possible artefacts induced by attempts to detect the process. One must remember that any measure of apoptosis is a snapshot in time, and it is difficult to assess the rate of apoptosis within a given system (19).

Visual methods

Microscopy is the original method of detection and is still useful. Light microscopy of cells is rapid and quantitative, enabling visualisation of nuclear changes and measurement of apoptotic frequency across the field. Problems are inevitable with light microscopy and a consensus between investigators as to the criteria for an apoptotic cell must be agreed as individual bias may influence results. Late stages of apoptosis may be difficult to distinguish from necrosis and morphology is not unambiguous evidence that cells are apoptotic (19, 20). Light microscopy should not be used alone, but combined with other methods the technique is still powerful. Electron microscopy provides the most definitive proof of apoptosis by visualising with exquisite detail the morphology of a cell at that precise time (Figure 2). Electron microscopy is not quantitative however and is difficult to apply for experimental and comparative use (20).

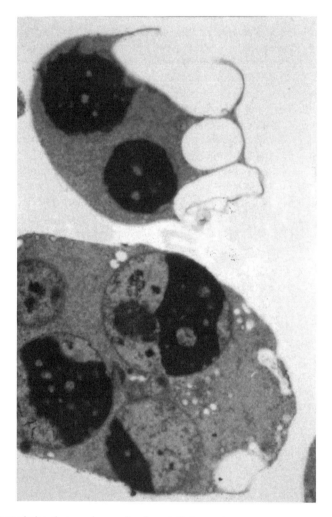

Figure 2 Transmission electronmicrographs of apoptotic leucocytes.

Vital dyes are another means of visual identification of cell death. This is based on the loss of membrane integrity of a cell on death, allowing access to dye that cannot penetrate a living cell. Examples are trypan blue (visible on light microscopy) and propidium iodine (visible on fluorescent microscopy) (20). However, these dyes are non-specific and stain necrotic cells and reliance on membrane permeability means that on late apoptotic cells stain making an underestimation of apoptosis in that tissue at that time. Like microscopy, this technique is better used in combination with others.

Nuclear stains can be used to locate condensed or segregated nuclear chromatin, the dyes available are fluorescent and include acridine orange, bisbenzimide (Hoechst 33258 and 33342) and propidium iodide. The latter requires fixation and permeation of the cell prior to staining (20). These dyes are rapid, easy to perform on many samples and can be used to quantify apoptotic death (20) and are often used with flow cytometry.

Further methods utilise chemical labelling and visualisation of internucleosomal DNA cleavage fragments. 'Terminal deoxynucleotidyl transferase-mediated dUTP-biotin nick end labelling' of DNA fragments or TUNEL incorporates biotinylated dUTP onto the 3' ends of DNA fragments by utilising the activity of terminal deoxynucleotidyl transferase, and was originally developed for detection of apoptotic cells in tissue sections (21). Subsequent modifications have enabled its use in tissue sections (22) and incorporation of an additional strand breakage induce by photolysis, which is proportional to DNA replication, allows both cell proliferation and apoptosis to be measured in a single step procedure (23, 24, 25). The second method is '*in situ* end labelling' or 'ISEL' and like TUNEL adds biotinylated dUTP to 3' ends of DNA using DNA polymerase I (Klenow fragment). ISEL has followed the same evolution as TUNEL (20, 26, 27). After labelling appropriate visualisation is achieved by the addition of fluorescent dyes or the perioxidase method (20). Both methods are sensitive for detecting early DNA fragmentation and enable quantification of apoptosis. They may be combined with other cell staining techniques such as cell specific markers to localise interest to one cell subset (20). The main drawback is that not all cells that are apoptotic undergo DNA cleavage, necrotic cells experience random cleavage and some forms of apoptosis in certain cells continues without cleavage (28, 29, 30, 31, 32, 33).

Clearance of apoptotic bodies depends on expression of membrane factors to highlight the body for phagocytosis; one example of such is phosphatidyl-serine (34, 35). Annexin V has a high-affinity binding to phosphatidyl-serine, making it a highly specific marker for apoptotic cells prior to and following membrane breakdown (23). Fluorescent labelling of annexin V enables visualisation, and such labelling by annexin V has been widely used to investigate and quantify apoptosis in various systems (23, 36, 37, 38).

Other methods are available and expanding rapidly; the most obvious is immunocytochemistry, the direct binding of antibodies to specific proteins to enable subsequent visualisation by fluorescence or peroxidase reactions. Such techniques have been applied to the study of apoptosis to identify cleavage sites for caspases, enzymes that disable other enzymes, e.g. poly(ADP-ribose) polymerase (PARP) that is involved in DNA repair (39) or Bcl-XL, a potent inhibitor of programmed cell death (40). As such, identification of specific proteins only expressed in apoptosis or the identification of caspase cleavage fragments by visual or biochemical means provides alternative apoptotic markers.

Indirect Methods

The principal indirect method used is 'flow cytometry', that can measure the mechanism and extent of cell death by measuring the light-scattering properties together with cellular ability to take up and retain dyes or labels (41, 42, 43). Such a technique is often combined with one or more visual methods described above. A further technique that is frequently used, involves the effect of nuclear condensation and loss of DNA fragments rendering apoptotic cells smaller and containing less DNA than a G_0/G_1 diploid cell following fixation and dying of cells (44, 45, 46, 47). The problems that exist include; particles that contain fractional DNA content are assumed to be apoptotic, however, these may be cellular fragments from artifact or necrotic lysis. This overestimates the apoptotic index (19). Adding compensation filters to only measure certain fragment sizes can underestimate the index (19). Not only these, but phagocytes that have ingested apoptotic bodies now contain altered DNA, abnormal plasma membranes and other characteristic apoptotic features. Thus if the flow cytometry is combined with a method that utilises these features, phagocytic cells will be falsely labelled as apoptotic. The apoptotic index generated by flow cytometry is only the percentage of cells within a population that are apoptotic and not a measure of the rate of apoptosis or a quantitative measure of cell death, it is not cumulative (19).

Biochemical Methods

Wyllie et al (7) described the biochemical hallmark of apoptosis in 1980, the cleavage of genomic DNA into multiples 180-200 base pair oligonucleotides. Various methods are available for isolating these oligonucleotides, and subsequently displaying the results on an ethidium bromide gel or autoradiographic detection after ^{32}P-labelling of the DNA fragments. The appearance seen has become known as DNA laddering. The identification of such is proof of cation-dependent endonuclease activity, that is energy requiring and specific to apoptosis and therefore an excellent method of identifying apoptosis per se. The process is semi-quantitative, in that relative amounts of low molecular weight DNA may be determined using computerised means (20). However, large numbers are cells are required, specific populations of cells cannot be examined (19, 20) and DNA fragmentation is not associated with all forms of apoptosis (19, 28, 29, 30, 31, 32, 33).

Enzyme linked immunoassays have been commercially produced using monoclonal antibodies against DNA and histones. These enable measurement of apoptosis by quantitating histone-associated DNA fragments released from cultured cells, these systems are quick but have the same disadvantages as the DNA laddering method (20).

An old method of detection of cell death relied on lactate dehydrogenase release on loss of plasma membrane integrity, which is common both to necrosis and late apoptotic processes, it is rapid, simple and quantitative (20, 48).

The MTT (3-(4,5-dimethylthiazol-2-yl)2,5-diphenyltetrazolium bromide)/XTT assay is an indirect measure of cell growth/cell death relying on the conversion of

MTT/XTT into a coloured formazan by mitochondria, allowing spectrophotometric measurement (20). Dead or dying cells cannot achieve this conversion, like measurement of lactate dehydrogenase, the assay is not specific and mitochondria remain functional until late in apoptosis (7) and artifacts arise in proliferating cultures as population levels are not static so percentages of cell death may become inaccurate (20).

COUNTING - THE SIGNIFICANCE OF NUMBERS

In many in vitro settings the frequency of apoptosis is high, so that counting individual cells is easy. Furthermore, in this situation it is relatively easy to demonstrate other biochemical properties that can be seen in apoptosis cells, such as nucleosomal ladders, caspase activation and cleavage of substrates such as PARP. However, in many clinical situations the rate of apoptosis may be much lower and perhaps be interpreted as evidence that apoptosis is not occurring (because no biochemical assay is positive) or that the amount of apoptosis is so small as to be insignificant. A powerful illustration of how this can lead to an underestimation of the importance of the phenomenon is provided from the field of immunology. Mice injected with a single dose of anti-CD4 antibody have a severe depletion of CD4 positive T lymphocytes that occurs within 24 hours. In fact after a single dose the number of cells is reduced by 50% at 48 hours. The death appears to be the result of apoptosis but despite this the maximal rate of apoptosis counted using morphological criteria on tissue sections is 1.3% (49). The explanation for this apparent discrepancy is the extremely rapid time course of apoptosis and phagocytosis in vivo. Conversely, in a situation where TUNEL appears to suggest a rate of apoptosis exceeding 10 or 20% in clinical material one is wise to exercise scepticism. Is apoptosis likely to be that frequent in a disease where the evolution of injury and destruction of cells occurs over a period measured in months or years, such as congestive cardiac failure?

RESOLUTION OF APOPTOSIS

Perhaps, one of the most striking differences between apoptosis and necrosis is the lack of an inflammatory response to death from apoptosis, in the vast majority of cases. As alluded to earlier the final stage of apoptosis is clearance; which is achieved by phagocytosis, both by the professional phagocyte such as the macrophage and the semi-professional phagocyte, the neighbouring cell (50). Early studies of phagocytosis implicated interactions of endogenous macrophage lectins with specific N-acetyl sugar moieties displayed on the surface of apoptotic cells with initiation of phagocytosis within resident macrophage tissue populations (5, 51). Subsequently, monocyte derived macrophages and neutrophils that rapidly take up large numbers of apoptotic cells employ a different recognition system, revolving around $\alpha_v\beta_3$ vitronectin receptor and CD36. Co-operation from thrombospondin (TSP)-1, a soluble adhesive glycoprotein produced by many cells, enables a bridge from the macrophage to markers expressed upon the apoptotic cell/body (50, 52, 53, 54). Such markers were shown to include phosphatidylserine, normally localised internally on the inner aspect of a membrane and are expressed externally in apoptosis (55), in addition to specific N-acetyl sugar moictics; it is this that annexin V binds to. In addition, the mammalian ATP-binding cassette transporter (56), scavenger receptors and specific phosphatidylserine receptors (involved in removal of apoptotic granulocytes in areas of inflammation) (53) have been associated with the initiation of the phagocytic pathway ending with engulfment of the apoptotic body. It has been hypothesised that in some circumstance inflammation may be an actively pursued course to bring in more phagocytes to a region of high apoptosis (52).

Therefore, the uptake of apoptotic bodies is dependent on the appropriate expression of surface markers on those bodies that shout 'eat me', failure to do so or failure of recognition allows the contents of these bodies to leak as they undergo secondary necrosis, initiating an inflammatory response. This may be important in the understanding of the pathogenesis of inflammatory and immune disease (50). An excellent example was the widespread hepatic apoptosis induced in murine models after exposure to anti-Fas antibody, the local phagocyte reserves were exceeded and severe liver damage occurred through inflammatory processes (57). Our observations of myocardia from autopsy subjects with a history of ischaemic heart disease has led to a postulation that the associated fibrosis commonly seen within the myocardium from repeated ischaemia may in fact be a similar apoptotic problem. The lack of capable phagocytes in the region or the poor phagocytic ability of the local myofibres may lead to a low grade inflammatory response that recruits phagocytes, but in turn initiates a fibrotic repair damaging tissue architecture.

SUMMARY

Apoptosis has become recognised as a very important basic biological process regulating tissue size and cell number in health and disease. In general terms there is a stereotyped set of morphological changes that are part of the apoptotic mechanism. These may have associated biochemical changes. However, it is increasingly recognised that within different tissues and after different types of injury a selection occurs. This implies a degree of heterogeneity within what is collectively known as apoptosis. As a result of this it is important to define precisely in any given setting what precisely is being investigated and to appreciate that there is no "gold standard" that defines apoptosis in every situation in which it might occur. Finally, apoptosis is a quiet killer! Very low apparent frequency in a tissue section may hide the fact that dramatic cell loss and tissue remodelling is occurring. The challenge of understanding apoptosis and its regulation in cardiovascular disease is still in its infancy.

References

1. Kerr JFR, Wyllie AH, Currie AR. Apoptosis: a basic biological phenomenon with wide-ranging implications in tissue kinetics. *Br J Cancer.* 1972;26:239-257.
2. Trump BF, Berezesky IK, Chang SH, Phelps PC. The pathways of cell death: oncosis, apoptosis, and necrosis. *Toxicologic Pathology.* 1997;25:82-88.

3. Majno G, Joris I. Apoptosis, oncosis and necrosis. An overview of cell death. *Am J Pathol.* 1995;146:3-15.
4. Von Recklinghausen F. Untersuchungen uber Rachitis und Osteomalacie. Jena: Verlag Gustav Fischer; 1910.
5. Webb S J, Harrison DJ, Wyllie AH. In: Kaufmann SH, ed. *Apoptosis: Pharmacological implications and therapeutic opportunities.* London: Academic Press; 1997:1-34.
6. Freude B, Masters TN, Kostin S, Robicsek F, Schaper J. Cardiomyocyte apoptosis in acute and chronic conditions. *Basic Res Cardiol.* 1998;93:85-89.
7. Wyllie AH. Glucocorticoid-induced thymocyte apoptosis is associated with endogenous endonuclease activation. *Nature.* 1980;284:555-556.
8. Columbano A. Cell death: current difficulties in discriminating apoptosis from necrosis in the context of pathological processes in vivo. *J Cellular Biochemistry.* 1995;58:181-190.
9. Leist M, Nicotera P. The shape of cell death. *Biochem Biophys Res Comm.* 1997;236:1-9.
10. Jacobson MD, Burne JF, Raff MC. Programmed cell death and Bcl-2 protection in the absence of a nucleus. *EMBO J.* 1994;13:1899-1910.
11. Schulze-Osthoff K, Walczak H, Droge W, Kramer PH. Cell nucleus and DNA fragmentation are not required for apoptosis. *J Cell Biol.* 1994;127:15-20.
12. Kaufmann SH. Induction of endonuclease DNA cleavage in human acute myelogenous leukaemia by etopiside, camptothecin, and other cytotoxic anticancer drugs: a cautionary note. *Cancer Res.* 1989;49:5870-5878.
13. Ucker DS, Meyers J, Obermiller PS. Activation-driven T cell death. II. Quantitative differences alone distinguish stimuli triggering non-transformed T cell proliferation or death. *J Immunol.* 1992;149:1583-1592.
14. Lazebnik YA, Cole S, Cooke CA, Nelson WG, Earnshaw WC. Nuclear events of apoptosis in vitro in cell-free mitotic extracts: A model system for analysis of the active phase of apoptosis. *J Cell Biol.* 1993;123:7-22.
15. Reipert S, Reipert BM, Hickman JA, Allen TD. Nuclear pore clustering is a consistent feature of apoptosis in vitro. *Cell Death Differ.* 1996;3:131-139.
16. Kroemer G, Petit P, Naofal Z, Vayssiere J-L, Mignotte B. The biochemistry of programmed cell death. *FASEB J.* 1995;9:1277-1287.
17. Fesus L, Thomazy V, Falus A. Induction and activation of tissue transaglutaminase during programmed cell death. *FEBS Lett.*1987;224:104-108.
18. Bursch W, Paffe S, Putz B, Barthel G, Schulte-Hermann R. Determination of the length of the histological stages of apoptosis in normal liver and in altered hepatic foci of rats. *Carcinogenesis.* 1990;11:847-853.
19. Darzynkiewicz Z, Bedner E, Traganos F, Murakami T. Critical aspects in the analysis of apoptosis and necrosis. *Human Cell.* 1998;11:3-12.
20. Loo DT, Rillema JR. Measurement of cell death. *Methods in Cell Biol.* 1998;57:251-264.
21. Gavrieli Y, Sherman Y, Ben-Sasson SA. Identification of programmed cell death in situ via specific labelling of nuclear DNA fragmentation. *J Cell Biol.* 1992;119:493-501.
22. Hotz MA, Gong J, Traganos F, Darzynkiewicz Z. Flow cytometric detection of apoptosis: comparison of the assays of in situ DNA degradation and chromatin changes. *Cytometry.* 1994;15:237-244.
23. Moore AM, Donahue CJ, Bauer KD, Mather JP. Simultaneous measurement of cell cycle and apoptotic cell death. *Methods in Cell Biol.* 1998;57:265-278.
24. Li X, Traganos F, Melamed MR, Darynkiewicz Z. Simultaneous analysis of DNA replication and apoptosis during treatment of HL-60 cells with camptothecin and hyperthermia and mitogen stimulation of human lymphocytes. *Cancer Res.* 1994;54:4289-4293.
25. Li X, Traganos F, Melamed MR, Darynkiewicz Z. Single-step procedure for labelling DNA strand breaks with fluorescein – or BODIPY – conjugated deoxynucleotides detection of apoptosis and bromodeoxyuridine incorporation. *Cytometry.* 1995;20:172-180.
26. Ansari B, Coates PJ, Greenstein BD, Hall PA. In situ end-labelling detects DNA strand breaks in apoptosis and other physiological and pathological states. *J Pathol.* 1993;170:1-8.
27. Laio Y, Tang Z-Y, Liu K-D, Ye S-L, Huang Z. Apoptosis of human BEL-7402 hepatocellular carcinoma cells released by antisense H-RAS DNA – in vitro and in vivo studies. *J Cancer Res Clin Oncol.* 1997;123:25-33.
28. Zakeri ZF, Quaglino D, Latham T, Locksin RA. Delayed internucleosomal DNA fragmentation in programmed cell death. *FASEB J.* 1993;7:470-478.

29.   Boe R, Gjersten BT, Vintermyr OK, Houge G, Lanotte M, Doskeland SO. The protein phosphatase inhibitor okadaic acid induces morphological changes of apoptosis in mammalian cells. *Exp Cell Res.* 1991;195:237-246.
30.   Oberhammer FA, Pavelka M, Sharma S, Tiefenbacher R, Purchio AF, Bursch W, Schulte-Hermann R. Induction of apoptosis in cultured hepatocytes and in regressing liver by growth factor beta 1. *Proc Natl Acad Sci USA.* 1992;89:5408-5412.
31.   Oberhammer FA, Bursch W, Parzefall W, Breit P, Erber E, Stadler M, Schulte HR. Effect of transforming growth factor beta on cell death of cultured rat hepatocytes. *Cancer Res.* 1991;51:2478-2485.
32.   Cohen GM, Sun X-M, Snowden RT, Dinsdale D, Skilleter DN. Key morphological features of apoptosis may occur in the absence of internucleosomal DNA fragmentation. *Biochem J.* 1992;286:331-334.
33.   Collins RJ, Harmon BV, Gobe GC, Kerr JFR. Internucleosomal DNA cleavage should not be the only criterion for identifying apoptosis. *Int J Radiat Biol.* 1992;61:451-453.
34.   Vermes I, Haanen C, Steffens-Nakken H, Reutelingsperger C. A novel assay for apoptosis. Flow cytometric detection of phosphatidylserine expression on early apoptotic cells using fluorescein labelled annexin V. *J Immunol Methods.* 1995;184:39-51.
35.   Martin SJ, Reutelingsperger CPM, McGahon AJ, Rader JA, Vanschie ECAA, Laface DM, Green DR. Early redistribution of plasma membrane phosphatidylserine is a general feature of apoptosis regardless of the initiating stimulus: inhibition by overexpression of Bcl-2 and Abl. *J Exp Med.* 1995;182:1545-1546.
36.   Boersma AWM, Nooter K, Oostrum RG, Stoter G. Quantification of apoptotic cells with fluorescein isothiocyanate-labelled annexin V in chinese hamster ovary cell cultures treated with cisplatin. *Cytometry.* 1996;24:123-130.
37.   Bennet MR, Gibson DF, Schwartz SM, Tait JF. Binding and phagocytosis of apoptotic vascular smooth muscle is mediated in part by exposure of phosphatidylserine. *Circul Res.* 1995;77:1136-1142.
38.   Pitti RM, Marsters SA, Ruppert S, Donahue CJ, Moore A, Ashkenazi A. Induction of apoptosis by APO-2 ligand, a new member of the tumor necrosis factor cytokine family. *J Biol Chem.* 1996;271:12687-12690.
39.   Sallmann FR, Bourassa S, Saint-Cyr J, Poirier GG. Characterization of antibodies specific for the caspase cleavage site on poly(ADP-ribose) polymerase: specific detection of apoptotic fragments and mapping of the necrotic fragments of poly(ADP-ribose) polymerase. *.Biochem Cell Biol.* 1997;75:451-456.
40.   Clem RJ, Cheng EH, Karp CL, Kirsch DG, Ueno K, Takahashi A, Kastan MB, Griffin DG, Earnshaw WC, Veliuona MA, Hardwick JM. Modulation of cell death by Bcl-XL through caspase interaction. *Proc Natl Acad Sci USA.* 1998;95:554-559.
41.   Dive C, Gregory CD, Phipps DJ, Evans DL, Milner AE, Wyllie AH. Analysis and discrimination of necrosis and apoptosis (programmed cell death) by multiparameter flow cytometry. *Biochim Biophys Acta* 1992;1133:275-285.
42.   Deckers CLP, Lyons AB, Samuels K, Sanderson A, Maddy AH. Alternative pathways of apoptosis induced by methylprednisolone and valinomycin analyzed by flow cytometry. *Exp Cell Res.*1993;208:362-370.
43.   Ormerod MG, Sun X-M, Brown D, Snowden RT, Cohen GM. Quantification of apoptosis and necrosis by flow cytometry. *Acta Oncol.* 1993;32:417-424.
44.   Nicoletti I, Migiorati G, Pagliacci MC, Grignani F, Riccardi C. A rapid and simple method for measuring thymocyte apoptosis by propidium iodide staining and flow cytometry. *J Immunol Meth.*1991;139:271-279.
45.   Telford WG, King LE, Fraker PJ. Comparative evaluation of several DNA binding dyes in the detection of apoptosis-associated chromatin degradation by flow cytometry. *Cytometry.* 1992;13:137-143.
46.   Telford WG, King LE, Fraker PJ. Rapid quantification of apoptosis in pure and heterogeneous cell populations using flow cytometry. *J Immunol Meth.* 1994;172:1-16.
47.   Afanasyev VN, Korol AB, Matylevich NP, Pechatnikov VA, Umansky SR. The use of flow cytometry for the investigation of cell death. *Cytometry.* 1993;14:603-609.
48.   Wroblewski F, LaDue JS. Lactate dehydrogenase activity in blood. *Proc Soc Exp Biol Med.* 1955;90:210-213.

49. Howie SEM, Sommerfield AJ, Gray E, Harrison DJ. Peripheral T lymphocyte depletion by apoptosis after CD4 ligation in vivo: selective loss of CD44- and 'activating' memory T cells. *Clin Exp Immunol*.1994;95:195-200.
50. Savill J. Phagocyte recognition of apoptotic cells. *Biochem Soc Trans*. 1996;24:1065-1069.
51. Duvall E, Wyllie AH, Morris RG. Macrophage recognition of cells undergoing programmed cell death (apoptosis). *Immunol*. 1985;56:351-358.
52. Savill J. Apoptosis in resolution of inflammation. *J Leukocyte Biol*. 1997;61:375-380.
53. Savill JS, Dransfield I, Hogg N, Haslett C. Vitronectin receptor-mediated phagocytosis of cells undergoing apoptosis. *Nature*. 1990;343:170-173.
54. Savill JS, Hogg N, Ren Y, Haslett C. Thrombospondin co-operates with CD36 and the vitronectin receptor in macrophage recognition of neutrophils undergoing apoptosis. *J Clin Invest*. 1992;90:1513-1522.
55. Fadok VA, Voelker DR, Campbell PA, Cohen JJ, Bratton DL, Henson PM. Exposure of phosphatidylserine on the surface of apoptotic lymphocytes triggers specific recognition and removal by macrophages. *J Immunol*.1992;148:2207-2216.
56. Flora PK, Gregory CD. Recognition of apoptotic cells by human macrophage: inhibition of a monocyte/macrophage-specific monoclonal antibody. *Eur J Immunol*. 1994;24:2625.
57. Ogasawara J, Waanabe-Fukunga R, Adachi M, Matsuzawa A, Kasgul T, Kitamura Y, Itoh N, Suda T, Nagata S. Lethal effect of the anti-Fas antibody in mice. *Nature*. 1993;364:806-809.

PART TWO:
Cellular targets in the cardiovascular system

II.1
Blood vessels

II.1.1
Apoptosis and cell cycle in endothelial cells

Ioakim Spyridopoulos, M.D.
Universität Tübingen, Tübingen, Germany

INTRODUCTION

Apoptosis is an active process of cell death that occurs both under physiologic and pathophysiologic conditions. Specifically, apoptosis has been involved in vasculogenesis and atherosclerosis, inflammation, as well as wound healing, respectively. Its hallmark is the cleavage of genomic DNA into nucleosomal fragments of 180 bp (1). Although it has not been established to what extent endothelial cell death occurs in vivo, there is increasing evidence that endothelium may become apoptotic in various disease states.

ENDOTHELIAL CELL APOPTOSIS AS A TRIGGER FOR ATHEROSCLEROSIS

Hypercholesterolemia is a major risk for development of atherosclerosis in humans, most likely due to oxidative modification of low density lipoproteins (LDL) (2). Both oxidatively modified LDL (oxLDL) and cholesterol oxidation products are found in atherosclerotic lesions and in the plasma (3). Experiments in animals support the hypothesis that injury to the endothelium might trigger the atherosclerotic process. Endothelial cell injury could result in cell death, either by necrosis or apoptosis. A mechanistic clue to this process has been postulated by the study group around A. Zeiher, who found the specific activation of CPP32-like caspases by oxLDL (4). Further studies found that cyclosporine A completely inhibited the oxLDL-induced release of cytochrome C from the mitochondrium into the cytoplasm (5). Apoptosis suppression by cyclosporin A correlated with prevention of mitochondrial dysfunction. While cytochrome C and CPP32-like caspases reflect relatively "late" events in the apoptotic cascade, little is known about the intermediate signals leading to oxLDL-induced apoptosis. Harada-Shiba et al. have found ceramide to be an important mediator of oxLDL-induced cell death in human umbilical vein endothelial cells (6). Inhibitors of acid sphingomyelinase, an enzyme converting sphingomyelin into ceramide, inhibited both generation of ceramide and cell death induced by oxLDL. The toxic effect of oxLDL was mainly due to the oxysterol-fraction. Controversy exists about the potency of lysophosphatidylcholine (LPC), another non-oxysterol component of oxLDL, to induce apoptosis in endothelial cells. We and others (6) have found little or no toxic effect of LPC in physiologically occuring doses, whereas apoptosis occured only at higher doses (>20 μg/ml). Sata et al. found increased expression of Fas ligand in LPC-treated endothelial cells, hence activating apoptosis via the Fas/Fas ligand system (7). A possible cause for the diversity of these results could lie in the heterogeneity of endothelial cells, including isolation, passage number and type of growth media.

TNF-ALPHA INDUCES PROGRAMMED CELL DEATH IN HUMAN ENDOTHELIAL CELLS

Disruption of the integrity of the endothelial barrier has been postulated as a mechanism for the initiation of atherogenesis (2, 3, 8). Recent data also suggest a role for tumor necrosis factor alpha (TNF) in the pathogenesis of atherosclerotic lesions and restenosis (9, 10). By using electron microscopy we found typical morphological features of apoptosis in human endothelial cells treated with TNF, such as condensation of chromatin at the periphery of the nucleus, and blebbing and fragmentation of the cytoplasm. Staining with acridine orange revealed similar results by usage of fluorescent microscopy. Biochemical features of apoptosis consisted of nucleosomal DNA fragmentation, which could be seen as a DNA laddering on agarose gels or as subdiploid DNA using flow-cytometric analysis of propidium iodide stained endothelial cells (Figure 1). Finally we established a dose-response relationship for TNF-α-induced cell death using the colorimetric MTS assay, which depends on the intact mitochondrial activity. After 24 hours of treatment at the highest dose of 40 ng/ml, 35% of cells died from apoptosis, whereas the lowest concentration of 0.1 ng/ml still induced 4% cell death over the same amount of time.

By Northern blot analysis we found 10-fold upregulation of ICE mRNA expression under treatment with TNF-α (11). This was consistent with the upregulation of ICE protein after 24 hours of TNF-α exposure. To provide further evidence of a functional role for ICE in human endothelial cell apoptosis, ICE protein expression was examined by immunofluorescence microscopy. Cells were simultaneously examined for biochemical features of apoptosis by use of the TUNEL method to fluorescently label DNA strand breaks. Finally, fluorescent counterstaining with Hoechst 33342 of human umbilical vein endothelial cell (HUVEC) nuclei was also performed to permit the examination of cells for morphological features of apoptosis.

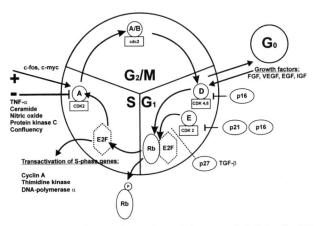

Figure 1 Biochemical features of apoptosis are shown in human endothelial cells: DNA laddering on the left (T= TNF, C= Control, M= Marker) as well as subdiploid DNA accumulation on the right side.

Expression of ICE protein localized to cells that also exhibited the morphological and biochemical features of apoptosis. The nuclei of cells that stained positive for ICE were shrunken and deformed. In addition, those cells showed evidence of DNA strand breaks manifested as green fluorescence, indicative of terminal deoxy transferase labeling of 3' DNA ends (TUNEL). The absence of ICE expression in the morphologically normal-appearing cells suggested that ICE expression was limited to cells undergoing apoptosis. Whether or not ICE is crucial in the signaling cascades of caspases still remains to be clarified. Dimmeler et al. have demonstrated the induction of CPP32 (caspase 3) by TNF-α in HUVEC cells (12). Our own studies showed that PARP, a substrate of CPP32, was also cleaved by TNF-treatment (13).

ESTROGEN AND ENDOTHELIAL CELL APOPTOSIS

Since TNF-α can induce apoptosis in human endothelial cells (11, 14), protection of endothelial cells from cytokine induced injury and apoptosis may therefore represent one potential mechanism for prevention of atherosclerosis.

Adherent HUVEC demonstrate typical cobblestone morphology under control conditions whereas after exposure to TNF-α, the cells become rounded and partially detach while demonstrating the lobulated appearance of apoptotic cells. At the same time the density of the adherent cells is decreased as compared with control conditions, indicating detachment of HUVEC exposed to TNF-α. The presence of 10^{-9} M oestradiol together with TNF-α reversed the apoptotic morphology in most of the cells, while cell density was increased as compared to HUVEC exposed to TNF-α. Two independent studies have demonstrated the presence of a functional estrogen receptor in human endothelial cells, including HUVECs, coronary artery and aortic endothelial cells (15, 16). Northern blots verified that human endothelial cells express abundant amount of mRNA for the ER. Ligand-binding studies estimated 2×10^4 to 6×10^4 receptors per endothelial cell and scatchard analysis of radioligand binding showed a K_d of ≈ 5 nmol/L. Nuclear extracts from HUVECs interacted with a consensus estrogen response element in an electrophoretic mobility shift assay and antibody against the ER supershifted the protein-DNA complex to prove specificity. We also found equal ER protein expression in HUVECs under control conditions and in TNF-α treated cells by Western blotting.

To assess cell viability we used a nonradioactive cell-proliferation assay containing the tetrazolium compound MTS and an electron coupling reagent, PMS. MTS is reduced by viable cells to formazan, whose yellow color can be measured with a spectrophotometer by the amount of 490-nm absorbance. Formazan production is time dependent and proportional to the number of viable cells (17). The advantage of this assay is its evaluation of mitochondrial function, which can detect cell death at earlier stages than other techniques (18). In the present study, TNF-α alone resulted in $35\pm4\%$ cell death after 24 hours, as assessed by the MTS assay. Simultaneous treatment with oestradiol demonstrated a dose-dependent increase in cell survival. At an estrogen concentration of 10^{-9} mol/L, the percentage of dying cells decreased to $18\pm2\%$ (p=0.0004 versus TNF-α alone; Figure 2). The specific estrogen-receptor antagonist ICI 182,780 completely abrogated the protective effect of estrogen. Treatment with estrogen alone for 24 hours did not result in a significant increase in cell number, which shows that the increase in survival due to estrogen is not based on cell proliferation over that short period of time.

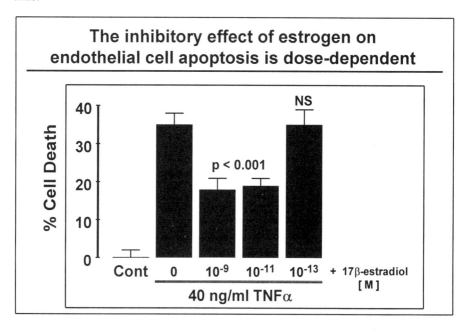

Figure 2 Protective effect of 17β-estradiol on endothelial cell apoptosis (HUVEC cells).

We have also used flow cytometry to determine the proportion of human endothelial cells in culture that are apoptotic. This method utilizes intact cells and results in highly quantitative information regarding the degree of apoptosis in this population. Fixing the cells in 70% ethanol gives best results for apoptotic cells due to the tendency of the cytoplasm of these cells to contract. Staining with propidium iodide, an intercalative DNA binding dye, allows excitation with the 488-nm beam of an argon laser and detection at 620-700 nm. Control HUVEC cells showed 6.5% apoptotic events after being in 20% charcoal-stripped growth media. Addition of 40 ng/ml TNF-α led to 39.3% apoptosis whereas simultaneous treatment with estrogen decreased apoptosis by over 50% to 16.6%. Cell counting of HUVEC exposed to study conditions in 24-well plates revealed similar findings: total cell count decreased from $18.7\pm3.7\times10^3$ cells per well under control conditions to $5.9\pm1.4\times10^3$ cells per well after 24 hours of TNF-α exposure. Treatment with estradiol (10^{-9} mol/L) resulted an increase in cell count to $11.2\pm4.0\times10^3$ ($p<0.001$ versus TNF-α alone). This beneficial effect was abolished when the specific estrogen-receptor antagonist ICI 182,780 (10^{-9} mol/L) was coincubated: the cell count decreased to $6.3\pm1.6\times10^3$ cells per well ($p<0.001$ versus TNF-α + estradiol, p=NS versus TNF-α alone).

NITRIC OXIDE - THE RESCUER?

Nitric oxide (NO) is a cellular messenger with numerous biological functions, including regulation of vascular tone, cellular signaling in the brain, and killing pathogens in nonspecific immune responses. NO is derived from the guanidino nitrogen atom of L-arginine through a reaction catalyzed by NO synthase (NOS). Up to now, three distinct NOS cDNAs have been cloned: neuronal NOS (nNOS), endothelial NOS (eNOS) and inducible NOS (iNOS).

Estrogen has been reported to increase endothelium-dependent relaxation, and female rabbit aorta seem to release more NO than that of male (19). The effect of estrogen on eNOS mRNA level is controversial in bovine and porcine endothelial cells. To determine whether functional recovery of the endothelium was accelerated by oestradiol, the production of nitric oxide by excised arterial segments was measured as previously described (20).

Further studies conducted by Krasinski et al. investigated the potential role of nitric oxide in the protective effect of estrogen. Excised arteries were placed in an organ bath and nitric oxide was measured after 15 min according to the Griess reaction. Nitric oxide production by the oestradiol-treated arteries was significantly greater than that of placebo-treated arteries 1 week after injury (8.55 ± 1.7 vs. 2.8 ± 0.18 μmol $\cdot$ L^{-1} $\cdot$ mm^{-2} per 15 minutes, $p<0.0001$) (21). The acceleration of anatomical recovery, as identified by Evans blue staining, was also accompanied by estrogen-induced acceleration of functional endothelial recovery.

The exact mechanism of the survival effect of estrogen on endothelial cells remains to be clarified, but the ability of estrogen to protect endothelial cells from cytokine-induced injury suggests another possible mechanism of its atheroprotective effect. The benefit of this effect in vivo has still to be shown, though nitric oxide is a strong contender as the anti-apoptotic mediator of estrogen. Again, nitric oxide can act as both, inducer (22) and inhibitor of apoptosis. Dimmeler et al. (12) have shown that NO inhibits TNF-induced apoptosis in human endothelial cells at physiologically relevant doses. They find 'high amounts of NO linked to proapoptotic effects under pathophysiological conditions, whereas the continuous release of endothelial NO inhibits apoptosis and may contribute to the antiatherosclerotic function of NO.' (23)

VEGF IN ANGIOGENESIS AND SURVIVAL

VEGF, also termed vascular permeability factor is an endothelial cell mitogen which also promotes angiogenesis (24-28). VEGF can also serve as a survival factor for endothelial cells by inhibiting programmed cell death induced by tumor-necrosis factor alpha (29), loss of adhesion (30), hyperoxia (31) or irradiation (32). Endothelial cells contain at least two high-affinity receptors for VEGF, Flk-1/KDR and Flt-1 (33, 34), both of which belong to the family of receptor-tyrosine kinases. Autophosphorylation of these receptors leads to association with phosphatidylinositol (PIP) 3-kinase and phospholipase C γ (PLC γ) (35-37). Subsequent production of DAG and IP_3 together with mobilization of calcium causes translocation of PKC to the cytoplasmic membrane and thereby activation. PKC represents a family of homologous subtypic kinases, which all contain an autoinhibitory domain with substrate-like properties (38), the so called pseudosubstrate domain. This domain keeps the enzyme inactive, supposedly by interacting with the substrate binding site in the catalytic domain. Although vascular endothelial cells contain various amounts of PKC isoforms α, $\beta 1$, $\beta 2$, δ, ϵ, ζ but not γ, only the calcium-dependent α- and β_2- isoforms are consistently translocated to the plasma membrane upon activation by VEGF (37). While activation of the PKC-β_2 isoform is predominantely responsible for the mitogenic effect of VEGF, adenoviral overexpression of PKC-α can enhance endothelial cell migration (39).

Several studies in the past have addressed the role of protein kinase C on endothelial function, vascular permeability and angiogenesis (40-47). Due to the fact that a) phorbolesters such as PMA strongly induce expression of VEGF themselves (48, 49), b) PKC inhibitors like staurosporine, H-7 and calphostin C are not specific for protein kinase C (50), c) staurosporine induces cell death at inhibitory concentrations (51), and d) prolonged stimulation with phorbolesters results in downregulation of PKC activity (52-56), it has been somewhat difficult to draw definitive conclusions about PKC-dependent effects of VEGF.

In order to investigate the role of PKC in the signaling of VEGF mediated effects, we used a novel compound to specifically inhibit the α- and β- isoforms of PKC. A myristoylated peptide (myr-φPKC) has previously been shown to be a highly selective and cell-permeable inhibitor of PKC (57, 58). Myr-φPKC contains a sequence of 13 amino acids identical with the pseudosubstrate domain in both isoforms and competes with other substrates for the catalytic subunit, whereas alanine residues prevent it from phosphorylation. Myristoylation greatly facilitates hazardless passage through the plasma membrane and makes it a potent inhibitor of both isoforms.

To separate different signaling pathways, we compared the influence of protein kinase C on the transduction of VEGFs principal biological activities: proliferation, angiogenesis, survival and NO production. Our results highlighted PKC as a major component in the signaling pathway required for VEGF induced proliferation and angiogenesis (59). This stands in sharp contrast to VEGFs abilities as an endothelial survival and vascular permeability factor. Surprisingly both properties were enhanced rather than abrogated by inhibiting PKC. Inhibition of calcium dependent PKC isoforms by itself lead to induction of nitric oxide and rendered human endothelial cells independent from growth factors in order to survive. Although nitric oxide synthase is a downstream target for VEGF-induced angiogenesis, its induction per se was not sufficient to promote neovascularization.

CELL CYCLE AND APOPTOSIS

Progression of the cell cycle and control of apoptosis are thought to be intimately linked processes, acting to preserve homeostasis and developmental morphogenesis (60, 61). Although proteins that regulate apoptosis have been implicated in restraining cell-cycle entry and controlling ploidy, the effector molecules at the interface between cell proliferation and cell survival have remained elusive. In this section some of the mechanisms that control EC proliferation and its implication in cardiovascular pathology will be discussed. Mature ECs display a very low proliferative index. However, EC proliferation plays an essential role during growth of new vessels from preexisting ones (angiogenesis) and during reendothelialization after acute mechanical vessel injury (i. e., after angioplasty). On the other hand, noxious stimuli such as oxidative stress or cytokines can impair cell cycle progression in otherwise healthy ECs. A general scheme of how the endothelial cell cycle is regulated is shown in Figure 3.

For all types of macro- and microvascular endothelial cells (EC) optimal growth and formation of a monolayer is observed when cultured on fibronectin or gelatin substrates in the presence of EC growth factor and heparin. Under such conditions macrovascular ECs reach maximal cell densities of 1400 - 1900 ECs/mm^2 (microvascular ECs 700-900 ECs/mm^2) (62). The cell cycle times calculated from the population-doubling time and the stathmokinetic index amounts to approximately 29 hours for arterial macrovascular ECs. When primary endothelial cells reach maximal cell density and therefore confluency, they stop further proliferation. In contact-inhibiting fibroblasts and endothelial cells, protein levels of the CDK-inhibitor p27^{Kip1} have been demonstrated to dramatically increase by a posttranscriptional mechanism (63, 64). Induction of p27 then leads to impaired association of the cyclin E/cdk2 kinase complex with the E2F/p107 complex, normally thethered to the E2F binding site in the cyclin A promoter (basepairs –37 to –33) (65). Since transactivation of cyclin A is required to control S phase entry (66, 67), the cell must arrest in G1 phase. Promoter studies in confluent bovine aortic endothelial cells show the importance of another DNA binding site in the cyclin A promoter, the cAMP response element (CRE or ATF) located at basepairs

−80/-73 (68). Under confluent conditions (2000 ECs/mm^2), the cyclin A promoter is about 30-fold repressed compared to subconfluent endothelial cells. Mutation of the CRE-binding site abolishes this difference. Another interesting aspect dependent on the state of confluence is the response of endothelial cells to nitric oxide (NO). Lopez-Farre et al. (69) found that inhibition of NO-production in subconfluent bovine endothelial cells lead to increased proliferation, accompanied by increased expression of the oncogene-encoding proteins c-myc and c-fos. Surprisingly, the same treatment leads to the induction of apoptosis when cells were confluent, emphasizing the importance of cell density in the regulation of survival and proliferation in endothelial cells.

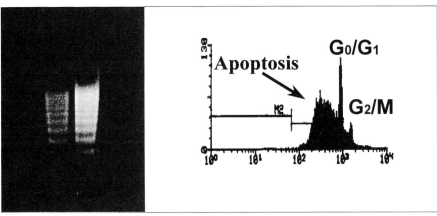

M T T C

DNA-laddering   **FACS analysis**

Figure 3 *Regulation of the endothelial cell-cycle.* Serumstarvation synchronizes cells in the G0 state, whereas supplement of growth factors induces Cyclin D1 thus allowing entrance into G1 phase. Cyclins (Circular shaped, grey colored) and Cyclin dependent kinases, also termed CDKs (rectangular shaped) have to associate in order to build a functional unit. CDK2 together with Cyclin E can phosphorylate the retinoblastoma gene product (Rb), leading to the liberation of the transcription factor E2F, which in turn activates synthesis of required S phase gene products, such as Cyclin A, DNA-polymerase-α and thymidine kinase. TNF interferes with the cell cycle through Cyclin A downregulation.

In addition to cyclins, whose expression in ECs fluctuates throughout the different phases of the cell cycle, other genes are also regulated in a cell cycle-dependent manner in ECs. Transglutaminase, for example, which catalyzes the covalent incorporation of polyamines into proteins and glutamine-lysine cross-links between proteins, is associated with cell growth, differentiation and malignant transformation. Transglutaminase mRNA levels are highest in G_0-synchronized bovine ECs, dropping rapidly in proliferating or G_2/M-arrested cells (70). In contrast, telomerase activity is high in proliferating human ECs and is repressed in G_0- and G_2/M-arrested cells (71). Similar kinetics are observed with exogenous FGF-1, which is constantly endocytosed by human ECs but translocates to the nucleus only at late G_1 (72). A good example for cell cycle-dependent signalling is protein kinase C, which exhibits a socalled "bimodal" regulatory mechanism (73, 74). Glucose on the other hand prolongs cell-cycle traversal of human ECs equally throughout all phases of the cell cycle when administered at high levels (75). Other agents exist which exhibit their effect only in specific phases of the cell cycle. The anti-inflammatory drug sulfasalazine inhibits S-phase progression in ECs by selective reduction of *de novo* synthesis of thymidine in a folate-dependent manner (76). Platelet factor-4 specifically inhibits entry into and progression through S-phase in ECs (77). Several cytotoxic agents also show cell cycle-dependent activity. For example, avian hemangiosarcoma virus-induced cytotoxicity in bovine aortic ECs is much stronger in G_0/G_1-arrested cells than in actively dividing cells (78).

INFLUENCE OF TNF ON ENDOTHELIAL CELL CYCLE REGULATION

TNF-α is an important cytokine which is secreted by SMCs and macrophages. TNF-α has been demonstrated in human coronary atherosclerotic lesions, as well as in the vessel wall following percutaneous transluminal coronary angioplasty (10, 79-81). TNF-α can induce programmed cell death (apoptosis) in ECs (11, 82, 83), although its cytotoxicity is regulated in a cell cycle-dependent manner so that starvation-synchronized or S- and G2/M-arrested ECs are resistant to TNF-α treatment (12). TNF-α-induced apoptosis in proliferating human ECs caused detachment from their underlying matrix (11). It has been shown that cell cycle progression and cyclin A expression is anchorage-dependent in fibroblasts (84, 85), raising the question as to whether loss of adhesion in apoptotic ECs is associated with inhibition of cyclin A expression.

We have observed that TNF-α treatment of ECs caused G_1 arrest and inhibition of ^{3}H-thymidine uptake (13). While protein expression of cyclin A was almost completely repressed, cyclin D and cyclin E levels remained unchanged in TNF-α-treated ECs. Promoter analysis revealed a 8-fold decrease in cyclin A promoter activity in ECs treated with TNF-α, and mutations affecting the E2F site located at position −37 to -32 (Figure 4) abrogated TNF-dependent downregulation of cyclin A promoter activity. These results indicate that loss of anchorage in TNF-treated ECs is associated with repression of cyclin A transcription in an E2F-dependent manner.

```
                                      Sp1
- 160   GTTTGTTTCT CCCTCCTGCC CCGCCCCTGC TCAGTTTCCT TTGGTTTACC
                                  -133

                                             ATF           Yc1-F
- 110   CTTCACTCGC CCTGACCCTG TCGCCTTGAA TGACGTCAAG GCCGCGAGCG
                                        -80

          Yc1-C                        CDE       CHR
-  60   CTTTCATTG GTCCATTTCA ATAGTCGCGG GATACTTGAA CTGCAAGAAC
                                  -35       -27

-  10   AGCCGCGCTC CAGCGGGCTG CTCGCTGCAT CTCTGGGCGT CTTTGGCTCG
                   +1

+  40   CCACGCTGGG CAGTGCCTGC CTGCGCCTTT CGCAACCTCC TCGGCCCTGC


+  90   GTGGTCTCGA GCTGGGTGA
                 +100
```

Figure 4   The Cyclin A promoter between bases −160 and +110 with its important DNA-binding sites is shown: Sp1 binds the transcription factor AP1, ATF the cyclic AMP response element binding site, and CDE the variant E2F site.

In our following experiment (Figure 5) we used a replication-defective adenovirus directing overexpression of E2F1 to determine whether restoration of E2F function would rescue the EC phenotype. Infection of bovine aortic endothelial cells (BAEC) with -E2F1-Adenovirus (Ad-E2F) resulted in a marked and dose-dependent 2.6-fold decrease in TNF-α induced EC apoptosis while progression into S phase was restored. Increased expression of E2F1 in the Ad-E2F infected cells was confirmed by immunoblotting, which also disclosed decreased E2F1 expression in control adenovirus–infected EC exposed to TNF-α. Furthermore, cyclin A expression, which was repressed by TNF-α exposure in all other cells, was restored in the Ad-E2F infected BAEC despite TNF exposure. Expression of cdc2 was also maintained at the level of normally cycling EC, implying that (in the E2F overexpressing cells) the cell cycle was progressing despite TNF-α exposure. Thus, our studies demonstrate that TNF-α is capable of inducing cell-cycle arrest in proliferating EC by a mechanism involving loss of E2F activity, culminating in programmed cell death. Moreover, adenovirus-mediated overexpression of E2F promotes cell-cycle progression and rescues EC from TNF-induced apoptosis. All together, these results suggest that mechanisms governing cell-cycle regulation and survival are tightly linked in endothelial cells and also define a previously unrecognized role for the cell cycle–regulated transcription factor E2F, that of a putative survival factor for EC under stress.

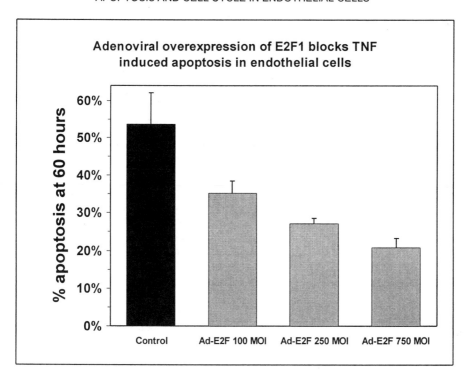

Figure 5 Restoration of E2F expression restores cell-cycle progression and abrogates TNF-α-induced EC apoptosis. BAEC were plated at equal densities and infected for 12 hours in 10% FCS-containing media. Cells were allowed to grow for an additional 24 hours before addition of TNF-α. Results are mean±SEM of 3 duplicate experiments. Restoration of E2F expression abrogated TNF-α-induced EC apoptosis: apoptosis was quantified after 60 hours of TNF-α exposure by FACS. Ad-E2F infection results in dose-dependent inhibition of TNF-α-induced EC apoptosis.

PRO- AND ANTI-APOPTOTIC FACTORS

Endothelial cell injury is a key event in the pathogenesis of atherosclerosis. We and others have established in-vitro and in-vivo models to assess pro- and anti-atherogenic factors. Using cultured human endothelial cells, it is possible to investigate in-vitro survival factors in parallel with 'artificial' injury, caused by cytokines, reactive oxygen species, oxidized LDL, or other noxious stimuli. The induction of endothelial cell injury by growth factor withdrawl also leads to apoptosis. This phenomenon occurs age-dependently, meaning a higher sensitivity in older-passage cells (86). Addition of phorbolester blocks apoptosis (87) and correlates with the induction of the zinc-finger protein A20 (86, 88, 89). Vascular endothelial growth factor (VEGF) and fibroblast growth factor (FGF) are solely capable of acting as survival factors (59, 90). VEGF can induce production of important matrix molecules such as fibronectin and β3 integrin (29), giving one possible mechanism to promote survival. Dimmeler et al. have reviewed several pro- and anti-apoptotic factors for endothelial cells (91). Table 1 updates their overview on the basis of our own experiments and todays literature, apologizing to all collegues whose work has not been cited due to space limitation.

Table 1   Pro- and anti-apoptotic factors in endothelial cells.

endothelial cell apoptosis	
Induction	Protection
TNF-α (11, 82) Ceramide (92) Oxidized LDL (4) Oxysterols (6) Angiotensin II (93) Glucose (94) Reactive oxygen species (95) Growth factor withdrawl (59) Nitric oxide (high dose)(12) G1 cell-cycle arrest (13) Irradiation (96)	VEGF, EGF, IGF, bFGF (29) Phorbolester (PMA) (86) A20 (Zinc finger protein) (86, 89) Nitric oxide (12) Laminar shear stress (12) Oestrogen (11) Antioxidants (95) E2F transcription factor, Cyclin A (13) bcl-2 (97) Cyclosporin A (5)

References

1. Kerr, JFR, Wyllie, AH Currie, AR. Apoptosis: a basic biologic phenomenon with wide-ranging implications in tissue kinetics. British Journal of Cancer 1972;26:239-257.
2. Ross, R. The pathogenesis of atherosclerosis: A perspective for the 1990s. Nature 1993;362:801-809.
3. Steinberg, D, Parthasarathy, S, Carew, TE, Khoo, JC Witztum, JL. Beyond cholesterol: modifications of low-density lipoproteins that increase its atherogenicity. New England Journal of Medicine 1989;320:915-924.
4. Dimmeler, S, Haendeler, J, Galle, J Zeiher, AM. Oxidized low-density lipoprotein induces apoptosis of human endothelial cells by activation of CPP32-like proteases. Circulation 1997;95:1760-1763.
5. Walter, DH, Haendeler, J, Galle, J, Zeiher, AM Dimmeler, S. Cyclosporin A inhibits apoptosis of human endothelial cells by preventing release of cytochrome C from mitochondria. Circulation 1998;98:1153-1157.
6. Harada-Shiba, M, Kinoshita, M, Kamido, H Shimokado, K. Oxidized low density lipoprotein induces apoptosis in cultured human umbilical vein endothelial cells by common and unique mechanisms. J Biol Chem 1998;273:9681-9687.
7. Sata, M Walsh, K. Oxidized LDL activates Fas-mediated endothelial cell apoptosis. J Clin Invest 1998;102:1682-1689.
8. Kugiyama, K, Kerns, SA, Morrisett, JD, Roberts, R Henry, PD. Impairment of endothelium-dependent arterial relaxation by lysolecithin in modified low-density lipoproteins. Nature 1990;344:160-162.
9. Kaartinen, M, Pentitilä, A Kovanen, PT. Mast cells in rupture-prone areas of human coronary atheromas produce and store TNF-alpha. Circulation 1996;94:2787-2792.

10. Barath, P, Fishbein, MC, Cao, J, Berenson, J, Helfant, RH Forrester, JS. Detection and localization of tumor necrosis factor in human atheroma. Am J Cardiol 1990;65:297-302.
11. Spyridopoulos, I, Sullivan, AB, Kearney, M, Isner, JM Losordo, DW. Estrogen-receptor-mediated inhibition of human endothelial cell apoptosis. Estradiol as a survival factor. Circulation 1997;95:1505-1514.
12. Dimmeler, S, Haendeler, J, Nehls, M Zeiher, AM. Suppression of apoptosis by nitric oxide via inhibition of interleukin-1β-converting enzyme (ICE)-like and cysteine protease protein (CPP)-32-like protease. J Exp Med 1997;185:601-607.
13. Spyridopoulos, I, Principe, N, Krasinski, K, Kearney, M, Isner, JM Losordo, DW. Restoration of E2F expression rescues vascular endothelial cells from TNF-induced apoptosis. Circulation 1998;98:2883-2890.
14. Spyridopoulos, I, Wang, J, Andres, V, Sullivan, A, Kearney, M Losordo, DW. TNF-induced apoptosis in endothelial cells is associated with cell cycle arrest and decreased expression of cdk inhibitor p27^{Kip1}. Circulation 1996;94:I-282.
15. Kim-Schulze, S, McGowan, KA, Hubchak, SC, Cid, MC, Martin, MB, Kleinman, HK, Greene, GL Schnaper, HW. Expression of an estrogen receptor by human coronary artery and umbilical vein endothelial cells. Circulation 1996;94:1402-1407.
16. Venkov, CD, Rankin, AB Vaughan, DE. Identification of authentic estrogen receptor in cultured endothelial cells. A potential mechanism for steroid hormone regulation of endothelial function. Circulation 1996;94:727-733.
17. Buttke, TM, McCubrey, JA Owen, TC. Use of an aqueous soluble tetrazolium/formazan assay to measure viability and proliferation of lymphokine-dependent cell lines. J Immunol Methods 1993;157:233-240.
18. Tepper, CG, Jayadev, S, Liu, B, Bielawska, A, Wolff, R, Yonehara, SH, YA Seldin, MF. Role for ceramide as an endogenous mediator of Fas-induced cytotoxicity. Proc Natl Acad Sci USA 1995;92:8443-8447.
19. Hishikawa, K, Nakabi, T, Marumo, T, Suzuki, H, Kato, R Saruta, T. Up-regulation of nitric oxide synthase by estradiol in human aortic endothelial cells. FEBS Lett 1995;360:291-293.
20. van der Zee, R, Murohara, T, Luo, Z, Zollmann, F, Passeri, J, Lekutat, C Isner, JM. Vascular endothelial growth factor (VEGF)/vascular permeability factor (VPF) augments nitric oxide release from quiescent rabbit and human vascular endothelium. Circulation 1997;95:1030-1037.
21. Krasinski, K, Spyridopoulos, I, Asahara, T, van der Zee, R, Isner, JM Losordo, DW. Estradiol accelerates functional endothelial recovery after arterial injury. Circulation 1997;95:1768-1772.
22. Hortelano, S, Dallaporta, B, Zamzami, N, Hirsch, T, Susin, SA, Marzo, I, Bosca, L Kroemer, G. Nitric oxide induces apoptosis via triggering mitochondrial permeability transition. FEBS Lett 1997;30:373-377.
23. Dimmeler, S Zeiher, AM. Nitric oxide and apoptosis: another paradigm for the double-edged role of nitric oxide. Nitric Oxide 1997;1:275-281.
24. Ferrara, N Henzel, W.J. Pituitary follicular cells secrete a novel heparin-binding growth factor specific for vascular endothelial cells. Biochem Biophys Res Commun 1989;161:851-855.
25. Keck, PJ, Hauser, SD, Krivi, G, Sanzo, K, Warren, T, Feder, J Connolly, DT. Vascular permeability factor, an endothelial cell mitogen related to PDGF. Science 1989;246:1309-1312.
26. Connolly, DT et al. Tumor vascular permeability factor stimulates endothelial cell growth and angiogenesis. J Clin Invest 1989;84:1470-1478.
27. Leung, DW, Cachianes, G, Kuang, WJ, Goeddel, DV Ferrara, N. Vascular endothelial growth factor is a secreted angiogenic mitogen. Science 1989;246:1306-1309.
28. Senger, DR, Galli, SJ, Dvorak, AM, Perruzzi, CA, Harvey, VS Dvorak, HF. Tumor cells secrete a vascular permeability factor that promotes accumulation of ascites fluid. Science 1983;219:983-985.
29. Spyridopoulos, I, Brogi, E, Kearney, M, Sullivan, AB, Cetrulo, C, Isner, JM Losordo, DW. Vascular endothelial growth factor inhibits endothelial cell apoptosis induced by tumor necrosis factor-α: balance between growth and death signals. J Mol Cell Cardiol 1997;29:1321-1330.
30. Watanabe, Y Dvorak, HF. Vascular permeability factor/vascular endothelial growth factor inhibits anchorage-disruption-induced apoptosis in microvessel endothelial cells by inducing scaffold formation. Exp Cell Res 1997;233:340-349.

31. Alon, T, Hemo, I, Itin, A, Pe'er, J, Stone, J Keshet, E. Vascular endothelial growth factor acts as a survival factor for newly formed retinal vessels and has implications for retinopathy of prematurity. Nat Med 1995;1:1024-1028.
32. Katoh, O, Tauchi, H, Kawaishi, K, Kimura, A Satow, Y. Expression of the vascular endothelial growth factor (VEGF) receptor gene KDR in hematopoietic cells and inhibitory effect of VEGF on apoptotic cells death caused by ionizing radiation. Cancer Res 1995;55:5687-5692.
33. Millauer, B, Wizigman-Voos, S, Schnurch, R, Martinez, R, Moller, NP, Risau, W Ullrich, A. High affinity VEGF binding and developmental expression suggest Flk-1 as a major regulator of vasculogenesis and angiogenesis. Cell 1993;72:835-846.
34. De Vries, C, Escobedo, JA, Ueno, H, Houck, K, Ferrara, N Williams, LT. The fms-like tyrosine kinase, a receptor for vascular endothelial growth factor. Science 1992;255:989-991.
35. Waltenberger, J, Claessonwelsh, L, Siegbahn, A, Shibuya, M Heldin, CH. Different signal transduction properties of KDR and FLT1, two receptors for vascular endothelial growth factor. J Biol Chem 1994;269:26988-26995.
36. Guo, D, Jia, Q, Song, HY, Warren, RS Donner, DB. Vascular endothelial cell growth factor promotes tyrosine phosphorylation of mediators of signal transduction that contain SH2 domains. Association with endothelial cell proliferation. J Biol Chem 1995;270:6729-6733.
37. Xia, P et al. Characterization of vascular endothelial growth factor's effect on the activation of protein kinase C, its isoforms, and endothelial cell growth. J Clin Invest 1996;98:2018-2026.
38. House, C Kemp, BE. Protein kinase C contains a pseudosubstrate prototype in its regulatory domain. Science 1987;238:1726-1728.
39. Harrington, EO, Löffler, J, Nelson, PR, Kent, KC, Simons, M Ware, JA. Enhancement of migration by protein kinase Cα and inhibition of proliferation and cell cycle progression by protein kinase Cδ in capillary endothelial cells. J Biol Chem 1997;272:7390-7397.
40. Ohgushi, M, Kugiyama, K, Fukunaga, K, Murohara, T, Sugiyama, S, Miyamoto, E Yasue, H. Protein kinase C inhibitors prevent impairment of endothelium-dependent relaxation by oxidatively modified LDL. Arterioscler Thromb Vasc Biol 1993;13:1525-1532.
41. Montesano, R Orci, L. Tumor-promoting phorbol esters induce angiogenesis in vitro. Cell 1985;42:469-477.
42. Tsopanoglou, NE, Pipili-Synetos, E Maragoudakis, ME. Protein kinase C involvement in the regulation of angiogenesis. J Vasc Res 1993;30:202-208.
43. Auerbach, W Auerbach, R. Angiogenesis inhibition: A review. Pharmac Ther 1994;63:265-311
44. Montesano, R. Regulation of angiogenesis in vitro. Eur J Clin Invest 1992;22:504-515.
45. Ramirez, MM, Kim, DD Duran, WN. Protein kinase C modulates microvascular permeability through nitric oxide synthase. Am J Physiol 1996;271:H1702-H1705.
46. Murray, MA, Heistad, DD Mayhan, WG. Role of protein kinase C in bradykinin-induced increases in microvascular permeability. Circ Res 1991;68:1340-1348.
47. Nagpala, PG, Malik, AB, Vuong, PT Lum, H. Protein kinase C β_1 overexpression augments phorbol ester-induced increase in endothelial permeability. J Cell Physiol 1996;166:249-255.
48. Murohara, T, Horowitz, JR, Silver, M, Tsurumi, Y, Chen, D, Sullivan, A Isner, JM. Vascular endothelial growth factor / vascular permeability factor enhances vascular permeability via nitric oxide and prostacyclin. Circulation 1997;97:99-107.
49. Enholm, B et al. Comparison of VEGF, VEGF-B, VEGF-C and Ang-1 mRNA regulation by serum, growth factors, oncoproteins and hypoxia. Oncogene 1997;14:2475-2483.
50. Hidaka, H Kobayashi, R. Use of protein (serine/threonine) kinase activators and inhibitors to study protein phosphorylation in intact cells. in Protein phosphorylation 1 edn Vol. 123 (ed. Hardie, D.G.) 87-107 (Oxford University Press, Oxford, GB, 1993).
51. Jarvis, WD, Turner, AJ, Povirk, LF, Traylor, RS Grant, S. Induction of apoptotic DNA fragmentation and cell death in HL-60 human promyelocytic leukemia cells by pharmacological inhibitors of protein kinase C. Cancer Res 1994;54:1707-1714.
52. Presta, M, Tiberio, L, Rusnati, M, Dell'Era, P Ragnotti, G. Basic fibroblast growth factor requires a long-lasting activation of protein kinase C to induce cell proliferation in transformed fetal bovine aortic endothelial cells. Cell Regul 1991;2:719-726.
53. Santell, L, Bartfeld, NS Levin, EG. Identification of a protein transiently phosphorylated by activators of endothelial cell function as the heat-shock protein HSP27. Biochem J 1992;284:705-710.

54. Kent, KC, Mii, S, Harrington, EO, Chang, JD, Mallette, S Ware, JA. Requirement for protein kinase C activation in basic fibroblast growth factor-induced human endothelial cell proliferation. Circ Res 1995;77:231-238.

55. Ohara, Y, Sayegh, HS, Yamin, JJ Harrison, DG. Regulation of endothelial constitutive nitric oxide synthase by protein kinase C. Hypertension 1995;25:415-420.

56. Daviet, I, Herbert, JM Maffrand, JP. Involvement of protein kinase C in the mitogenic and chemotaxis effects of basic fibroblast growth factor on bovine cerebral cortex capillary endothelial cells. FEBS Lett 1990;259:315-317.

57. Eichholtz, T, de Bont, DBA, de Widt, J, Liskamp, RMJ Ploegh, HL. A myristoylated pseudosubstrate peptide, a novel protein kinase C inhibitor. J Biol Chem 1993;268:1982-1986.

58. Ward, NE O'Brian, CA. Inhibition of protein kinase C by N-myristoylated peptide substrate analogs. Biochemistry 1993;32:11903-11909.

59. Spyridopoulos, I, Chen, D, Murohara, T, Principe, N, Isner, JM Losordo, DW. Inhibition of protein kinase C by a myristoylated pseudosubstrate peptide suppresses VEGF-induced angiogenesis, but promotes survival and activation of nitric oxide synthase in endothelial cells. submitted to Circulation.

60. Bates, S Vousden, KH. p53 in signaling checkpoint arrest or apoptosis. Current Opinion in Genetics & Development 1996;6:12-19.

61. Wang, J Walsh, K. Resistance to apoptosis conferred by cdk inhibitors during myocyte differentiation. Science 1996;273:359-361.

62. Beekhuizen, H van Furth, R. Growth characteristics of cultured human macrovascular venous and arterial and microvascular endothelial cells. J Vasc Res 1994;31:230-239.

63. Hengst, L Reed, SI. Translational control of p27^{Kip1} accumulation during the cell cycle. Science 1996;271:1861-1864.

64. Wang, J, Chen, D Walsh, K. Regulation of Cdk2 activity in proliferating versus contact-inhibited endothelial cells: The role of the p27 cyclin kinase inhibitor. Circulation 1996;95:I-524 (abstract).

65. Zerfass-Thome, K, Schulze, A, Zwerschke, W, Vogt, B, Helin, K, Bartek, J, Henglein, B Jansen-Dürr, P. p27^{Kip1} blocks cyclin E-dependent transactivation of cyclin A gene expression. Molecular and Cellular Biology 1997;17:407-415.

66. Henglein, B, Chenivesse, X, Wang, J, Eick, D Brechot, C. Structure and cell cycle-regulated transcription of the human cyclin A gene. Proc Natl Acad Sci USA 1994;91:5490-5494.

67. Schulze, A, Zerfass-Thome, K, Spitkovsky, D, Middendorp, S, Berges, J, Helin, K, Jansen-Dürr, P Henglein, B. Cell cycle regulation of the cyclin A gene promotor is mediated by variant E2F site. Proc Natl Acad Sci USA 1995;92:11264-11268.

68. Yoshizumi, M, Hsieh, CM, Zhou, F, Tsai, JC, Patterson, C, Perrella, MA Lee, ME. The ATF site mediates downregulation of the cyclin A gene during inhibition in vascular endothelial cells. Molecular and Cellular Biology 1995;15:3266-3272.

69. Lopez-Fabre, A et al. Role of nitric oxide in autocrine control of growth and apoptosis of endothelial cells. Am J Physiol 1997;272:H760-H768.

70. Nara, K, Aoyama, Y, Iwata, T, Hagiwara, H Hirose, S. Cell cycle-dependent changes in tissue transglutaminase mRNA levels in bovine endothelial cells. Biochem Biophys Res Commun 1992;187:14-17.

71. Hsiao, R, Sharma, HW, Ramakrishnan, S, Keith, E Narayanan, R. Telomerase activity in normal endothelial cells. Anticancer Research 1997;17:827-832.

72. Imamura, T, Oka, S, Tanahashi, T Okita, Y. Cell cycle-dependent nuclear localization of exogenously added fibroblast growth factor-1 in BALB/c 3T3 and human vascular endothelial cells. Exp Cell Res 1994;215:363-372.

73. Zhou, W, Takuwa, M, Kumada, M Takuwa, Y. Protein kinase C-mediated bidirectional regulation of DNA synthesis, Rb protein phosphorylation, and cyclin-dependent kinases in human vascular endothelial cells. J Biol Chem 1993;268:23041-23048.

74. Zhou, W, Takuwa, N, Kumada, M Takuwa, Y. E2F1, b-myb and selective members of cyclin/cdk subunits are targets for protein kinase C-mediated biomodal growth regulation in vascular endothelial cells. Biochem Biophys Res Commun 1994;199:191-198.

75. Lorenzi, M, Nordberg, JA Toledo, S. High glucose prolongs cell-cycle traversal of cultured human endothelial cells. Diabetes 1987;36:1261-1267.

76. Sharon, P, Drab, EA, Linder, JS, Weidman, SW, Sabesin, SM Rubin, DB. The effect of sulfasalazine on bovine endothelial cell proliferation and cell cycle phase distribution. Comparison

with olsalazine, 5-aminosalicylic acid, and sulfapyridine. Journal of Laboratory & Clinical Medicine 1992;119:99-107.

77. Gupta, SK Singh, JP. Inhibition of endothelial cell proliferation by platelet factor-4 involves a unique action on S phase progression. J Cell Biol 1994;127:1121-1127.

78. Eldor, A, Sela-Donenfeld, D, Korner, M, Pick, M, Resnick-Roguel, N Panet, A. Injury models of the vascular endothelium: apoptosis and loss of thromboresistance by a viral protein. Haemostasis 1996;26:37-45.

79. Tipping, PG Hancock, WW. Production of tumor necrosis factor and interleukin-1 by macrophages from human atheromatous plaques. Am J Pathol 1993;142:1721-1728.

80. Clausell, N, de Lima, VC, Molossi, S, Liu, P, Turley, E, Gotlieb, AI, Adelman, AG Rabinovitch, M. Expression of tumor necrosis factor α and accumulation of fibronectin in coronary artery restenotic lesions retrieved by atherectomy. Br Heart J 1995;73:534-539.

81. Tanaka, H, Sukhova, G, Schwartz, D Libby, P. Proliferating arterial smooth muscle cells after ballon injury express TNF-alpha but not interleukin-1 or basic fibroblast growth factor. Arterioscler Thromb Vasc Biol 1996;16:12-18.

82. Robaye, B, Mosselmanns, R, Fiers, W, Dumont, JE Galand, P. Tumor necrosis factor iduces apoptosis (programmed cell death) in normal endothelial cells in vitro. Am J Pathol 1991;138:447-453.

83. Polunovsky, VA, Wendt, CH, Ingbar, DH, Peterson, MS Bitterman, PB. Induction of endothelial cell apoptosis by TNFα : modulation by inhibitors of protein synthesis. Exp Cell Res 1994;214:584-594.

84. Assoian, RK Marcantonio, EE. The extracellular matrix as a cell cycle control element in atherosclerosis and restenosis. J Clin Invest 1996;98:2436-2439.

85. Assoian, RK. Anchorage-dependent cell cycle progression. J Cell Biol 1997;136:1-4.

86. Varani, J, Dame, MK, Taylor, CG, Sarma, V, Merino, R, Kunkel, RG, Nunez, G Dixit, VM. Age-dependent injury in human umbilical vein endothelial cells: relationship to apoptosis and correlation with a lack of A20 expression. Lab Invest 1995;73:851-858.

87. Araki, S, Shimada, Y, Kaji, K Hayashi, H. Role of protein kinase C in the inhibition by fibroblast growth factor of apoptosis in serum-depleted endothelial cells. Biochem Biophys Res Commun 1990;172:1081-1085.

88. Jaattela, M, Mouritzen, H, Elling, F Bastholm, L. A20 zinc finger protein inhibits TNF and IL-1 signaling. Journal of Immunology 1996;156:1166-1173.

89. Opipari Jr., AW, Hu, HM, Yabkowitz, R Dixit, VM. The A20 zinc finger protein protects cells from tumor necrosis factor cytotoxicity. J Biol Chem 1992;267:12424-12427.

90. Araki, S, Shimada, Y, Kaji, K Hayashi, H. Apoptosis of vascular endothelial cells by fibroblast growth factor deprivation. Biochem Biophys Res Commun 1990;168:1194-1200.

91. Dimmeler, S, Hermann, C Zeiher, AM. Apoptosis of endothelial cells. Contribution to the pathophysiology of atherosclerosis. Eur Cytokine Netw 1998;9:697-698.

92. Slowik, MR, De Luca, LG, Min, W Pober, JS. Ceramide Is not a signal for tumor necrosis factor-induced gene expression but does cause programmed cell death in human vascular endothelial cells. Circ Res 1996;79:736-747.

93. Dimmeler, S, Rippmann, V, Weiland, U, Haendeler, J Zeiher, AM. Angiotensin II induces apoptosis of human endothelial cells: protective effect of nitric oxide. Circ Res 1997;81:970-976.

94. Baumgartner-Partzer, SM, Wagner, L, Pettermann, M, Grillari, J, Gessl, A Waldhusl, W. High glucose-triggered apoptosis in cultured endothelial cells. Diabetes 1995;44:1323-1327.

95. Dimmeler, S, Hermann, C, Galle, J Zeiher, AM. Upregulation of superoxide dismutase and nitric oxide synthase mediates the apoptosis-suppressive effects of shear stress on endothelial cells. Arterioscler Thromb Vasc Biol 1999;19:656-664.

96. Fuks, Z et al. Basic fibroblast growth factor protects endothelial cells against radiation-induced programmed cell death in vitro and in vivo. Cancer Res 1994;54:2582-2590.

97. Karsan, A, Yee, E Harlan, JM. Endothelial cell death induced by tumor necrosis factor-α is blocked by the bcl-2 family member A1. J Biol Chem 1997.

II.2
Myocardium

II.2.1
Endurance under stress and cardioprotective functions by cardiac fibroblasts

Mahboubeh Eghbali-Webb, Ph.D.
Yale University, New Haven, CT, USA

INTRODUCTION

In the interstitium, the majority of cells are fibroblasts (1,2). Apoptosis or programmed cell death is an essential stage of cell cycle in cardiac morphogenesis during development and of central importance in maintaining homeostasis by eliminating the damaged and dysfunctional fibroblasts which will be replaced by new generation of cells. The mechanisms of apoptosis in cardiac fibroblasts are vastly unknown and in depth examination of various intracellular pathways responsible for apoptosis in response to environmental stress are yet to be performed. Relatively more is known on signals controlling apoptosis in cardiac myocytes than in cardiac fibroblasts. This issue is discussed in detail in separate chapter. Based on as yet limited information on both systems it is evident that the intracellular mechanisms and extracellular inducers of apoptosis in cardiac fibroblasts are not similar to those in post-mitotic cardiac myocytes. It is also evident that under environmental stress, such as hypoxia, which would cause apoptosis and cell death in cardiac myocytes, cardiac fibroblasts survive if not indefinitely, at least longer. This resilience lends support to the notion that cardiac fibroblasts may indeed have a mission to protect other cardiac cells or to compensate for their loss. In the past decade a growing body of evidence demonstrating various functions of cardiac fibroblasts has emerged and their role in the regulation of biological responses of other cardiac cells during development, normal growth, aging, ventricular hypertrophy and heart failure after myocardial infarction has been recognized. An in depth analysis of the biological properties of cardiac fibroblasts reveals that their collective function may best be described as "cardioprotective". This chapter summarizes reports on the properties of cardiac fibroblasts which may directly or indirectly provide protection to other cells in the heart under normal and stressful conditions.

CARDIAC FIBROBLASTS IN CULTURE

Cardiac fibroblasts have multiple functions ranging from the synthesis of almost all proteins of the extracellular matrix to release of a vast array of growth factors and cytokines necessary for cell growth and differentiation (1-4). A significant portion of data on their properties was obtained as the result of studies on rodent cells. These cells share many characteristics, including synthesis of fibrillar collagens with fibroblasts from other tissues (5). They express types I, III and IV collagens and almost 80% of total newly synthesized collagen is collagen type I (5,6). They also express laminin, fibronectin, cytoskeletal actin, transforming growth factor-beta (TGF-β_1) (5-8), connexin-43 (8) all three types of TGF-β_1 receptors (9) and basal and TGF-β_1-stimulated collagenase activity (10). Rodent cardiac fibroblasts express angiotensin II receptor type AT1 (11-13) which is developmentally regulated (14) and is involved in angiotensin II-induced stimulation of growth and proliferation (15). The fibroblasts in failing myopathic hamster express AT2 receptors which exerts anti-AT1 effect on the progression of fibrosis by inhibiting collagen synthesis and cell proliferation (16). In two- and three-dimensional collagen gels angiotensin II induces contraction of collagen gel by cardiac fibroblasts and this effect is mediated by beta$_1$-integrin (17). Wang and Brecher (18) reported that angiotensin II induces activation of mitogen-activated protein (MAP) kinases and TGF-β_1 expression in rat cardiac fibroblasts and that nitric oxide and N-acetylcystein inhibit this effect of angiotensin II. Recent studies demonstrated that oxytocin is expressed in the rat heart in cardiac fibroblasts (19).

Differences between human and rodent cardiac fibroblasts

Human cardiac fibroblasts in culture may serve as an in vitro model system that would allow studies aimed at understanding the underlying molecular and cellular mechanisms involved in normal and pathologic performance of the human heart. Although the number of studies on human cardiac fibroblasts is on the rise, most studies have been performed on cells obtained from rodent heart. Increasingly, comparison of the results obtained with rodent and human cells reveals major differences in biological properties of both systems. In human cardiac fibroblasts, basic fibroblast growth factor (bFGF) stimulates collagenase gene expression and TGF-β_1 suppresses this effect (20). Whereas, TGF-β_1 is a stimulator of collagenase activity in rabbit cardiac fibroblasts (10). In our laboratory, a comparative study revealed important dissimilarities between human and rabbit cardiac fibroblasts (21). Human cells had significantly larger surface area per cell than rabbit cells. They had lower rate of DNA synthesis and a longer doubling time compared with rabbit cells. Similar to rabbit cells human cardiac fibroblasts express types I, II and III TGF-β_1 receptors. However, the values for type III/ type I and type II/ type I ratios were higher in human cells than in rabbit cells. These differences in the TGF-β_1 receptor profile were compatible with the relatively moderate effect of TGF-β_1 on DNA synthesis and on collagen type I mRNA transcripts in human cardiac fibroblasts compared with that in rabbit cells. The mitogenic effects of bFGF, angiotensin II and thyroid hormones had a lower magnitude in human cardiac fibroblasts compared with rabbit cells. The level of mRNA for pro α_1 (l) collagen was relatively lower in human cells. These results clearly demonstrate that there are significant differences in biological properties of human and rodent cardiac fibroblasts in culture. These variations may reflect dissimilarities in their in vivo behavior and which may be accentuated under pathophysiological conditions. A relatively lower basal level of DNA synthesis in human cardiac fibroblasts may be the result of differential expression and availability of local growth factors with either positive or negative effects on cell proliferation. The observed differences between the response of human cardiac fibroblasts to bFGF, angiotensin II, thyroid hormone and TGF-β_1, and that of rodent cells point to potential variations in specific receptors (density, subtype, affinity) or in downstream response pathways for these factors. Studies by Neuss et al (22) support this notion by showing that human cardiac fibroblasts express an unusual type of angiotensin II receptor that has not been reported in rodent cells. Consistently, studies by Villarreal et al (23) demonstrated that there is few angiotensin II receptors in human cardiac fibroblasts compared with that in rodent cells. Hafizi et al (24) reported the expression of AT1 receptor and functional angiotensin-converting enzyme in human cardiac fibroblasts and showed that the angiotensin II-induced collagen synthesis is mediated by AT1 receptor. Gallagher et al (25) showed that the density of AT1 receptors in human neonatal cardiac fibroblasts is fewer than that in rat cells. Together, these variations suggest that not all results of studies in rodents may predict the biology of human cells and that in an in vivo context, over-production or deficiency of a given factor may not produce signals of comparable intensity in human and rodent hearts, although this requires further study.

CARDIOPROTECTIVE ROLE OF CARDIAC FIBROBLASTS

In the heart cardiac fibroblasts interact with other cell types both via the extracellular matrix and by releasing soluble factors (Figure 1). As the result, their cardio-protective effects may emerge in several ways:

Protective effects provided by extracellular matrix

Their most-evident protective effect is the one brought about by the synthesis and deposition of the extracellular matrix. It is established that cardiac fibroblasts are the cellular source of fiber-forming collagen types I and III (1-2). Scanning electron microscopy has shown that the collagen matrix of the heart is an intricate and highly organized structure that serves to interconnect cardiac myocytes to one another and to their neighboring capillaries (26). The highly specialized arrangement of matrix provides support for cardiac myocytes, prevents their slippage and maintains their alignment during a cardiac cycle.

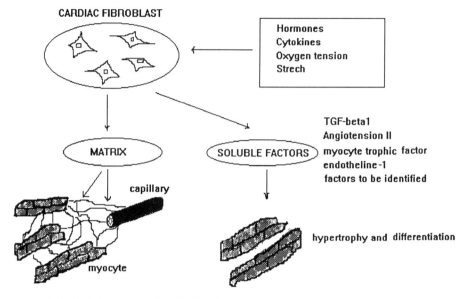

Figure 1   Biological properties of cardiac fibroblasts.

In addition to this important role, collagen matrix of the heart may also act as a link between the contractile element of adjacent cardiac myocytes and as a conduit of information that is necessary for cell function. This assumption is supported by data demonstrating that the interaction of collagen fibers with cardiac myocytes occurs at regions near the Z band and that the cell attachment is mediated by specific molecules belonging to the family of integrins (27). Furthermore, expression of gap junction-specific proteins by cardiac fibroblasts and their active participation in the myocardial cell communication has been demonstrated by electrophysiological studies in which neonatal rat cardiac fibroblasts were shown to make conductance-dependent electrical coupling with cardiac myocytes and with cardiac fibroblasts (28). A variety of growth factors and hormones have been found to alter matrix production in cardiac fibroblasts either by a direct effect on collagen gene expression or indirectly by their effect on the cardiac fibroblast proliferation. For example, norepinephrine, a biogenic amine which induces cardiac fibrosis in experimental models of pressure overload, does not induce changes in collagen type I gene expression in cardiac fibroblasts (7). In contrasts, TGF-ß$_1$ for which cardiac fibroblasts are both the source and the target (4,9) stimulates collagen type I gene expression in cardiac fibroblasts and this effect is dependent on de novo synthesis of proteins (29) and suggested to be at the transcriptional level similar to effect of TGF-ß$_1$ on collagen gene expression in other cells.

Of all known forms of pathological hypertrophy, thyroid hormone-induced hypertrophy is unique in that it lacks fibrosis and is completely reversible. We established, using rats with hyperthyroidism (30), thyroidectomized rats (31) and tight skin mouse, a genetic model of cardiac fibrosis (32), that circulating thyroid hormones down-regulate collagen type I biosynthesis in the heart. Our in vitro studies showed decreased levels of collagen type I mRNA with moderate changes in mRNA stability and a significant decrease in the activity of collagen type I promoter in thyroid hormone-treated cells (30). Thyroid hormones act through the intracellular receptor types α and ß which belong to the superfamily of ligand-activated transcription factors and bind to thyroid hormone response elements on the target promoters and act as activator or repressor of transcription (33). In addition to their receptor-mediated effects, thyroid hormones exert regulatory effects via cross-talk with other transcription factors. An example is their interaction with jun and fos proto-oncogenes (34), the components of AP-1 (activator protein factor 1 in Hella cells). Similar to phorbol myristate acetate, an inducer of AP-1, thyroid hormone causes down-regulation of collagen type I gene expression and expression of c-fos and c-jun mRNAs in cardiac fibroblasts (30). The role of AP-1 in regulation of collagen type I gene expression in cardiac fibroblasts of the tight skin (TSK) mouse is well established. It is shown that a reduced interaction of negative regulatory sequences on pro α_1 (l) collagen gene with AP-1 is responsible for increased collagen type I gene expression in TSK cells (35). We showed that sequences on the 5'flanking regions of pro α_1(l) collagen gene are responsible for the inhibitory effect of thyroid hormones on promoter activity (36) and that thyroid hormone receptor type ß binds to proximal (-15/+115) sequences of the promoter and that an AP-1 response element located at +92/+97 is necessary for the T_3-induced inhibition of pro α_1(l) collagen promoter activity in cardiac fibroblasts. These data show that binding of ß receptor to collagen type I promoter in the absence of AP-1 binding is not sufficient for T_3-induced inhibition of promoter activity.

The association of AT2 angiotensin II receptors with collagen production is shown in failing human and hamster heart (16,37). Cardiac fibroblasts from cardiomyopathic hamsters have significantly higher level of collagen types I, III, IV and V synthesis compared to cells from normal hamsters and captopril, an ACE inhibitor, causes decrease in collagen synthesis in those fibroblasts (38). The role of angiotensin II in collagen production by cardiac fibroblasts has also been demonstrated by studies on cardiac fibroblasts from spontaneously hypertensive rats (SHR) and their normotensive counterparts, Wistar-Kyoto (WKY) rats (39). Kawaguchi and kitabataki (40) showed that the basal levels of collagen synthesis in cardiac fibroblasts from SHR is higher than that in WKY cells and the stimulation of collagen synthesis in SHR cells by angiotensin II is significantly enhanced compared to that in WKY cells. Basal and angiotensin II-induced realease of Prostacyclin from cardiac fibroblasts caused a decrease in collagen types I and III gene expression, suggesting a role for eicosanoids in modulating collagen deposition (39). The release of prostacyclines by cardiac fibroblasts is also involved in bradykinin-induced reduction in collagen synthesis (41).

Exogenous substances can also cause changes in the collagen matrix. We showed that nicotine decreases mRNA levels for Pro α_1(I) but not pro α_2(I) collagen and causes a decrease in collagenase activity in cardiac fibroblasts (42). Mimosine, a prolyl-4-hydroxylase inhibitor also inhibits synthesis and secretion of mature collagen type I and causes intracellular accumulation of procollagen which leads to a loss of coordinated monomeric procollagen synthesis and secretion of triple helical mature collagen.   Mimosine also elevated the activity of matrix metalloprotease, MMP-9 (43).

Changes in physical tension and pressure, brought about by various pathophysiological conditions, could have a significant impact on the biological responses of cardiac fibroblasts. Lee and McCulloch (44) used multiaxial strain to demonstrate that biological responses in adult rat cardiac fibroblasts is correlated with the magnitude and two-dimensional pattern of strain.   Cultured cardiac fibroblasts on stretchable membrane provide a suitable system to study the effect of mechanical stretch on collagen gene expression (45). Using this system, it has been shown that the ratio of collagen type III/I increases in mechanically stretched cells and that this was due to increase in type III mRNA levels in response to cyclic stretch.   Stretch also affects the expression and activity of transmembrane matrix metalloproteinases and tissue plasminogen activator (46). In rat cardiac fibroblasts 4% static biaxial stretch caused activation of integrin-dependent ERK1/2 and c-Jun NH2 terminal kinases (47).   Study indicated that integrins act as mechanotransducers, converting mechanical stimuli into biochemical signals (47). Separate studies utilizing cyclic mechanical stretch indicated that cardiac fibroblasts may mediate the stretch-induced hypertrophic effect on cardiac myocytes by increasing endothelin-1 production (48). Gudi et al (49) identified G proteins as a mediator in the signaling pathways in cardiac fibroblasts that transforms mechanical stretch into biochemical response. They showed that equibiaxial strain and the rate at which the strain is applied stimulates early activation of G proteins in cardiac fibroblasts.

Hypoxia which is caused as the result of myocardial ischemia, is a powerful regulator of gene expression for multiple regulatory proteins including growth factors (50), enzymes (51) and stress proteins (52-53) which, in turn, regulate gene expression, growth, proliferation and differentiation in cardiac cells.   We determined the effect of hypoxia on collagen type I production in human cardiac fibroblasts under basal conditions of cell culture and in response to growth factors. Hypoxia caused an increase in the basal level of pro $\alpha_1(l)$ collagen mRNA and protein (54). The TGF-ß$_1$-induced increase in the level of pro $\alpha_1(l)$ collagen mRNA was not observed under hypoxia. But, the T$_3$-induced decrease in pro $\alpha_1(l)$ collagen mRNA was reversed under hypoxia.   TGF-ß$_1$ and T$_3$ under ambient conditions caused decrease in collagen type I. Under hypoxia, effects of both factors were reversed (54). These results provide evidence that hypoxia by increasing the basal level and by reversing the factor-induced inhibition of collagen type I gene expression in human cardiac fibroblasts can enhance overall collagen type I production. Combinatorial effects of hypoxia on proliferation (discussed below) and collagen production can contribute to the post-infarct remodeling of the collagen matrix in failing heart.   Tamamori et al (55) reported hypoxia-induced enhanced expression of collagen type I and III in cardiac fibroblasts and attenuation of this effect by atrial natriuretic factor (ANF) and suggested that paracrine effects of ANF which is produced by cardiac myocytes may play a role in prevention of cardiac fibrosis in ischemic heart diseases.

Protective effects brought about by soluble factors

The most intriguing property of cardiac fibroblasts is the protection that they provide from various injuries to cardiac myocytes and possibly to cells in vessel wall (Figure 2). A significant body of evidence in support of such role has been accumulated and the in vitro influence of cardiac fibroblasts on several biological responses of cardiac myocytes has been demonstrated. Neonatal cardiac fibroblasts when co-cultured with cardiac myocytes from the same tissue enhanced the surface area of myocytes and suppressed their beating rate. Both phenomena are characteristic features associated with growth and differentiation of cardiac myocytes during development. Thus cardiac fibroblasts may play an important role in modulation of cardiac myocyte growth in developing heart (56).

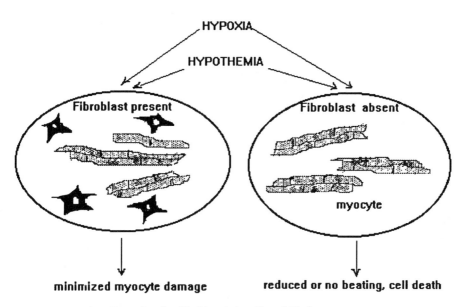

Figure 2 Protective effects of cardiac fibroblasts induced by soluble factors.

This role is also evident by studies in which co-culture of cardiac myocytes with cardiac fibroblasts led to increased protein synthesis in cardiac myocytes and this effect was potentiated in the presence of angiotensin II, but angiotensin II alone did not have the same trophic effect on cardiac myocytes (57). Later studies showed that cardiac fibroblasts release endothelin-I and TGF-$_1$ in response to angiotensin II stimulation (58-60) and that endothelin-1 acts in a paracrine fashion as a hypertrophic factor for cardiac myocytes. These results demonstrated that cardiac fibroblasts regulate the development of myocyte hypertrophy at least partially via endothelin-1 secretion. Bhat and Baker (61) showed that in cardiac fibroblasts a cross-talk between angiotensin II and IL-6 is mediated through Stat3 transcription factor which may have relevance in ventricular hypertrophy. We demonstrated that while the beating rate of cardiac myocytes decreases under hypoxia, the presence of cardiac fibroblast-conditioned medium prevents the hypoxia-induced inhibition of beating rate (Agocha and Eghbali-Webb, 1997, unpublished data). Guo et al (62) reported that co-culturing cardiac myocytes with fibroblasts or in cardiac fibroblast-conditioned medium leads to decreased expression of the voltage-gated potassium channel alpha subunit Kv1.5 in cardiac myocytes and that this effect as well as trophic effect on cardiac myocytes were abolished by the presence of Losartan, an angiotensin II AT1 receptor blocker. Protective role of cardiac fibroblasts can extend beyond promoting growth and maintenance of beating rate under hypoxia. This assumption is based on studies that have shown that cardiac fibroblasts in neonatal rat heart protect cardiac myocytes from hypothermic injury (63). These studies showed that the hypothermia-induced decrease in the beating rate was considerably less pronounced in cardiac myocytes which were co-cultured with cardiac fibroblasts. In addition, the release of creatine phosphokinase and lactate dehydrogenase from cardiac myocytes in response to hypothermic stimulus was significantly lower in the presence of cardiac fibroblasts than in their absence (63). It is suggested that cardiac fibroblasts may play an important role in protection of cardiac myocytes during hypothermic conditions of pre-transplant preservation of cardiac tissue. Cardiac fibroblasts are also implicated in inhibition of angiogenesis in three-dimensional fibrin gels, where they induced contact-inhibition of endothelial sprouting (64).

CELL CYCLE REGULATION IN CARDIAC FIBROBLASTS

Proliferation

Proliferation of cardiac fibroblasts is an important event associated with myocardial remodeling under physiopathological conditions including development, ventricular hypertrophy and heart failure post-myocardial infarction. As indicated earlier, in addition to matrix proteins, a vast array of growth factors and cytokines are produced by cardiac fibroblasts and their altered number will cause an overall change in the microenvironment in the myocardium. Many factors to which cardiac fibroblasts are exposed can regulate their proliferative response. Thyroid hormones, for example, stimulate DNA synthesis in cardiac fibroblasts (30). Platelet-derived growth factor is also a potent mitogen for cardiac fibroblasts and this effect is not associated with MAP-kinase pathway (65). An important regulator of cell cycle, TGF-β_1, regulates proliferative capacity of cardiac fibroblasts. In vitro, TGF-β_1 changes proliferative response of cardiac fibroblasts and alters their phenotype from fibroblastic into muscle cell-like (66,9). Both changes are specifically induced by TGF-β_1 and seem to be cardiac-specific, because they are not induced by other trophic factors including thyroid hormones and angiotensin II and do not occur in human skin fibroblasts. The proliferative effects of TGF-β_1 varies with its dose and depends on the cell density as the result of density-dependent expression of TGF-β_1 receptors. In addition to the effect of exogenous TGF-β_1, the autocrine effect of this growth factor influences proliferation in cardiac fibroblasts (67). Modified anti-sense oligonucleotides complementary to translation initiation site on TGF-β_1

mRNA could block TGF-ß$_1$ synthesis in cardiac fibroblasts. We showed that treatment of cardiac fibroblasts with these oligonucleotides leads to a significant enhancement of DNA synthesis. It also appears that the autocrine effect of TGF-ß$_1$ regulates the response of cardiac fibroblasts to other growth factors such as bFGF and angiotensin II, as demonstrated by increased bFGF- and angiotensin II-induced DNA synthesis in anti-sense-treated cells (67).

Although norepinephrine does not alter collagen gene expression it enhances DNA synthesis in cardiac fibroblasts (7). Therefore, norepinephrine-induced cardiac fibroblast proliferation may indirectly contribute to an overall change in collagen content of the heart (7). However, data by Fisher and Absher (68) which showed that norepinephrine induces augmentation of TGF-ß$_1$ release, may provide an alternative mechanism by which norepinephrine may indirectly stimulate collagen production in cardiac fibroblasts. They also attributed the growth-enhancing effects of norepinephrine to the release of TGF-ß$_1$. Calderone et al (69) reported that nitric oxide and atrial natriuretic peptide attenuate the growth-promoting effects of norepinephrine by a cyclic GMP-mediated inhibition of norepinephrine-stimulated Ca2+ influx. Zheng et al (70) showed that extracellular ATP inhibits the norepinephrine-induced stimulation of DNA synthesis. Cloning the adrenergic receptors from rat heart showed that the adrenergic receptor system in cardiac fibroblasts is the type beta and the type alpha is absent (71).

Compelling evidence support a regulatory role for angiotensin II in proliferation of cardiac fibroblasts independent of hemodynamic effects. Angiotensin II causes stimulation of DNA synthesis in neonatal rat cardiac fibroblasts via AT1 receptor (72). It also causes a rapid induction of c-fos, c-jun, c-myc, jun B, and Egr-1 in cardiac fibroblasts (15). We demonstrated that angiotensin II-induced DNA synthesis in human cardiac fibroblasts is potentiated under hypoxia (54). Nitric oxide donors are shown to inhibit the angiotensin-induced DNA synthesis in cardiac fibroblasts (73). Angiotensin II receptor on cardiac fibroblasts is G protein-coupled and has been shown to activate the signal transducers and activators of transcription (STAT) signal transduction pathway (74). Angiotensin II also appears to activate MAP kinases (ERKs) via tyrosine kinase, but not protein kinase C activation (72,75). The presence of local angiotensin converting enzyme (ACE) seems to be necessary for the stimulatory effect of angiotensin II on proliferation because inhibition of ACE in cardiac fibroblasts led to inhibition of angiotensin II-induced stimulation of DNA synthesis (76).

The role of female hormones in the prevalence of cardiac diseases are recognized but not fully explored. We investigated the effect of estrogen (17ß-estradiol) on proliferative capacity of cardiac fibroblasts from female rat heart. Basal DNA synthesis increased in estrogen-treated cells and this effect was abolished by tamoxifen. Estrogen caused induction of MAP kinases ERK1/2 and in the presence of a synthetic inhibitor of MAP kinase pathway, PD98059, failed to stimulate DNA synthesis. We also showed that type ß receptor is the predominant type of estrogen receptor in cardiac fibroblasts with both cytoplasmic and nuclear localization and that estrogen-treatment induces the translocation of receptor to the nucleus (77). These data provide evidence that cardiac fibroblasts are cellular targets for estrogen and that this hormone regulates their proliferative response via estrogen receptor-

and MAP kinase-dependent mechanisms (77). Dubey et al (78) demonstrated that in both female and male cardiac fibroblasts, 17ß-estradiol inhibits the serum-induced stimulation of DNA synthesis, estrogen metabolites were more potent than estrogen and that the effect of estrogen was potentiated in the presence of progesterone. Grohe et al(79) demonstrated that oestrone stimulates DNA synthesis in cardiac fibroblasts. These findings suggest that estrogen, by its effect on cardiac fibroblast proliferation, can affect the remodeling of the extracellular matrix and alter the microenvironment of cardiac cells, hence affect the integrity of myocardial function.

Cell cycle termination

Termination of cell cycle progression in cardiac fibroblasts is as important as their proliferation. Although the extracellular inhibitors of cell cycle and the intracellular signal transduction pathways responsible for the exit of cardiac fibroblasts from cell cycle are vastly unexplored, the available data indicate that several biological factors to which cardiac fibroblasts are naturally exposed along with hemodynamic stimuli play an important role in the inhibition of cardiac fibroblast proliferation. Long's group have demonstrated that IL-1ß, a pleiotropic hormone-like polypeptide which is produced in the heart under inflammatory myocardial injury, is an inhibitor of cardiac fibroblast proliferation (80). They further demonstrated that IL-1ß exerts its inhibitory effects at the G1/S phase of cell cycle by preventing the phosphorylation of retinoblastoma (Rb) gene. This action of IL-1ß involves cyclines, cycline-dependent kinases and the cycline kinase inhibitor p27 (81). Other natural factors with an inhibitory effect on cardiac fibroblasts are natriuretic pepetides. Cao et al (82) demonstrated that natriuretic peptides inhibit basal and stretch-induced stimulation of DNA synthesis in cardiac fibroblasts and that this effect is amplified by co-treatment with phosphodiesterase inhibitors. Natriuretic peptides also inhibit angiotensin II-induced proliferation of cardiac fibroblasts by blocking endothelin-1 gene expression (83). Adenosine, a nucleoside produced in cardiac fibroblasts, inhibits proliferation of cardiac fibroblasts in response to serum via activation of A2 adenosine receptor (84). We showed that adenosine inhibits the stimulation of DNA synthesis by angiotensin II and that A2 receptor agonists are more potent in this respect than A1 receptor agonists (85).

Hypoxia is a known inducer of apoptosis in a variety of cell types including cardiac myocytes. But it appears that cardiac fibroblasts are more resilient under hypoxia. We determined the effect of hypoxia on growth and proliferation of cardiac fibroblasts under basal conditions of cell culture and in response to TGF-ß$_1$, thyroid hormone, angiotensin II and bFGF. The cell viability, as examined by light microscopy and analysis of DNA did not change by hypoxia. Hypoxia caused a decrease in the basal but not growth factor-induced protein synthesis. Basal level of DNA synthesis decreased significantly under hypoxia. The TGF-ß$_1$-induced inhibition of DNA synthesis was reversed under hypoxia and this growth factor induced stimulation of DNA synthesis (54). Under ambient condition, thyroid hormone, angiotensin II and bFGF stimulated DNA synthesis and their effects enhanced under hypoxia (54). Despite inhibition of protein synthesis and proliferative response and dissimilar to the effect of hypoxia in cardiac myocytes (86), hypoxia did not induce apoptosis in cardiac fibroblasts as determined by DNA fragmentation and morphological criteria of apoptosis (54). These findings were also consistent with the results obtained by Long et al (86) which showed the absence of hypoxia-induced apoptosis-associated transcription factor, P53, in cardiac fibroblasts. In another model of cellular apoptosis, induced by a specific inhibitor of vacuolar proton ATPase, cardiac fibroblasts did not undergo apoptosis as evidenced by the absence of DNA fragmentation and P53 expression (87). Identical cellular intervention in cardiac myocytes induced apoptosis (87).

An exit from cell cycle in cardiac fibroblasts may also result in their entrance into the myogenic pathways. This assumption is based on their demonstrated plasticity and their predisposition to phenotypic modulation (66). We showed that cardiac fibroblasts, when exposed to TGF-ß$_1$, undergo phenotypic modulation based on four key items of evidence: 1) appearance of morphological features characteristic of cardiac myocytes in TGF-ß$_1$-treated cells; 2) induction of sarcomeric actin mRNA and sarcomeric filaments in cardiac fibroblasts; 3) disappearance of intermediate filament vimentin, as evidenced by immunofluorescent light microscopy; and 4) continued expression of muscle-specific morphological features and sarcomeric actin filaments in the second generation of cells stemmed from TGF-ß$_1$-treated cells, even in the absence of TGF-ß$_1$. This effect of TGF-ß$_1$ on cardiac fibroblasts seems to be specific to these cells since they were not induced in other fibroblasts and did not occur by other factors to which cardiac fibroblasts are naturally exposed. Furthermore, as noted earlier, these changes in phenotype coincided with the inhibition of proliferative response. In an in vivo context, however, this effect of TGF-ß$_1$ could be affected by the antagonistic or cooperative effects of other growth factors and hormones. To date, little is known about the myogenesis of cardiac muscle in postnatal periods. Stem cells have not been identified and no cell lines have been found to terminally differentiate into cardiac myocytes. Effects of TGF-ß$_1$ on cardiac fibroblast phenotype may prove to be part of yet to be identified myogenic pathways through which a terminal differentiation of cardiac fibroblasts into cardiac myocytes is possible. There are also differences in proliferation and collagen synthesis in cardiac fibroblasts obtained from different regions of the myocardium as shown in developing chick myocardium (epicardium vs atrioventricular valves). These differences, however, are suggested to be caused by the impact of the micro-environment rather than differences in phenotype (88). Klett et al (89) showed that two subsets of cardiac fibroblasts were isolated from ventricular tissue which differed in growth rate, angiotensin II receptor and angiotensin II responsiveness and suggested that these differences could be due to differences in phenotype. Studies by Reiss et al (90) demonstrated that insulin-like growth factor receptors are expressed by fetal cardiac fibroblasts, their expression reduces in postnatal period and this reduction is associated with reduced proliferative response in postnatal cardiac fibroblasts (90). Exogenous substances may also cause an inhibition of cell cycle progression in cardiac fibroblasts as seen by nicotine which causes decreased DNA synthesis in cardiac fibroblasts in the absence of morphological evidence of cytoxicity as determined by light microscopy (42).

SUMMARY

Cardiac fibroblasts produce matrix, cytokines, growth factors and hormones and their role in maintaining the integrity of myocardial function under physiopathological conditions is established. Although the mechanisms of physio-pathological apopotosis in cardiac fibroblasts is vastly unexplored, their relative resilience under stressful conditions is recognized and lends support to the notion that cardiac fibroblasts may play a role in protecting other cardiac cells. In depth study of their properties increasingly reveals that cardiac fibroblasts provide protection to cardiac myocytes and other non-fibroblastic cells in the heart. The underlying mechanisms of many of their biological properties still remain to be identified. Among these are mechanisms of apoptosis, their resilience and survival under stress, their phenotypic modulation and finally mechanisms responsible for transformation of mechanical stimuli into biochemical response.

References

1. Eghbali M, Czaja MJ, Zeydel M, Weiner FR, Zern MA, Seifter S, Blumenfeld OO. Collagen mRNAs in isolated adult heart cell. J Mol Cell Cardiol 1988; 20:267-276.
2. Eghbali M, Blumenfeld 00, Seifter S, Buttrick PM, Leinwand LA, Robinson TF, Zern MA, Giambrone MA. Localization of types I, III and IV collagen mRNAs in rat heart cells by in situ hybridization. J Mol Cell Cardiol 1989; 21:103-113.
3. Long CS, CJ Henrich, PC Simpson. A growth factor for cardiac myocytes is produced by cardiac non-myocytes. Cell Regulation 1991; 2:1081-1095.
4. Eghbali M. Cellular origin and distribution of transforming growth factor-β_1 in the normal rat myocardium.Cell Tiss Res 1989; 256:553-558.
5. Zeydel M, Puglia K, Eghbali M, Fant J, Seifter S, Blumenfeld OO. Heart fibroblasts of adult rats: Properties and relation to deposition of collagen. Cell Tiss Res 1991; 265: 353-359.
6. Bashey RI, Donnelly M, Insinga F, Jimenez SA. Growth properties and biochemical characterization of collagens synthesized by adult rat heart fibroblasts in culture. J Mol Cell Cardiol 1992; 24:691-700.
7. Bhambi B, Eghbali M. Effect of norepinephrine on myocardial collagen gene expression and response of cardiac fibroblasts following norepinephrine treatment. Am J Pathol 1991; 139:1131-1142.
8. Eghbali M. Cardiac fibroblasts: function, regulation of gene expression and phenotype modulation. In: Holtz J, Drexler H, Just H (eds). Cardiac Adaptation in Heart Failure. Steinkopff Verlag Darmstadt, 1992: 182-189.
9. Sigel VA, Centrella M and Eghbali-Webb M. Regulation of Proliferative Response of Cardiac Fibroblasts by Transforming Growth Factor-β_1. J Mol Cell Cardiol 28:1921-
10. Yao J, Tomek R, Bell F, Eghbali-M. Regulation of collagenase gene expression in cardiac fibroblasts by transforming growth factor-β. The FASEB J 1992; 6:A939. 1929, 1996.
11. Crabos M, Roth M, Hahn AW, Erne P. Characterization of angiotensin II receptors in cultured adult rat cardiac fibroblasts. Coupling to signaling systems and gene expression. J Clin Invest 1994; 93:2372-2378.
12. Villarreal FJ, Kim NN, Ungab GD, Printz MP, Killmann WH. Identification of functional angiotensin II receptors on rat cardiac fibroblasts. Circulation 1993; 88:2849-2861.
13. Sano H. Effect of angiotensin II on collagen metabolism in cultured rat cardiac fibroblasts: its relation to cardiac hypertrophy. J Med Sci 1994; 69:25-34.
14. Matsubara H, Kanasaki M, Murasawa S, Tsukaguchi Y, Nio Y, Inada M. Differential gene expression and regulation of angiotensin II receptor subtypes in rat cardiac fibroblasts and cardiomyocytes in culture. J Clin Invest 1994; 93:1592-1601.
15. Sadoshima J, Izumo S. Molecular characterization of angiotensin II--induced hypertrophy of cardiac myocytes and hyperplasia of cardiac fibroblasts. Critical role of the AT1 receptor subtype. Circ Res 1993; 73:413-423.

16. Ohkubo N, Matsubara H, Nozawa Y, Mori Y, Murasawa S, Kijima K, Maruyama K, Masaki H, TsutumiY, Shibazaki Y, Iawasaka T, Inada M. Angiotensin type 2 receptors are reexpressed by cardiac fibroblasts from failing myopathic hamster hearts and inhibit cell growth and fibrillar collagen metabolism. Circulation 1997; 96:3954-3962.

17. Burgess ML, Carver WE, Terracio L, Wilson SP, Wilson MA, Borg TK. Integrin-mediated collagen gel contraction by cardiac fibroblasts. 'Effects of angiotensin II. Circ Res 1994; 74:291-298.

18. Wang D, Yu X, Brecher P. Nitric oxide and N-acetylcysteine inhibit the activation of mitogen-activated protein kinases by angiotensin II in rat cardiac fibroblasts. J Biol Chem 1998; 273:33027-33034.

19. Jankowski M, Hajjar F, Kawas SA, Mukaddam-Daher S, Hoffman G, McCann SM, Gutkowska J. Rat Heart: a site of oxytocin production and action. Proc Natl Acad Sci 1998; 95: 14558-14563.

20. Chua CC, Chua BH, Zhao ZY, Krebs C, Diglio C, Perrin E. Effect of growth factors on collagen metabolism in cultured human heart fibroblasts. Connective Tiss Res 1991; 26:271-281.

21. Agocha A, Sigel VA and Eghbali-Webb M. Characterization of adult human heart fibroblasts in culture: a comparative study of growth, proliferation and collagen production in human and rabbit cardiac fibroblasts. Cell and Tissue Res 288:87-93, 1997.

22. Neuss M, Regitz-Zagrosek V, Hildebrandt A, Fleck E. Human cardiac fibroblasts express an angiotensin receptor with unusual binding characteristics which is coupled to cellular proliferation. Biochem Biophys Res Comm 1994; 204:1334-1339.

23. Villarreal FJ, Kim NN, Ungab GD, Printz MP, Dillmann WH. Identification of functional angiotensin II receptors on rat cardiac fibroblasts. Circulation 1993; 88(6):2849-2861.

24. Hafizi S, Wharton J, Morgan K, Allen SP, Chester AH, Catravas JD, Polak JM, Yacoub MH. Expression of functional angiotensin-converting enzyme and AT1 receptors in cultured human cardiac fibroblasts. Circulation 1998; 98(23): 2553-2559.

25. Gallagher AM, Bahnson TD, Yu H, Kim NN, Printz MP. Species variability in angiotensin receptor expression by cultured cardiac fibroblasts and the infarcted heart. Am J Physiol 1998; 274: H801-809.

26. Robinson TF, Cohen-Gould L, Factor SM, Eghbali M, and Blumenfeld OO. Structure and function of connective tissue in cardiac muscle: Collagen type III in endomysial struts and pericellular fibers. Scanning Microscopy 1988; 2:1005-1015.

27. Terracio L, Rubin T, Gullberg D, Balog ED, Carver W, Jyring R, Borg TK. Expression of collagen binding integrins during cardiac development and hypertrophy. Circ Res 1991; 68:734-744.

28. Rook MB, van Ginneken AC, de Jonge B, el Aoumari A, Gros D, Jongsma HJ. Differences in gap junction channels between cardiac myocytes, fibroblasts, and heterologous pairs. Am J Physiol 1992; 263:C959-C977.

29. Eghbali M, Tomek R, Sukhatme VP, Woods C, Bhambi B. Differential effects of transforming growth factor-ß₁ and phorbol mirystate acetate on cardiac fibroblasts: Regulation of fibrillar collagen mRNAs and expression of early transcription factors. Circ Res 1991; 69:483-490.

30. Yao J, Eghbali M. Decreased collagen gene expression and absence of fibrosis in thyroid hormone-induced myocardial hypertrophy: Response of cardiac fibroblasts to thyroid hormone in vitro. Circ Res 1992; 71:831-839.

31. Klein LE, Sigel VA, Douglas JA, and Eghbali-Webb M. Up-regulation of collagen type I gene expression in the ventricular myocardium of thyroidectomized rats of both genders. J Mol Cell Cardiol 28:33-42, 1996.

32. Yao J, Eghbali M. Decreased collagen mRNA and regression of cardiac fibrosis in the ventricular myocardium of the tight skin mouse following thyroid hormone treatment. Cardiovasc Res 1992; 26:603-607.

33. Samuels HH, Forman BM, Horowitz ZD, Ye ZS. Regulation of gene expression by thyroid hormone. J Clin Invest 1988; 81:957-967.

34. Zhang X-K, Wills KN, Husmann M, Hermann T, Pfahl M. Novel pathway for thyroid hormone receptor action through interaction with jun and fos oncogene activities. MolCell Biol 1991; 11:6016-6025.

35. Phillips N, Bashey RI, Jimenez SA. Increased α₁(I) procollagen gene expression in tight skin mice myocardial fibroblasts is due to a reduced interaction of a negative regulatory sequence with AP-1 transcription factor. J Biol Chem 1995; 270:9313-9321.

APOPTOSIS IN CARDIAC BIOLOGY

36. Lee H-W, Klein LE, Raser J, Eghbali-Webb M. An activator protein-1 (AP-1) response element on pro α_1(l) collagen gene is necessary for thyroid hormone-induced inhibition of promoter activity in cardiac fibroblasts. J Mol Cell Cardiol 30:2495-2506, 1998.

37. Tsutsumi Y, Matsubara H, Ohkubo N, Mori Y, Nozawa Y, Murasawa S, Kijima K, Maruyama K, Masaki H, Moriguchi Y, Shibasaki Y, Kamihata H, Inada M, Iwasaka T. Angiotensin II type 2 receptor is upregulated in human heart with interstitial fibrosis, and cardiac fibroblasts are the major cell type for its expression. Circ Res 1998; 83:1035-1046.

38. Shinohara T, Shimizu M, Yoshio H, Ino H, Taguchi T, Mabuchi H. Collagen synthesis by cultured cardiac fibroblasts obtained from cardiomyopathic hamsters. Jpn Heart J 1998; 39:97-108.

39. Yu H, Gallagher AM, Garfin PM, Printz MP. Prostacyclin release by rat cardiac fibroblasts: inhibition of collagen expression. Hypertension 1997; 30(5):1047-1053.

40. Kawaguchi H, Kitabatake A. Altered signal transduction system in hypertrophied myocardium: angiotensin II stimulates collagen synthesis in hypertrophied hearts. J Card Fail 1996; 2(4 Suppl):S13-S19.

41. Gallagher AM, Yu H, Printz MP. Bradykinin-induced reductions in collagen gene expression involve prostacyclin. Hypertension 1998; 32(1): 84-88.

42. Tomek RJ, Rimar S, Eghbali-Webb M. Nicotine regulates collagen gene expression, collagenase activity, and DNA synthesis in cultured cardiac fibroblasts: In vivo impact on myocardial collagen matrix. Mol Cell Biochem 136: 97-103, 1994.

43. Ju H, Hao J, Zhao S, Dixon IMC. Antiproliferative and antifibrotic effects of mimosine on adult cardiac fibroblasts. Biochem Biophys Acta 1998; 1448(1): 51-60.

44. Lee AA, McCulloch AD. Multiaxial myocardial mechanics and extracellular matrix remodeling: mechanochemical regulation of cardiac fibroblast function. Adv Exp Med Biol 1997; 430: 227-240.

45. Carver W, Nagpal ML, Nachtigal M, Borge TK, Terracio L. Collagen expression in mechanically stimulated cardiac fibroblasts. Circ Res 1991; 69:116-122.

46. Tyagi SC, Lewis K, Pikes D, Marcello A, Mujumdar VS, Smiley LM, Moore CK. Stretch-induced membrane type matrix metalloproteinase and tissue plasminogen activator in cardiac fibroblast cells. J Cell Physiol 1998; 176: 374-382.

47. MacKenna DA, Dolfi F, Vuori K, Ruoslahti E. Extracellular signal-regulated kinase and c-jun NH2-terminal kinase activation by mechanical stretch is integrin-dependent and matrix-specific in rat cardiac fibroblasts. J Clin Invest 1998;101:301-310.

48. Harada M, Saito Y, Nakagawa O, Miyamoto Y, Ishikawa M, Kuwahara K, Ogawa E, Nakayama M, Kamitani S, Hamanaka I, Kajiyama N, Masuda I, Itoh H, Tanaka I, Nakao K. Role of cardiac nonmyocytes in cyclic mechanical stretch-induced myocyte hypertrophy. Heart Vessels 1997; Suppl 12:198-200.

49. Gudi SR, Lee AA, Clark CB, Frangos JA. Equibiaxial strain and strain rate stimulate early activation of G proteins in cardiac fibroblasts. Am J Physiol 1998; 274: C1424-1428.

50. Helfman T, Falanga V. Gene expression in low oxygen tension. Am J Med Sci 306:37-41, 1993.

51. Webster K, Murphy B. Regulation of tissue-specific glycolytic isozyme genes: coordinate response to oxygen availability in myogenic cells. Can J Zool 1988; 66:1046.

52. Williams RS, Thomas JA, Fina M, German Z, Benjamin IJ. Human heat shock protein 70 (hsp70) protects murine cells from injury during metabolic stress. J Clin Invest 1993;92:503-508.

53. Heacoke CS, Sutherland RM. Enhanced synthesis of stress proteins caused by hypoxia and relation to altered cell growth and metabolism. Br J Cancer 1990; 62:217-225.

54. Agocha A, Eghbali-Webb M. Hypoxia Regulates DNA Synthesis and Collagen Type I Production in Human Cardiac Fibroblasts: Effects of Transforming Growth Factor-beta$_1$, Thyroid hormone, Angiotensin II and Basic Fibroblast Growth Factor. J Mol Cell Cardiol 1997;29:2233-2244.

55. Tamamori M, Ito H, Hiroe M, Marumo F, Hata RI. Stimulation of collagen synthesis in rat cardiac fibroblasts by exposure to hypoxic culture conditions and suppression of the effect of natriuretic peptides. Cell Biol Int 1997;21:175-180.

56. Orita H, Fukasawa M, Hirooka S et al. Modulation of cardiac myocyte beating rate and hypertrophy by cardiac fibroblasts isolated from neonatal rat ventricle. Jap Circ J - English Ed 1993; 57:912-920.

57. Kim NN, Villarreal FJ, Printz MP, Lee AA, Dillmann WH. Trophic effects of angiotensin II on neonatal rat cardiac myocytes are mediated by cardiac fibroblasts. Am J Physiol 1995; 269:E426-E437.

58. Lee AA, Dillmann WH, McCulloch AD, Villarreal FJ. Angiotensin II stimulates the autocrine production of transforming growth factor-beta 1 in adult rat cardiac fibroblasts. J Mol Cell Cardiol 1995; 27(10):2347-2357.

59. Gray MO, Long CS, Kalinyak JE, Li HT, Karliner JS. Angiotensin II stimulates cardiac myocyte hypertrophy via paracrine release of TGF-beta 1 and endothelin-1 from fibroblasts. Cardiovasc Res 1998; 40(2): 352-363.

60. Harada M, Itoh H, Nakagawa O, Ogawa Y, Miyamoto Y, Kuwahara K, Ogawa E, Igaki T, Yamashita J, Masuda I, Yoshimasa T, Tanaka I, Saito Y, Nakao K. Significance of venticular myocytes and nonmyocytes interaction during cardiocyte hypertrophy: evidence for endothelin-1 as a paracrine hypertrophic factor from cardiac nonmyocytes. Circulation 1997; 96:3737-3744.

61. Bhat GJ, Baker KM. Cross-talk between angiotensin II and interleukin-6-induced signaling through Stat3 transcription factor. Basic Res Cardiol 1998; 93 Suppl 3:26-29.

62. Guo W, Kamiya K, Kada K, Kodama I, Toyama J. Regulations of cardiac Kv1.5K+ channel expression by cardiac fibroblasts and mechanical load in cultured newborn rat ventricular myocytes. J Mol Cell Cardiol 1998; 30(1): 157-166.

63. Orita H, Fukasawa M, Hirooka S, Fukui K, Kohi M, Washio M., Sasaki H. Protection of cardiac myocytes from hypothermic injury by cardiac fibroblasts isolated from neonatal rat ventricle. J Surg Res 1993; 55:654-658.

64. Nehls V, Herrmann R, Huhnken M, Palmetshofer A. Contact-dependent inhibition of angiogenesis by cardiac fibroblasts in three-dimentional fibrin gels in vitro: implications for microvascular network remodeling and coronary collateral formation. Cell Tissue Res 1998: 293:479-488.

65. Simm A, Nestler M, Hoppe V. PDGF-AA, a potent mitogen for cardiac fibroblasts from adult rats. J Mol Cell Cardiol 1997; 29: 357-368.

66. Eghbali M, Tomek R, Woods C, Bhambi B. Cardiac fibroblasts are predisposed to convert into myocyte phenotype: Specific effects of transforming growth factor-beta. Proc Natl Acad Sci 1991; 88:795-799.

67. Sigel A, Eghbali M. Autocrine transforming growth factor beta regulates DNA synthesis in cardiac fibroblasts. The FASEB J 1994; 8:A50 (Abs).

68. Fisher SA, Absher M. Norepinephrine and ANG II stimulate secretion of TGF-beta by neonatal rat cardiac fibroblasts in vitro. Am J Physiol 1995; 168(4 Pt 1): C910-917.

69. Calderone A, Thaik CM, Takahashi N, Chang DLF, Colucci WS. Nitric oxide, atrial natriuretic peptide, and cyclic GMP inhibit the growth-promoting effects of norepinephrine in cardiac myocytes and fibroblasts. J Clin Invest 1998; 101: 812-818.

70. Zheng JS, O'Neill L, Long X, Webb TE, Barnard EA, Lakatta EG, Boluyt MO. Stimulation of P2Y receptors activates c-fos gene expression and inhibits DNA synthesis in cultured cardiac fibroblasts. Cardiovasc Res 1998; 37: 718-728.

71. Stewart AF, Rokosh DG, Bailey BA, Karns LR, Chang KC, Long CS, Kariya K, Simpson PC. Cloning of the rat alpha 1C-adrenergic receptor from cardiac myocytes. alpha1C, alpha1B, and alpha1D mRNAs are present in cardiac myocytes but not in cardiac fibroblasts. Circ Res 1994; 75:796-802.

72. Schorb W, Booz GW, Dostal DE, conrad KM, Chang KC, Baker KM. Angiotensin II is mitogenic in neonatal rat cardiac fibroblasts. Circ Res 1993; 72:1245-1254.

73. Toshikazu Takizaw1; Miaofen Gu; Aram V. Chobanian; Peter Brecher. Effect of Nitric Oxide on DNA Replication Induced by Angiotensin II in Rat Cardiac Fibroblasts. Hypertension 1997; 30: 1035-1040.

74. Bhat GJ, Thekumkara TJ, Thomas WG, Conrad KM, Baker KM. Angiotensin II stimulates sis-inducing factor-like DNA binding activity: Evidence that the AT1A receptor activates transcription factor p91/or a related protein. J Biol Chem 1994; 269:31443-31449.

75. Zou Y, Komuro I, Yamazaki T, Kudoh S, Aikawa R, Zhu W, Shiojima I, Hiroi Y, Tobe K, Kadowaki T, Yazaki Y. Cell type-specific angiotensin II-evoked signal transduction pathways: critical roles of G betagamma subunit, Src family, and Ras in cardiac fibroblasts. Circ Res 1998; 82:337-345.

76. Grohe C, Kahlert S, Lobbert K, Neyses L, van Eickels M, Stimpel M, Vetter H. Angiotensin converting enzyme inhibition modulates cardiac fibroblast growth. J Hypertens 1998; 16(3):377-384.

77. Lee H-W, Eghbali-Webb M. Estrogen enhances proliferation of cardiac fibroblasts via mitogen-activated protein kinase- and estrogen receptor-dependent pathways. J Mol Cell Cardiol. 30:1359-1368, 1998.

78. Dubey RK, Gillespie DG, Jackson EK, Keller PJ. 17Beta-estradiol, its metabolites, and progesterone inhibit cardiac fibroblast growth. Hypertension 1998; 31(1 Pt 2): 522-528.
79. Grohe C, Kahlert S, Lobbert K, van Eickels M, Stimpel M, Vetter H, Neyses L. Effects of moexiprilat on oestrogen-stimulated cardiac fibroblast growth. Br J Pharm 1997; 121:1350-1354.
80. Palmer JN, Hartogensis WE, Patten M, Fortuin FD, Long CS. Interleukin-1 beta induces cardiac myocyte growth but inhibits cardiac fibroblast proliferation in culture. J Clin Invest 1995; 95: 2555-2564.
81. Farid Koudssi, Javier E. Lopez, Sonia Villegas, and Carlin S. Long. Cardiac Fibroblasts Arrest at the G1/S Restriction Point in Response to Interleukin (IL)-1beta. J Biol Chem 1998; 273: 25796-25803.
82. Cao L, Gardner DG. Natriuretic peptides inhibit DNA synthesis in cardiac fibroblasts. Hypertension 1995; 25: 227-234.
83. Fujisaki H, Ito H, Hirata Y, Tanaka M, Hata M, Lin M, Adachi S, Marumo F, Hiroe M. Natriuretic peptides inhibit angiotensin II-induced proliferation of rat cardiac fibroblasts by blocking endothelin-1 gene expression.
84. Dubey RK, Gillespie DG, Mi Z, Jackson EK. Exogenous and endogenous adenosine inhibits fetal calf serum-induced growth of rat cardiac fibroblasts: role of A2B receptors. Circulation 1997; 96: 2656-2666.
85. Smith MA, Eghbali-Webb M. Effect of selective adenosine receptor agonists on bFGF and angiotensin II-stimulated DNA synthesis in adult rat cardiac fibroblasts. FASEB J 1998; 12: A948.
86. Long X, Boluyt MO, Hipolito ML, Lundberg MS, Zheng JS, O'Neill L, Cirielli C, Lakatta EG, Crow MT. p53 and the hypoxia-induced apoptosis of cultured neonatal rat cardiac myocytes. J Clin Invest 1997; 99: 2635-2643.
87. Long X, Crow MT, Sollott SJ, O'Neill L, Menees DS, de Lourdes Hipolito M, Boluyt MO, Asai T, Lakatta EG. Enhanced expression of p53 and apoptosis induced by blockade of the vacuolar proton ATPase in cardiomyocytes. J Clin Invest 1998;101: 1453-1461.
88. Choy M, Oltjen S, Ratcliff D, Armstrong P. Fibroblast behavior in the embryonic chick heart. Develop Dynam 1993: 198:97-107.
89. Klett CP, Palmer AA, Dirig DM, Gallagher AM, Riosecco-Camacho N, Printz MP. Evidence for differences in cultured left ventricular fibroblast populations isolated from sponatneously hypertensive and Wistar-Kyoto rats. J Hypertens 1995;13:1421-1431.
90. Reiss K, Cheng W, Kajstura J, Sonnenblick EH, Meggs LG, Anversa P. Fibroblast proliferation during myocardial development in rats is regulated by IGF-1 receptors.Am J Physiol 1995; 269: H943-951.

II.2.2
Cardiac myocytes

Armin Haunstetter, M.D., Markus Haass, M.D., and Seigo Izumo, M.D.
Universität Heidelberg, Heidelberg, Germany
Harvard Medical School, Boston, MA, USA

INTRODUCTION

In recent years myocyte loss due to apoptosis has gained increasing attention in the field of cardiovascular research, as myocyte apoptosis was observed in several disease states suggesting a potential pathophysiological role. Whereas initial studies were mostly observational verifying the occurrence of apoptotic myocytes in the heart, increasingly efforts are being made to disentagle the intracellular mechanisms that induce or inhibit myocyte apoptosis. As other chapters of this book deal with the more general aspects of apoptosis, the scope of this article will be limited to summarize current knowledge of the role of apoptosis in myocardial disease and the regulatory mechanisms known to be involved in myocyte apoptosis.

MYOCYTE APOPTOSIS IN CARDIOVASCULAR DISEASE

Apoptosis of cardiac myocytes has been reported in many diseases of the myocardium with varying degrees of incidence. Most evidence has been provided for ischemic heart disease where apoptosis might be induced by three independent mechanims: (a) by a direct effect of either transient or persistent ischemia, (b) by reperfusion injury, and (c) during remodeling of the non-infarcted myocardium (1). In a series of pathological studies of human hearts, apoptotic myocytes were detected after myocardial infarction with predominant location in the border zone between the central infarct region and the non-compromised myocardium (2-5). However, other oberservations in rodent animal models suggested that apoptosis occurs at a subendocardial location and might even contribute significantly to cell death within the central infarct core (6,7). From a pathophysiological standpoint, a location within the central infarct core seems less plausible, as rapid and irreversible loss of energy-rich phosphates (creatine phosphate, ATP) is expected to result in cell swelling and early necrotic cell death before the apoptotic death program can be executed. In contrast, cells in the border zone between normal and infarcted myocardium or in the subendocardium might receive additional nutritional support from collaterals or by diffusion and thus may maintain a basic metabolic activity to undergo apoptosis. Actually, there is some evidence that apoptosis might depend on adequate levels of ATP (8,9).

Although one paper suggested a predominant role for reperfusion in myocyte apoptosis, most experimental protocols do not allow to distinguish between the relative importance of transient ischemia versus reperfusion (7,10-12). Pathophysiology of the two conditions might be different, as reperfusion injury may predominantly involve oxidative damage and calcium overload, whereas metabolic derangement might be the main inducer of apoptosis during the ischemic period. In most of the studies, an ischemic time of 30-45 min is followed by 2-24 hours of reperfusion to induce apoptosis in the experimental setting. Interestingly, preconditioning by short (5 min) repetitive ischemic periods reduced myocyte apoptosis induced by a longer period of ischemia (15 min) and reperfusion (120 min) (13). In addition, myocyte apoptosis was also detected after chronic hypoperfusion (myocardial hibernation) (14).

Of major importance is whether apoptosis during myocardial ischemia constitutes more or less an epiphenomenon or whether it substantially contributes to myocyte loss and secondary heart failure after myocardial ischemia. In a rat model of coronary ligation (30 min) and reperfusion (24 hours), infarct size was reduced significantly and both systolic and diastolic function were improved by treatment with a caspase inhibitor (15). However, the long-term benefit of reduced apoptosis due to caspase inhibition is not yet known.

Heart failure constitutes another major myocardial disease entity with strong evidence for apoptotic myocyte loss. The occurrence of myocyte apoptosis seems to be independent from the etiology of the heart failure, as both ischemic and dilated cardiomyopathy have been shown to be associated with myocyte loss in patients (16,17). In addition, in arrhythmogenic right ventricular dysplasia foci of apoptotic myocytes were detected in the right ventricular wall (18). The mechanisms leading to myocyte apoptosis in the failing heart are not well characterized. Based on observations in animal models and isolated ventricular myocytes, several potential inducers (stretch of myocytes, pressure overload, norepinephrine, atrial natriuretic peptide, angiotensin II) have been suggested (19-23), although firm evidence for a major pathogenetic role of these factors in myocyte apoptosis during clinical heart failure is lacking. In addition, apoptosis due to remodeling of the normal myocardium after myocardial infarction or due to pressure overload are gaining increasing attention as potentially important mechanisms in the transition from compensated cardiac disease to heart failure (1,20).

Quantitative analysis of apoptotic myocytes in heart failure varies over a wide range from 0.2 % to 35.5 % (16,17). It is obvious that some of the quantitative data only apply to small focal areas of increased apoptosis, as a uniform apoptosis rate of that magnitude would eliminate all cardiac myocytes within a short period. Therefore, the true amount of apoptotic myocytes in heart failure is still controversial. However, it has to be kept in mind that even a low apoptotic index could contribute substantially to disease progression, although currently no long-term data are available to confirm the pathophysiologic significance of apoptosis in heart failure.

MORPHOLOGY OF MYOCYTE APOPTOSIS

Current classification of cell death is quite strictly categorized into two separate entities, namely necrosis and apoptosis. Some authors advocate the term "oncosis" instead of "necrosis", as the latter is considered to denote tissue alterations after massive cell loss (24). In contrast to apoptosis, oncosis is characterized by the loss of energy-rich phosphates (creatine phosphate and ATP) and dysregulation of the transmembrane transport of solutes with secondary cell and organelle swelling. The rupture of intracellular and extracellular membranes finally leads to the demise of the myocyte.

Defining criteria for cell apoptosis include both morphological and biochemical markers that reflect a distinct pathophysiological mechanism of cell death. Morphologically, cells appear to be shrunken with intact membranes (24). At an advanced stage, several membrane blebs become visible that finally detach to form individual apoptotic bodies. The nucleus diminishes in size and the chromatin condenses to high density clumps with primarily marginal localization as evidenced by electron microscopy. At the biochemical level, the central feature of apoptosis is the activation of caspases, a distinct class of aspartate-specific cysteine proteases, and the appearance of fragments of cellular target proteins for caspases (e.g. PARP, lamin, fodrin). Secondary consequences of caspase activation are the exposure of phosphatidylserine on the outer leaflet of the plasma membrane and the internucleosomal cleavage of the genomic DNA. The latter feature is the basis for the two most widespread tests, TUNEL staining and the demonstration of DNA laddering on agarose gels, used to provide evidence for apoptotic loss of cardiomyocytes in several myocardial diseases.

Many of these features have been observed in isolated cardiac myocytes (25,26). However, most studies of apoptosis done in animals or in human myocardial specimens are limited to TUNEL staining and the demonstration of genomic DNA fragmentation on agarose gel electrophoresis. Therefore, knowledge of morphological alterations specific for myocyte apoptosis in tissues is more limited. In a study using electron microscopy evidence for myocyte shrinkage, cell fractionation and nuclear condensation in myocardial tissue was provided (14).

Interestingly, many of the myocytes shown in published myocardial tissue sections with positive TUNEL staining exhibit normal morphology of both the nucleus and the cytoplasm on light microscopy. It is not known whether this represents an early stage of myocyte apoptosis that will be followed by other cytosolic and nuclear morphologic alterations typical for apoptosis or whether under certain conditions, myocytes do not exhibit all typical alterations of apoptosis. A more recent study in reperfused rabbit hearts lends additional support to the notion that the dichotomy between apoptotic (TUNEL-positive myocytes) and necrotic (swollen and ruptured myocytes) may be oversimplified (27). By modification of the TUNEL technique to detect DNA fragmentation with electron microscopy, the authors showed that myocytes with DNA fragmentation actually had ultrastructural features suggestive of necrosis (cell swelling, dense bodies in mitochondria and cell rupture) and not for apoptosis. Interestingly, the time course of positive TUNEL staining both in light microscopy and electron microscopy went in parallel with the appearance of DNA laddering on agarose gel electrophoresis, indicating internucleosomal DNA cleavage. Therefore, positive TUNEL staining and even DNA laddering might not necessarily be associated with typical morphological alterations of apoptosis in cardiac myocytes. It is not known whether under these circumstances activation of caspases or anti-apoptotic regulatory mechanisms (e.g. Bcl-2) play any functional role.

MOLECULAR MECHANISMS INVOLVED IN MYOCYTE APOPTOSIS

Studies in isolated neonatal and adult ventricular myocytes as well as in some *in vivo* animal models have helped to delineate several potential signaling and regulatory pathways that may exert either a pro-apoptotic or an anti-apoptotic effect. Experimental models and stimuli that were used to induce and study myocyte apoptosis are summarized in Table 1. The role of mitogen-activated protein kinases, growth factors, cell cycle regulation, the p53 oncogene, nitric oxide, the death receptors and mitochondria will be discussed in more detail below.

Role of mitogen- and stress-activated protein kinases

Mitogen-activated and stress-activated protein kinases are part of parallel multi-step signaling cascades that propagate signals from cell membrane receptors or cellular stress signals (Fig. 1). This class of intracellular kinases includes the extracellular signal regulated kinases 1 and 2 (ERK 1/2), c-Jun amino-terminal kinase (JNK), and the α and β isoforms of p38. Downstream substrates in the signaling cascade are mostly transcription factors that regulate the cellular response by modifying gene transcription (e.g c-Jun, ATF).

Although experimental evidence in cardiac myocytes is limited, activation of ERK appears to exert an anti-apoptotic effect. Stimulation of isolated cardiac myocytes with cardiotrophin-1 can activate the JAK/STAT and ERK signaling pathways. However, only pharmacologic inhibition of the ERK kinase cascade blocked the anti-apoptotic activity of cardiotrophin-1 in serum-deprived neonatal cardiac myocytes (38). Similarly, both baseline apoptosis and apoptosis induced by hydrogen peroxide were augmented by inhibition of MEK, the upstream regulator of ERK (34). As for p38, overexpression of a constitutively active form of MKK3, the upstream activator of p38α, increased cell loss (40,41). Furthermore, myocyte survival was improved by overexpressing a dominant-negative mutant of the downstream kinase p38α, indicating a pro-apoptotic effect of the MKK3/p38α pathway. On the other hand, the signaling pathway involving MKK6 and p38β appears to protect against chemically-induced apoptosis (40).

Table 1   Experimental model systems used to study apoptosis in cardiac myocytes. The list comprises studies in isolated cultured myocytes (NRVM, neonatal rat ventricular myocytes; ARVM, adult rat ventricular myocytes), isolated heart preparations and interventional studies in intact animals.

Apoptotic stimulus	Model	Ref.
Pathologic clinical conditions		
Infarction	rat heart	(6)
	mouse heart	(7,28)
Ischemia/reperfusion	rat heart	(11,15,29)
	rabbit heart	(10)
Hypoxia	NRVM	(30,31)
Preconditioning	rat heart	(13)
Myocyte stretch	ARVM	(19)
Ischemic cardiomyopathy	dog heart	(32)
Pressure overload	rat heart	(20)
Transplant rejection	rat heart	(33)
Paracrine mediators or toxins		
Hydrogen peroxide	NRVM	(34)
Angiotensin II	ARVM	(23)
Sphingosine	NRVM	(26)
Staurosporine	NRVM	(25)
Daunorubicin	NRVM	(35)
Tumor necrosis factor α	NRVM	(26)
Atrial natriuretic peptide	NRVM	(22)
Norepinephrine	ARVM	(21)
Cytokines (IL1, TNF-α, IFN-γ)	NRVM	(36)
Endotoxin	ARVM	(37)
Serum withdrawal	NRVM	(38)
Intracellular signaling mechanisms		
Gsα overexpression	mouse heart	(39)
MEKK1 overexpression	NRVM	(40)
MKK3 overexpression	NRVM	(41)
p53 overexpression	NRVM	(42)
E1A overexpression	NRVM	(43)
E2F-1 overexpression	NRVM	(44)
E2F-1 overexpression	mouse heart	(45)

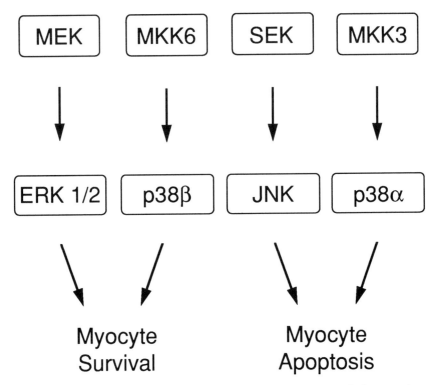

Figure 1 Schematic diagram summarizing current evidence for the involvement of mitogen- and stress-activated protein kinase cascades in the regulation of myocyte apoptosis. Signaling through MEK (MAPK/ERK kinase) and MKK6 (mitogen-activated protein kinase kinase 6) was shown to mediate anti-apoptotic protection in isolated cardiac myocytes. In contrast, activation of SEK (SAPK/ERK kinase), JNK (c-Jun N-terminal kinase), MKK3 (mitogen-activated protein kinase kinase 3) and the α isoform of p38 has been implicated in pro-apoptotic signaling in myocytes.

Interestingly, apoptosis and caspase activation were diminished by a non-specific p38 kinase inhibitor in an ischemia model in neonatal myocytes (46). Similar to overexpression of MKK3, constitutively active SEK/MEKK1 (the upstream activator of JNK) induced apoptosis in isolated myocytes (40). Although one study showed a correlation between JNK activation and apoptosis induced by ischemia/reperfusion in the rabbit heart (47), further studies are required to elucidate the role of these signaling cascades in myocyte apoptosis in clinically relevant myocardial disorders.

Growth factors

Culture of most tumor cell lines requires the presence of growth factors that promote cell proliferation and at the same time prevent apoptotic cell death. That these two functions can be separated was shown in cells overexpressing the anti-apoptotic regulator Bcl-2, where the lack of growth factor inhibited cell proliferation, yet cell viability was maintained (48). It seemed therefore attractive that growth factor treatment might protect post-mitotic cardiac myocytes from apoptosis induced by other stimuli. In isolated neonatal cardiac myocytes that were kept under serum-free conditions, apoptosis was induced as indicated by TUNEL staining and agarose gel electrophoresis of genomic DNA (38). Apoptosis was inhibited by the growth factors cardiotrophin-1, leukemia inhibitory factor and insulin-like growth factor I (IGF-1). The receptors for cardiotrophin-1 and leukemia inhibitory factor contain a common gp130 subunit, suggesting a similar anti-apoptotic mechanism for these two growth factors. Insulin-like growth factor I was also shown to reduce apoptosis and caspase-3 activation after combined serum withdrawal and doxorubicin treatment, although the protective effect was only partial (49). In IGF-1-transgenic mice and in rats pretreated with IGF-1, the number of apoptotic cells in the ischemic area after coronary ligation was significantly reduced compared to control animals (28,29). In contrast, the extent of myocyte loss due to cell necrosis was not affected (28). Intracellular signaling by IGF-1 involves activation of phosphatidylinositol 3-kinase and the downstream kinase Akt. In non-myocytes, this intracellular signaling pathway has been implicated in mediating the anti-apoptotic effect of growth factors by phosphorylating and thus inactivating the pro-apoptotic regulator Bad. However, it is not known whether this pathway mediates the anti-apoptotic effect of growth factors in cardiac myocytes, and further studies are required to determine the role of this pathway.

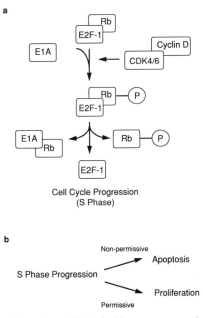

Figure 2 Role of the cell cycle regulators Rb (retinoblastoma gene product) and E2F-1 in cell cycle progression. (a) Overexpression of E2F-1 or inactivation of Rb by phosphorylation or interaction with the adenoviral E1A protein will force myocytes into the S phase of the cell cycle. (b) Depending on the cell type (e.g. terminally differentiated cell lineage) or environment (e.g. contact inhibition in cultured cells) forced cell cycle progression will induce apoptotic cell death.

Cell cycle

Adult cardiac myocytes are post-mitotic cells that are arrested in the G0/G1 phase of the cell cycle. Initial observations in other cell types indicated that cells undergo apoptosis when they are forced into cell cycle progression under conditions where they are normally quiescent. Progression into the S phase (DNA synthesis) of the cell cycle is tightly controlled by phosphorylation events. The cyclin-dependent kinases 4 and 6, activated by the association with D cyclins, phosphorylate the retinoblastoma protein, thus inducing its proteasome-mediated degradation. As the retinoblastoma protein inactivates the positive cell cycle regulator E2F-1, its degradation promotes progression into the S phase of the cell cycle (Fig. 2). Likewise, the adenoviral E1A protein interacts with the retinoblastoma protein also promoting the release of E2F-1. Overexpression of E1A or E2F-1 itself induces DNA synthesis in isolated neonatal cardiac myocytes (43,44). Cell cycle progression is associated with extensive myocyte apoptosis. Adenoviral gene transfer of E2F-1 into adult myocardium exerts a similar effect (45). However, at this point, the mechanisms that link forced cell cycle progression to the apoptotic death program are not well understood.

p53 and myocyte apoptosis

The p53 protein plays a central role in the regulation of DNA repair and as a transcription factor it controls the expression of the apoptosis-associated genes Bax and Fas. In some cellular models that involve DNA damage such as radiation-induced apoptosis in thymocytes, apoptosis depends on functional p53 (50). In a recently proposed model, p53 strongly induces the genes for pro-oxidant factors that cause mitochondrial damage with subsequent initiation of the caspase cascade (51). Infection of neonatal rat ventricular myocytes with an adenoviral construct containing p53 induces apoptosis, suggesting that all other components necessary for p53-mediated apoptosis are functional in myocytes (31,42). However, although hypoxia-induced p53 upregulation precedes myocyte apoptosis, the apoptotic rate in p53-deficient mouse hearts was not reduced compared to wild-type mice after ligation of the left coronary artery (7,31). Likewise, apoptosis induced by forced progression into the S phase of the cell cycle was not attenuated in the myocardium of p53 knockout mice (45). So far, stringent evidence is lacking to show that apoptosis in myocardial disease states depends on p53. However, it cannot be excluded that the p53-related genes p51 or p73 can functionally substitute for p53 in p53-deficient cells (52).

NO and reactive oxygen species

Nitric oxide functions as a paracrine mediator that is produced by the three NO synthases, inducible NO synthase (iNOS), endothelial cell NO synthase (eNOS) and the neuronal NO synthase (nNOS) (53). Although in some cell types NO appears to exert an anti-apoptotic function, there is increasing evidence that NO may actually have a cytotoxic effect on myocytes. Initial observations in isolated adult rat ventricular myocytes indicated that combined treatment with the cytokines γ-interferon, interleukin-1β and tumor necrosis factor α causes expression of iNOS and increased NO production (54). Myocyte death could be blocked by the NOS inhibitor L-NMMA, although it was not clear whether myocyte death was due to apoptosis. Using the same combination of cytokines in neonatal cardiomyocytes, evidence for myocyte apoptosis such as internucleosomal DNA cleavage, apoptotic nuclear changes and cleavage of caspase substrates was provided in another study (36). *In vivo* gene transfer by injecting a vector containing the endothelial type of NOS into the ventricular wall of the rat heart induced cell shrinkage and the regional appearance of TUNEL-positive cells (55). However, local eNOS expression was associated with a mononuclear cell infiltrate and it is not known whether apoptosis of myocytes was due to a direct cytotoxic effect of increased NO production or whether it was mediated by infiltrating mononuclear cells. In addition, the relative contribution of myocytes and non-myocytes to the total number of apoptotic cells was not clear, as no cell type-specific analysis was performed.

In animal models of rat and mouse cardiac transplantation, rejection was associated with apoptosis of infiltrating immune cells, myocytes and endothelial cells (33,56). When hearts were transplanted into iNOS-deficient mice, the total degree of apoptosis was reduced with similar reductions in all cell types (56). A correlation between reduced apoptosis and a decrease of caspase-1, caspase-3 and p53 expression and an increase in the Bcl-2/Bax ratio was provided. Other suggested mechanisms of NO-induced myocytes apoptosis include a cGMP-mediated effect and direct oxidative damage due to peroxynitrite formed by the interaction of the two radicals NO and superoxide (22,36). Treatment of myocytes with the atrial natriuretic peptide, which activates guanylate cyclase caused myocyte apoptosis in neonatal rat ventricular myocytes (22). Likewise, a membrane-permeable homolog of cGMP also induced myocyte apoptosis (22). On the other hand, myocytes are also known to undergo apoptosis in response to the pro-oxidant hydrogen peroxide, indicating that both mechanisms might be involved in NO-induced apoptosis (34).

Death receptor pathways

Death receptors constitute a subgroup of the major class of tumor necrosis factor receptors that are characterized by a distinct subcellular domain, the death domain. Stimulation of death receptors with their cognate ligands induces the interaction with the intracellular adaptor proteins TRADD, FADD or RAIDD and the subsequent activation of the upstream caspase FLICE (caspase-8). Death receptors include the receptors for Fas ligand (Fas), tumor necrosis factor (TNFR1) and TRAIL (death receptors 4 and 5). Cardiac myocytes are known to express Fas and TNFR1 and possibly also the death receptors 4 and 5 (57-59). Interestingly, death receptor expression in the heart can be modulated under certain pathophysiologic conditions. For example, TNFR1 expression is reduced at the protein level in failing human hearts due to either dilated cardiomyopathy or ischemic heart disease (60). In contrast, Fas expression is elevated from a low basal level during permanent ischemia or ischemia/reperfusion and after stretching of myocytes (6,19), indicating a potential role of Fas-mediatcd myocyte loss in ischemic heart disease and cardiac dilation. However, in a porcine model of myocardial hibernation, Fas expression was not altered (61).

As for the functional consequences of death receptor expression in the heart, available data are more limited. Tumor necrosis factor α has a negative inotropic effect on isolated cardiac myocytes and when overexpressed in the myocardium (62). Similarly, Fas stimulation in isolated mouse ventricular myocytes diminished resting membrane potential and the duration of the action potential, and it increased diastolic intracellular calcium concentrations (63). Apart from its functional effect, tumor necrosis factor α was shown to induce myocyte apoptosis in isolated neonatal and adult rat ventricular myocyes (26). At this point, it is not clear to which degree death receptor-mediated myocyte apoptosis contributes to myocyte loss in cardiac disease. Death receptor expression itself might not be sufficient to induce myocyte apoptosis, as intracellular anti-apoptotic mechanisms might protect myocytes against apoptotic cell death. Inhibitory proteins of Fas-induced apoptosis such as FLAME-1 and ARC show a high level of expression in the heart (64,65). In fact, ARC is predominantly expressed in heart and skeletal muscle suggesting an important role in myocytes.

Evidence for a special role of the death receptor pathway in cardiac development comes from knockout studies in mice. Deficiency of the intracellular adaptor protein FADD that links activation of Fas, TNFR1 and death receptor 3 to caspase-8 activation causes embryonic death with thinning of the myocardium and poorly developed trabeculation (66). An almost identical cardiac phenotype was observed in caspase-8 knockout mice indicating an important role of this intracellular pathway during cardiac development (67). However, as neither Fas deficiency, nor deficiency of TNFR1 induces a similar cardiac dysmorphology, it is presently not known which receptor acts as a central upstream regulator in the developing heart.

Mitochondria and myocyte apoptosis

Recent observations provide firm evidence that mitochondria play an important role in the induction of apoptosis (68). Essential for a mitochondrial induction of apoptosis is the translocation of pro-apoptotic proteins from the intermembranous space between the inner and outer mitochondrial membranes into the cytosol. Most evidence has been provided for the release of cytochrome c which in conjunction with Apaf-1 activates caspase-9 in the cytosol, and the apoptosis-inducing factor (AIF) that can induce nuclear changes typical for apoptosis independently from caspase activation (69,70). Furthermore, mitochondria are the site of action for both the pro- and anti-apoptotic members of the Bcl-2 family of apoptosis regulatory proteins.

Mitochondria are abundant in adult cardiac myocytes where they are densely packed between myofibrils to provide ATP for sarcomere contraction and relaxation. In addition, myocardial ischemia is associated with marked morphological alterations of mitochondria such as swelling, formation of amorphous matrix densities, and fragmentation of cristae (71). However, at this point there is only indirect evidence for an involvement of mitochondria in myocyte apoptosis. For example, for some stimuli of apoptosis that are known to induce apoptosis in cardiomyocytes, such as staurosporine, reactive oxygen species or overexpression of p53, mitochondria were suggested as essential mediators (25,34,42,51). In addition, the regulatory protein Bcl-2, which is predominantly localized to mitochondria, was shown to inhibit apoptosis in isolated neonatal rat ventricular myocytes (42). Definitely, further research is needed to characterize the role of the mitochondrial pro-apoptotic regulators Bax and Bak, release of cytochrome c or AIF, and the activation of caspase-9 in cardiac myocytes.

ACKNOWLEDGEMENT

Armin Haunstetter was supported by a grant of the Deutsche Forschungs-gemeinschaft (Ha 2606/1-1). Seigo Izumo was supported by a grant from NIH (USA).

References

1. Olivetti G, Quaini F, Sala R, Lagrasta C, Corradi D, Bonacina E, Gambert SR, Cigola E Anversa P. Acute myocardial infarction in humans is associated with activation of programmed myocyte cell death in the surviving portion of the heart. *J Mol Cell Cardiol* 1996;28:2005-16.
2. Itoh G, Tamura J, Suzuki M, Suzuki Y, Ikeda H, Koike M, Nomura M, Jie T, Ito K. DNA fragmentation of human infarcted myocardial cells demonstrated by the nick end labeling method and DNA agarose gel electrophoresis. *Am J Pathol* 1995;146:1325-31.
3. Bardales RH, Hailey LS, Xie SS, Schaefer RF, Hsu SM. In situ apoptosis assay for the detection of early acute myocardial infarction. *Am J Pathol* 1996;149:821-9.
4. Saraste A, Pulkki K, Kallajoki M, Henriksen K, Parvinen M, Voipio-Pulkki LM. Apoptosis in human acute myocardial infarction. *Circulation* 1997;95:320-3.
5. Veinot JP, Gattinger DA, and Fliss H. Early apoptosis in human myocardial infarcts. *Hum Pathol* 1997;28:485-92.
6. Kajstura J, Cheng W, Reiss K, Clark WA, Sonnenblick EH, Krajewski S, Reed JC, Olivetti G, Anversa P. Apoptotic and necrotic myocyte cell deaths are independent contributing variables of infarct size in rats. *Lab Invest* 1996;74:86-107.
7. Bialik S, Geenen DL, Sasson IE, Cheng R, Horner JW, Evans SM, Lord EM, Koch CJ, Kitsis RN. Myocyte apoptosis during acute myocardial infarction in the mouse localizes to hypoxic regions but occurs independently of p53. *J Clin Invest* 1997;100:1363-72.
8. Li P, Nijhawan D,Budihardjo I, Srinivasula SM, Ahmad M, Alnemri ES, Wang X. Cytochrome c and ATP-dependent formation of Apaf-1/Caspase-9 complex initiates an apoptotic protease cascade. *Cell* 1997;91:479-89.
9. Leist M, Single B, Castoldi AF, Kuhnle S, Nicotera P. Intracellular adenosine triphosphate (ATP) concentration: a switch in the decision between apoptosis and necrosis. *J Exp Med* 1997;185:1481-6.
10. Gottlieb RA, Burleson KO, Kloner RA, Babior BM, Engler RL. Reperfusion injury induces apoptosis in rabbit cardiomyocytes. *J Clin Invest* 1994;94:1621-8.
11. Fliss H, Gattinger D. Apoptosis in ischemic and reperfused rat myocardium. *Circ Res* 1996;79:949-56.
12. Black SC, Huang JQ, Rezaiefar P, Radinovic S, Eberhart A, Nicholson DW, Rodger IW. Co-localization of the cysteine protease caspase-3 with apoptotic myocytes after in vivo myocardial ischemia and reperfusion in the rat. *J Mol Cell Cardiol* 1998;30:733-42.
13. Maulik N, Yoshida T, Engelman RM, Deaton D, Flack III JE, Rousou JA, Das DK. Ischemic preconditioning attenuates apoptotic cell death associated with ischemia/reperfusion. *Mol Cell Biochem* 1998;186:139-45.

APOPTOSIS IN CARDIAC BIOLOGY

14. Elsasser A, Schlepper M, Klovekorn WP, Cai WJ, Zimmermann R, Muller KD, Strasser R, Kostin S, Gagel C, Munkel B, Schaper W, Schaper J. Hibernating myocardium: an incomplete adaptation to ischemia. *Circulation* 1997;96:2920-31.
15. Yaoita H, Ogawa K, Maehara K, Maruyama Y. Attenuation of ischemia/reperfusion injury in rats by a caspase inhibitor.*Circulation* 1998;97:276-81.
16. Olivetti G, Kajstura J, Cheng W, Nitahara JA, Quaini E, Di Loreto C, Beltrami CA, Krajewski S, Reed JC, Anversa P. Apoptosis in the failing human heart. *N Engl J Med* 1997;336:1131-41.
17. Narula J, Haider N, Virmani R, DiSalvo TG, Kolodgie FD, Hajjar RJ, Schmidt U, Semigran MJ, Dec GW, Khaw BA. Apoptosis in myocytes in end-stage heart failure. *N Engl J Med* 1996;335:1182-9.
18. Mallat Z, Tedgui A, Fontaliran F, Frank R, Durigon M, Fontaine G. Evidence of apoptosis in arrhythmogenic right ventricular dysplasia . *N Engl J Med* 1996;335:1190-6.
19. Cheng W, Li B, Kajstura J, Li P, Wolin MS, Sonnenblick EH, Hintze TH, Olivetti G, Anversa P. Stretch-induced programmed myocyte cell death. *J Clin Invest* 1995;96:2247-59.
20. Teiger E, Than VD, Richard L, Wisnewsky C, Tea BS, Gaboury L, Tremblay J,Schwartz K, Hamet P. Apoptosis in pressure overload-induced heart hypertrophy in the rat. *J Clin Invest* 1996;97:2891-7.
21. Communal C, Singh K, Pimentel DR, Colucci WS. Norepinephrine stimulates apoptosis in adult rat ventricular myocytes by activation of the b-adrenergic pathway. *Circulation* 1998;98:1329-1334.
22. Wu CF, Bishopric NH, and Pratt RE. Atrial natriuretic peptide induces apoptosis in neonatal rat cardiac myocytes. *J Biol Chem* 1997;272:14860-6.
23. Kajstura J, Cigola E, Malhotra A, Li P, Cheng W, Meggs LG, Anversa P. Angiotensin II induces apoptosis of adult ventricular myocytes in vitro. *J Mol Cell Cardiol* 1997;29:859-70.
24. Majno G, Joris I. Apoptosis, oncosis, and necrosis. An overview of cell death. *Am J Pathol* 1995;146:3-15.
25. Yue TL, Wang C, Romanic AM, Kikly K, Keller P, DeWolf WE, Hart TK, Thomas HC, Storer B, Gu JL, Wang X, Feuerstein GZ. Staurosporine-induced apoptosis in cardiomyocytes: A potential role of caspase-3. *J Mol Cell Cardiol* 1998;30:495-507.
26. Krown KA, Page MT, Nguyen C, Zechner D, Gutierrez V, Comstock KL, Glembotski CC, Quintana PJ, Sabbadini RA. Tumor necrosis factor alpha-induced apoptosis in cardiac myocytes. Involvement of the sphingolipid signaling cascade in cardiac cell death. *J Clin Invest* 1996;98:2854-65.
27. Ohno M, Takemura G, Ohno A, Misao J, Hayakawa Y, Minatoguchi S, Fujiwara T, Fujiwara H. "Apoptotic" myocytes in infarct area in rabbit hearts may be oncotic myocytes with DNA fragmentation. *Circulation* 1998;98:1422-30.
28. Li Q, Li B, Wang X, Leri A, Jana KP, Liu Y, Kajstura J, Baserga R, Anversa P. Overexpression of insulin-like growth factor-1 in mice protects from myocyte death after infarction, attenuating ventricular dilation, wall stress, and cardiac hypertrophy. *J Clin Invest* 1997;100:1991-9.
29. Buerke M, Murohara T, Skurk C, Nuss C, Tomaselli K, Lefer AM. Cardioprotective effect of insulin-like growth factor I in myocardial ischemia followed by reperfusion. *Proc Natl Acad Sci U S A* 1995;92:8031-5.
30. Tanaka M, Ito H, Adachi S, Akimoto H, Nishikawa T, Kasajima T, Marumo F, Hiroe M. Hypoxia induces apoptosis with enhanced expression of Fas antigen messenger RNA in cultured neonatal rat cardiomyocytes. *Circ Res* 1994;75:426-33.
31. Long X, Boluyt MO, Hipolito ML, Lundberg MS, Zheng JS, O'Neill L, Cirielli C, Lakatta EG, Crow MT. p53 and the hypoxia-induced apoptosis of cultured neonatal rat cardiac myocytes. *J Clin Invest* 1997;99:2635-43.
32. Sharov VG, Sabbah HN, Shimoyama H, Goussev AV, Lesch M, Goldstein S. Evidence of cardiocyte apoptosis in myocardium of dogs with chronic heart failure. *Am J Pathol* 1996;148:141-9.
33. Szabolcs M, Michler RE, Yang X, Aji W, Roy D, Athan E, Sciacca RR, Minanov OP, Cannon PJ. Apoptosis of cardiac myocytes during cardiac allograft rejection. Relation to induction of nitric oxide synthase. *Circulation* 1996;94:1665-73.
34. Aikawa R, Komuro I, Yamazaki T, Zou Y, Kudoh S, Tanaka M, Shiojima I, Hiroi Y, Yazaki Y. Oxidative stress activates extracellular signal-regulated kinases through src and ras in cultured cardiac myocytes of neonatal rats [In Process Citation]. *J Clin Invest* 1997;100:1813-21.

35. Sawyer DB, Fukazawa R, Arstall MA, Kelly RA. Daunorubicin-induced apoptosis in rat cardiac myocytes is inhibited by dexrazoxane. *Circ Res* 1999;84:257-65.
36. Ing DJ, Zang J, Dzau VJ, Webster KA, Bishopric NH. Modulation of cytokine-induced cardiac myocyte apoptosis by nitric oxide, Bak, Bcl-x. *Circ Res* 1998;84:21-33.
37. Comstock KL, Krown KA, Page MT, Martin D, Ho P, Pedraza M, Castro EN, Nakajima N, Glembotski CC, Quintana PJE, Sabbadini RA. LPS-induced TNF-a release from and apoptosis in rat cardiomyocytes: Obligatory role of CD14 in mediating the LPS response. *J Mol Cell Cardiol* 1998;30:2761-75.
38. Sheng Z, Knowlton K, Chen J, Hoshijima M, Brown JH, Chien KR. Cardiotrophin 1 (CT-1) inhibition of cardiac myocyte apoptosis via a mitogen-activated protein kinase-dependent pathway. Divergence from downstream CT-1 signals for myocardial cell hypertrophy. *J Biol Chem* 1997;272:5783-91.
39. Geng Y, Ishikawa Y, Vatner DE., Wagner TE, Bishop SP, Vatner SF, Homcy CJ. Apoptosis of cardiac myocytes in Gsa transgenic mice. *Circ Res* 1998;84:34-42.
40. Zechner D, Craig R, Hanford DS, McDonough PM, Sabbadini RA, Glembotski CC. MKK6 activates myocardial cell NF-kB and inhibits apoptosis in a p38 mitogen-activated protein kinase-dependent manner. *J Biol Chem* 1998;273:8232-9.
41. Wang Y, Huang S, Sah VP, Ross J, Brown JH, Han J, Chien KR. Cardiac muscle cell hypertrophy and apoptosis induced by distinct members of the p38 mitogen-activated protein kinase family. *J Biol Chem* 1998;273:2161-8.
42. Kirshenbaum LA, de Moissac D. The bcl-2 gene product prevents programmed cell death of ventricular myocytes. *Circulation* 1997;96:1580-5.
43. Kirshenbaum LA, Schneider MD. Adenovirus E1A represses cardiac gene transcription and reactivates DNA synthesis in ventricular myocytes, via alternative pocket protein- and p300-binding domains. *J Biol Chem* 1995;270:7791-4.
44. Kirshenbaum LA, Abdellatif M, Chakraborty S, Schneider MD. Human E2F-1 reactivates cell cycle progression in ventricular myocytes and represses cardiac gene transcription. *Dev Biol* 1996;179:402-11.
45. Agah R, Kirshenbaum LA, Abdellatif M, Truong LD, Chakraborty S, Michael LH, Schneider MD. Adenoviral delivery of E2F-1 directs cell cycle reentry and p53- independent apoptosis in postmitotic adult myocardium in vivo. *J Clin Invest* 1997;100:2722-8.
46. Mackay K, Mochly-Rosen D. An inhibitor of p38 mitogen-activated protein kinase protects neonatal cardiac myocytes from ischemia. *J Biol Chem* 1999;274:6272-9.
47. Yue TL, Ma XL, Wang X, Romanic AM, Liu GL, Louden C, Gu JL, Kumar S, Poste G, Ruffolo RR, Feuerstein GZ. Possible involvement of stress-activated protein kinase signaling pathway and Fas receptor expression in prevention of ischemia/reperfusion-induced cardiomyocyte apoptosis by carvedilol. *Circ Res* 1998;82:166-74.
48. Fairbairn LJ, Cowling GJ, Reipert BM Dexter TM. Suppression of apoptosis allows differentiation and development of a multipotent hemopoietic cell line in the absence of added growth factors. *Cell* 1993;74:823-32.
49. Wang L, Ma W, Markovich R, Chen J, Wang PH. Regulation of cardiomyocyte apoptotic signaling by insulin-like growth factor I. *Circ Res* 1998;83:516-22.
50. Lowe SW, Schmitt EM, Smith SW, Osborne BA, Jacks T. p53 is required for radiation-induced apoptosis in mouse thymocytes. *Nature* 1993;362:847-9.
51. Polyak K, Xia Y, Zweier JL, Kinzler KW, Vogelstein B. A model for p53-induced apoptosis. *Nature* 1997;389:300-5.
52. Jost CA, Marin MC, Kaelin WG. p73 is a human p53-related protein that can induce apoptosis. *Nature* 1997;389:191-4.
53. Michel T, Feron O. Nitric oxide synthases: Which, where, how, and why? *J Clin Invest* 1997;100:2146-52.
54. Pinsky DJ, Cai B, Yang X, Rodriguez C, Sciacca RR, Cannon PJ. The lethal effects of cytokine-induced nitric oxide on cardiac myocytes are blocked by nitric oxide synathase antagonism or transforming growth factor b. *J Clin Invest* 1995;95:677-85.
55. Kawaguchi H, Shin WS, Wang Y, Inukai M, Kato M, Matsuo-Okai Y, Sakamoto A, Uehara Y, Kaneda Y, Toyo-oka T. In vivo gene transfection of human endothelial cell nitic oxide synthase in cardiomyocytes causes apoptosis-like cell death. *Circulation* 1997;95:2441-7.

56. Koglin J, Granville DJ, Glysing-Jensen T, Mudgett JS, Carthy CM, McManus BM, Russell ME.Attenuated acute cardiac rejection in NOS2 -/- recipients correlates with reduced apoptosis. *Circulation* 1999;99:836-42.
57. Torre-Amione G, Kapadia S, Lee J, Bies RD, Lebovitz R, Mann DL. Expression and functional significance of tumor necrosis factor receptors in human myocardium. *Circulation* 1995;92:1487-93.
58. Pan G, O'Rourke K, Chinnaiyan AM, Gentz R, Ebner R, Ni J, Dixit VM. The receptor for the cytotoxic ligand TRAIL. *Science* 1997;276:111-3.
59. Sheridan JP, Marsters SA, Pitti RM, Gurney A, Skubatch M, Baldwin D, Ramakrishnan L, Gray CL, Baker K, Wood WI, Goddard AD, Godowski P, Ashkenazi A. Control of TRAIL-induced apoptosis by a family of signaling and decoy receptors. *Science* 1997;277:818-21.
60. Torre-Amione G, Kapadia S, Lee J, Durand JB, Bies RD, Young JB, Mann DL. Tumor necrosis factor-alpha and tumor necrosis factor receptors in the failing human heart. *Circulation* 1996;93:704-11.
61. Bartling B, Hoffmann J, Holtz J, Schulz R, Heusch G, Darmer D. Quantification of cardioprotective gene expression in porcine short-term hibernating myocardium. *J Mol Cell Cardiol* 1999;31:147-58.
62. Kubota T, McTiernan CF, Frye CS, Slawson SE, Lemster BH, Koretsky AP, Demetris AJ, Feldman AM. Dilated cardiomyopathy in transgenic mice with cardiac-specific overexpression of tumor necrosis factor-alpha. *Circ Res* 1997;81:627-35.
63. Felzen B, Shilkrut M, Less H, Sarapov I, Maor G, Coleman R, Robinson RB, Berke G, Binah O. Fas (CD95/Apo-1)-mediated damage to ventricular myocytes induced by cytotoxic T lymphocytes from perforin-deficient mice. *Circ Res* 1998;82:438-50.
64. Srinivasula SM, Ahmad M, Ottilie S, Bullrich F, Banks S, Wang Y, Fernandes-Alnemri T, Croce CM, Litwack G, Tomaselli KJ, Armstrong RC, Alnemri ES. FLAME-1, a novel FADD-like anti-apoptotic molecule that regulates Fas/TNFR1-induced apoptosis. *J Biol Chem* 1997;272:18542-5.
65. Koseki T, Inohara N, Chen S, Nunez G. ARC, an inhibitor of apoptosis expressed in skeletal muscle and heart that interacts selectively with caspases. *Proc Natl Acad Sci U S A* 1998;95:5156-60.
66. Yeh WC, Pompa JL, McCurrach ME, Shu HB, Elia AJ, Shahinian A, Ng M, Wakeham A, Khoo W, Mitchell K, El-Deiry WS, Lowe SW, Goeddel DV, Mak TW. FADD: essential for embryo development and signaling from some, but not all, inducers of apoptosis. *Science* 1998;279:1954-8.
67. Varfolomeev EE, Schuchmann M, Luria V, Chiannilkulchai N, Beckmann JS, Mett IL, Rebrikov D, Brodianski VM, Kemper OC, Kollet O Lapidot T, Soffer D, Sobe T, Avraham KB, Goncharov T, Holtmann H, Lonai P, Wallach D. Targeted disruption of the mouse Caspase 8 gene ablates cell death induction by the TNF receptors, Fas/Apo1, and DR3 and is lethal prenatally. *Immunity* 1998;9:267-76.
68. Green DR, Reed JC. Mitochondria and apoptosis. *Science* 1998; 281:1309-12.
69. Li P, Nijhawan D, Budihardjo I, Srinivasula SM, Ahmad M, Alnemri ES, Wang X. Cytochrome c and ATP-dependent formation of apaf-1/caspase-9 complex initiates an apoptotic protease cascade. *Cell* 1997;91:479-89.
70. Susin SA, Lorenzo HK, Zamzami N, Marzo I, Snow BE, Brothers GM, Mangion J, Jacotot E, Costantini P, Loeffler M, Larochette N, Goodlett R, Aebersold R, Siderovski DP, Penninger JM, Kroemer G. Molecular characterization of mitochondrial apoptosis-inducing factor. *Nature* 1999;397:441-6.
71. Schmiedl A, Schnabel PA, Mall G, Gebhard MM, Hunnemann DH, Richter J, Bretschneider HJ. The surface to volume ratio of mitochondria, a suitable parameter for evaluating mitochondrial swelling. Correlations during the course of myocardial global ischemia. *Virchows Arch A Pathol Anat Histopathol* 1990;416:305-15.

II.2.3
Cardiac myocytes and fibroblasts exhibit differential sensitivity to apoptosis-inducing stimuli

Edward G. Lakatta, M.D., Ph.D., Xilin Long, M.D.,
Alan Chesley Ph.D., and Michael Crow, Ph.D.

National Institute of Health, Baltimore, MD, USA

INTRODUCTION

Cell death in the cardiovascular system by apoptosis has received considerable attention in recent years. Cardiac and vascular cell death by apoptosis is not only a feature of embryologic and neonatal development, but can be elicited by a variety of diverse stimuli (Table I) and has been linked to virtually every major cardiovascular disease or disorder (Table II). In many of these disorders, particularly those leading to chronic heart failure, myocyte cell death/loss is usually accompanied by an increase in fibrous tissue content (1). Excessive fibrosis in the presence of myocyte loss has been advocated as a basis for impaired myocardial function in these disease states. The spontaneous hypertensive rat presents a clear example of the imbalance that exists as heart failure evolves (2). In this experimental model, increased cardiac myocyte apoptosis (Figure 1C) can be linked to the reduction in myocyte fractional mass (Figure 1A) as the hearts progress to failure. During this same time, there is a substantial increase in the fibrotic fractional area of the heart (Figure 1B).

This increase in fibrotic tissue mass in the face of increasing myocyte loss might result, in part, from a differential susceptibility of myocytes and fibroblasts to undergo apoptosis elicited by specific stimuli, such as those in Table 1 or others yet to be identified. Our recent studies have tested this hypothesis by examining the susceptibility of cultured cardiac myocytes and fibroblasts derived from rat neonatal hearts to some of these stimuli, namely hypoxia, intracellular acidosis, and forced expression of the tumor suppressor gene p53 or growth arrest-inducing gene, p21.

Table 1 STIMULI FOR CARDIOVASCULAR APOPTOSIS

- Mechanical Factors-Stretch
- Hypoxia/acidosis
- Growth Factors, e.g. AII: AT_1-Cardiac Myocytes; AT_2-VSM, Fb
- Growth Factor Withdrawal, e.g., serum removal from cells
- Cytokines, e.g., TNFα, IL_1, FAS/APO-1/TRAIL/APO-2
- matrix disconnect, e.g., Blockade of Integrin Signalling
- Tumor/cell cycle suppressors, e.g., p53, p73, p21
- Oncogenes, e.g., bcl_2, bax, bad
- Drugs, e.g., ACEI, ATII R Antagonists
- Mitochrondia-PTP

Table 2 SETTINGS FOR CARDIOVASCULAR APOPTOSIS

- Cardiac Development/Embryogenesis
- Cardiac Aging
- Acute Cardiac Ischemia-Hypoxia, Acidosis
- Chronic Ischemia-Neovascularization
- Chronic Heart Failure
      Idiopathic, Dilated--Hypertensive--Ischemic
- Atherosclerosis
- Vascular Injury (Restenosis)–VSM, Endothelial Cells
- Drug Therapy for Hypertension, e.g., ACEI, AT_1 R Blockers

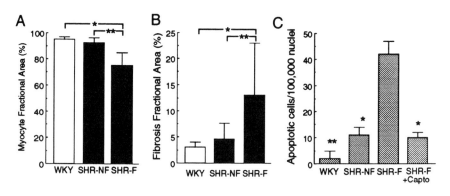

Figure 1. Changes in myocyte (**A**) fractional area and fibrosis (**B**) fractional area during the transition from stable hypertrophy to heart failure. Data are mean±SD for 7-12 preparations per group; *P<0.05; ** P<0.01. **C**. Average relative apoptotic cell number/100,000 nuclei in the section from hearts of each study group [Wistar-Kyoto (WKY), non-failing SHR (SHR-NF), and failing SHR (SHR-F) with and without captopril (Capto)]. Apoptotic cells in SHR-F are significantly higher than those of WKY or SHR-NF: **P<0.01, SHR-F vs WKY and SHR-F + Capto; *P<0.05, SHR-F vs SHR-NF (Ref. 2).

THE CELL MODEL

Neonatal ventricular myocytes were prepared from the digested hearts of 1-3 day old Wistar rat pups and cultured as previously described (3). Myocytes were routinely purified on a discontinuous Percoll gradient and plated on gelatin-coated dishes at an initial density of approximately 10^5 cells/cm^2. The myocyte composition of the cultures was monitored 48 hours after plating by immunocytochemistry with monoclonal antibodies to either sarcomeric α-actin or myosin heavy chains and was typically above 90 % (94±4% in 15 independent preparations).

During the initial 24 h after plating, myocytes were cultured in media consisting of four parts (by volume) of DMEM containing 4.5 g/liter glucose and one part medium 199 (Earle's salts; GIBCO BRL, Gaithersburg, MD) supplemented with 10% preselected, heat-inactivated horse serum, 5% heat-inactivated FBS, penicillin (100 U/ml), and streptomycin (100 µg/ml). After that, both the horse and fetal calf serum were removed and replaced with 1 µmol/liter insulin, 5 µmol/liter transferin, and 10 nmol/liter selenium. In the initial series of experiments, cultured myocytes were maintained in high levels of bromodeoxyuridine (10^{-4} M) to inhibit replication of the small percentage of fibroblasts that were present. However, neither the presence of bromodeoxyuridine nor contaminating fibroblasts affected the results presented.

Fibroblasts were isolated from the neonatal heart by two methods. The first involved taking cells from the 1.050 g/ml band of the Percoll gradient used to obtain purified myocytes and passaging the cells three times in culture. The second involved culturing cells that adhered to untreated tissue culture plastic during a one hour preplating of the heart digestion. These cells were then passaged a minimum of three times before use. Both methods produced cultures that failed to stain with antibodies to sarcomeric α-actin, sarcomeric myosin heavy chains, or smooth muscle actin. Cardiac fibroblasts were cultured in 4:1 DMEM:F12 supplemented with 10% fetal calf serum, penicillin (100 U/ml), and streptomycin (100 µg/ml).

THE RESPONSE OF CARDIAC MYOCYTES AND FIBROBLASTS TO PROLONGED HYPOXIA

Both acute and chronic myocardial ischemia lead to cardiac cell loss and scar formation, resulting in reduced pumping capacity and eventually to congestive heart failure and death (4). In vivo studies in the rabbit heart have reported that the cell death that follows the reperfusion of ischemic areas is due primarily to apoptosis, while that which occurs during prolonged ischemia is due to necrosis (5). On the other hand, studies in the rat indicate that cell death from prolonged ischemia can occur by both apoptotic and necrotic mechanisms (6). One of the many components of ischemic stress is hypoxia. Recent studies have shown that hypoxia of cultured neonatal cardiomyocytes causes morphological and biochemical changes characteristic of cell death by apoptosis (7,8).

To expose cells to hypoxia, cultures were placed in a plexiglas chamber and a constant stream of water-saturated 95% N_2/5% CO_2 was maintained over the culture. The partial pressure of oxygen (PO_2) of the culture media under these conditions decreased in an exponential fashion after the culture dish was placed in the equilibrated chamber and a steady state PO_2 of < 15 Torr was achieved after 8 hours (Figure 2). The hypoxia produced under the above conditions produced a substantial stress on the myocytes as indicated by induction of heme oxygenase (HO-1), a stress-induced protein involved in the conversion of heme to biliverdin and carbon monoxide (CO) (9). As early as 6 hours after the onset of hypoxia, there was a 3-fold increase in the level of HO-1 mRNA, and by 48 hours the level of HO-1 mRNA was increased 30-fold compared to normoxic cells. The increase in HO-1 mRNA was accompanied by increased expression of HO-1 protein (6.7 and 8.7-fold increased over normoxic controls at 24 and 48 hours of hypoxia, respectively) as demonstrated by Western blotting and immunofluorescence staining. Hypoxia also significantly increased the production of CO in cardiac myocytes by 2.5 and 8 fold at 24 and 48 hours, respectively (9).

Cultured neonatal rat cardiac myocytes exposed to hypoxia exhibited intranucleosomal cleavage of genomic DNA characteristic of apoptosis. The extent of cleavage increased with time and was readily visible with conventional DNA laddering methods at 48 hours of hypoxia. Normoxic time-matched controls showed markedly less DNA fragmentation at this time (Figure 3A). Using ligation mediated-PCR (LM-PCR) to increase the sensitivity of detection, evidence for cleavage as early as 24 hours after placement in the chamber was routinely observed (Figure 3B). Increased end-labeling of DNA among individual hypoxia-treated myocytes was also detected by the TUNEL method and the time course of the changes in end-labeling in normoxic and hypoxic myocytes is shown in Figure 4.

Time Course of PO₂ Change in the Culture Medium

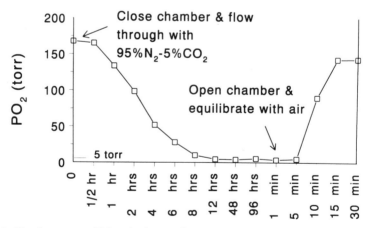

Figure 2 The time course of PO_2 reduction and final levels of PO_2 achieved in neonatal cell cultures. At time zero, cell cultures were placed in a humidified Plexiglass chamber at 37°C and a continuous stream of 95%N_2/5%CO_2 was maintained over the cultures. The partial pressure was measured with an oxygen electrode and a dual differential oxygen electrode amplifier (Instech Lab., Plymouth MA). (Ref. 8).

These data show that while there was a significant increase in the number of TUNEL-positive cells during the first day of exposure to hypoxia, an even greater increase occurred over the next 24 hours with > 60% of the remaining cells in the culture scored as TUNEL-positive after 48 hours of hypoxia. While some myocytes maintained under normoxic conditions were TUNEL positive (11.3±1.5% at 48 hr), it was clear that hypoxia markedly increased cardiomyocyte apoptosis even after only 24 hours of exposure.

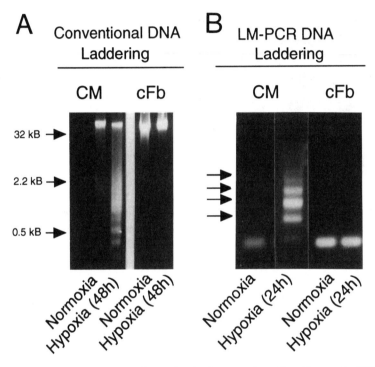

Figure 3 Chronic exposure to hypoxia results in fragmentation of cardiomyocyte DNA. **A.** Conventional DNA laddering assay of 5 μg genomic DNA fromcardiac myocytes (CM) and cardiac fibroblasts (cFb). **B.** Nucleosomal fragmentation detected by ligation-mediated PCR. Arrows identify PCR-generated nuclesomal fragments from a total of 500 ng genomic DNA.

The myocytes treated with the protocol described above and in more detail elsewhere (8) remained metabolically active during at least the first 24 hours of exposure to hypoxia. At later times of exposure (48 hours), however, the pH of the media decreased significantly and there were fewer contracting myocytes. This acidification was attributed to the buildup of glycolytic endproducts (e.g., lactic acid), since glucose and insulin had been provided in the culture media. This was consistent with the observation that the time at which media acidification appeared was dependent on the number of cells in the dishes and the volume of the culture media added to the dishes. Under the conditions established in the laboratory, acidification is not a factor in the apoptosis after 24 hours of exposure to hypoxia, but is likely to contribute to cell death at later times.

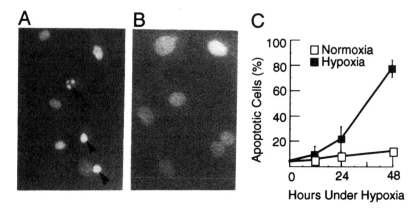

Figure 4 Staining of myocytes (**A**) and fibroblasts (**B**) for nuclear fragmentation as detected by the Hoechst dye 33342 after exposure to hypoxia. Condensed and fragmented nuclei are observed only in myocytes and are indicated by the black arrow. **C**. Quantitative analysis of the percent myocytes undergoing apoptosis as measured by the TUNEL technique.

Interestingly, the effect of hypoxia in the experimental model described above was confined to cardiomyocytes isolated from the heart. Cardiac fibroblasts isolated from the same hearts and exposed to hypoxia showed no sign of increased DNA fragmentation (Figure 3 A,B).

INHIBITION OF THE VACUOLAR PROTON ATPASE (VPATPASE) STIMULATES APOPTOSIS

Although the mechanisms underlying cardiac apoptosis are still largely unclear, evidence from recent studies has implicated the VPATPase in the regulation of apoptotic cell death in other cell types. The VPATPase is localized to the membranes of the plasma and various intracellular compartments of eukaryotic cells and is likely to be responsible for extrusion of protons from the cytosol and the preservation of the pH gradient between the cytoplasmic and intracellular compartments (10,11). It has been reported, for example, that granulocyte colony-stimulating factor delays apoptosis in neutrophils by upregulating the VPATPase (12). It has also been suggested that cardiomyocyte preconditioning reduces apoptosis in adult cardiac myocytes by activating the VPATPase (13). Likewise, the inhibition of the VPATPase by the macrolide antibiotic, bafilomycin A1, results in acidification of the cytoplasm and has been shown to induced apoptotic cell death in lymphoma cells (14). Our recent study has made use of the potency and apparent specificity of bafilomycin A1 to examine the role of VPATPase in apoptosis of isolated neonatal cardiomyocytes and fibroblasts (15). If, as expected, bafilomycin A1 can be shown to induce intracellular acidification in myocytes, it could be a useful experimental treatment to study the effects of intracellular acidification independently of other factors associated with ischemia.

Cardiac myocytes treated with either 50 or 100 nM bafilomycin A1 for 24 h exhibited increased DNA fragmentation compared to vehicle (DMSO)-treated myocyte cultures (Figure 5A). In contrast, cardiac fibroblasts isolated from neonatal rat hearts showed no sign of DNA fragmentation when treated with bafilomycin A1 (Figure 5B). Compared with untreated controls, bafilomycin A1-treated myocytes exhibited a number of the morphological changes characteristic of programmed cell death or apoptosis, including cell shrinkage, chromatin compaction, cytoplasmic condensation or loss of cytoplasm. Using the in situ end-labeling method to identify fragmented DNA, it was observed that >80% of the cardiomyocytes were positively stained after 24 h of treatment with 100 nM bafilomycin A1, while only 12% staining was detected in time-matched vehicle (DMSO)-treated cardiomyocytes (Figure 5D) and that the response to bafilomycin A1 was dose-dependent (Figure 5C).

Changes in pH_i were measured in cardiac myocytes and fibroblasts after treatment with bafilomycin A1 and are shown in Figures 5E and 5F, respectively. Bafilomycin A1 caused biphasic changes in myocyte pH_i. In myocytes. there was a slight elevation between 3 and 18 hr after treatment, followed by a sharp and marked decline in pH_i between 18 and 21 hr that continued up to the final timepoint measured (24 hr). In the absence of bafilomycin, there was no significant change in myocyte pH_i over the experimental time period. In contrast to myocytes, there was no change in pH_i in cardiac fibroblasts exposed to bafilomycin A1 (Figure 5F). The resistance of cardiac fibroblasts to the apoptosis-inducing effects of bafilomycin A1 may, therefore, be due to their ability to maintain pH_i during exposure to bafilomycin A1, although other mechanisms may also be responsible.

Overall, the results in Figure 5 demonstrate that bafilomycin A1 is sufficient to cause massive and nearly complete death of isolated cardiomyocytes by apoptosis. This effect is likely to be a specific one in that the dose required to induce apoptosis is 10,000 times lower than that needed to inhibit other ATPases (11).

It seems likely that bafilomycin A1 causes apoptosis through its ability to alter pH_i as a result of VPATPases inhibition. This presumption is supported by the observations that intracellular acidification is known to be a general feature of apoptotic cell death (12, 16-22) and is thought to contribute to the activation of endogenous endonucleases, leading to DNA cleavage (23,24). Furthermore, apoptosis in neutrophils (12) and in Jurkat cells (17) is preceded by intracellular acidification and in the experiments on cardiomyocytes shown in figure 4 is temporally associated with the period of massive cell death (15).

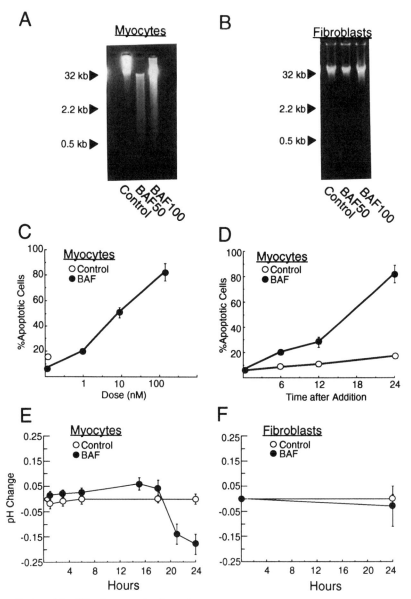

Figure 5 A and B. DNA fragmentation in cardiac myocytes (A) or fibroblasts (B) exposed for 24 h to either vehicle (Control), 50 nM (BAF50), or 100 nM bafilomycin (BAF100). **C and D.** Dose (**C**)- and time (**D**)-dependent induction of apoptosis in cardiomyocytes by bafilomycin as measured by the TUNEL technique. Dose-response was performed for 24 h. Values are mean±SEM, n=6; *P<0.05 (ANOVA). The time course of cells undergoing apoptosis was performed with 100 nM bafilomycin A1. Values are mean±SEM, n=6; *P<0.05 (ANOVA). **E and F.** pH$_i$ changes in vehicle- and bafilomycin A1-treated cardiomyocytes (E) and fibroblasts (F) as previously described (15).   Individual cell groups (1-4 cells) were analyzed by fluorescence microscopy with excitation at 530 nm and emission at 590 and 694 nm.

Finally, cells, such as cardiac fibroblasts, that are resistant to the apoptotic-inducing effects of bafilomycin A1 fail to undergo changes in intracellular pH when treated with bafilomycin A1 (15).

p53 AND CARDIOMYOCYTE APOPTOSIS INDUCED BY HYPOXIA OR BAFILOMYCIN A1

In the course of seeking to identify potential mechanisms for myocyte apoptosis caused by hypoxia and bafilomycin A1, additional studies focused on the expression of p53 and the pathways it utilizes to cause apoptosis. p53 is a tumor suppresor gene whose mutational inactivation is a common event in a variety of human tumors (reviewed in 25). While work on p53 originally focused on its ability to control cell proliferation, the product of the p53 gene has more recently received considerable attention as an important regulator of apoptosis. In fact, mutations that affect the ability of p53 to induce apoptosis are as critical to tumor formation as those that affect its ability to suppress cellular proliferation (26). Because the development of p53 null (-/-) mice appears normal (27), one important function of p53 may be to act as a surveillance factor to induce apoptosis in response to cellular damage or stress, while normal developmental pathways of apoptosis are regulated independently of p53.

In cells other than cardiomyocytes, protein levels of p53 have been shown to increase in response to a number of apoptotic-inducing stimuli, including oxidative stress (28), DNA damage (29), and hypoxia (30). Furthermore, an increase in expression and activity of p53 can increase the transcription of the pro-apoptotic gene *bax* while suppressing transcription of the anti-apoptotic gene *BCL-2* (31,23). Introduction of p53 into the myeloid leukemia cell line M1, which has no endogenous p53 expression, induces apoptosis (33), while in other myeloid cell lines the expression of a dominant negative p53 gene can prevent apoptosis that results from growth factor withdrawal (34).

A role for p53 in cardiomyocyte apoptosis has also been demonstrated (35) in isolated adult heart cells and is consistent with a study on cellular localization of p53 in a dog model of heart failure using conformation-specific antibodies to detect active and inactive forms of p53 (36). This study showed that expression of an active form of p53 occurred in cardiomyocytes undergoing apoptosis within the borders of infarction zones, while conformationally inactive p53 was present in regions away from the infarct. One could speculate that expression of conformationally inactive p53 may serve to shield myocytes outside the infarct zone from stress-induced apoptosis occurring in the infarct.

In neonatal cardiomyocytes, prolonged (24-48 hours) to hypoxia is accompanied by increased p53 protein levels (Figure 6A and C) and an increase in p53 DNA binding/transactivation as measured with a luciferase reporter construction driven by multiple p53 DNA binding sites (8). Hypoxia also increases the expression of p21/WAF-1/cip1, a well-characterized downstream target of p53 sequence-specific transactivation (8). p53 protein levels also increased in bafilomycin-treated cardiomyocytes. Significant increases in protein accumulation were detected as early as 6 h after administration of bafilomycin A1, continued to increase at 12 h, and remained elevated even after 24 h (Figure 6C and E). The increased protein accumulation was accompanied by parallel increases in p53 mRNA levels (15). Consistent with the increase in p53 protein levels, the treatment of myocytes with bafilomycin A1 also resulted in increased p53-dependent gene transactivation as measured by p53-dependent reporter gene expression (15). In contrast to the effects of bafilomycin A1 on myocytes, there was no change in p53 protein levels in cardiac fibroblasts after 12 and 24 h of exposure to the VPATPase inhibitor (Figures 6B and E).

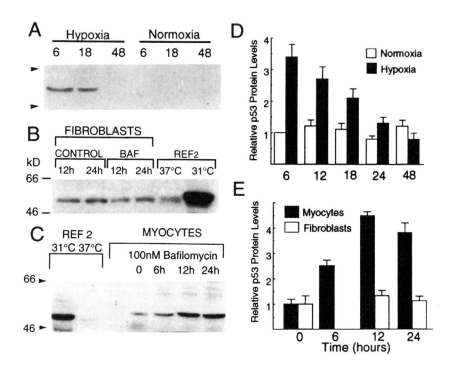

Figure 6 A and B. Expression of p53 protein in cardiac myocytes exposed to hypoxia Representative Western blot (A) prepared and analyzed as described in (8). Extracts from REF2 cells grown at the permissive (31°C) and restrictive (37°C) temperature for expression of a stably transfected mutant p53 were used a controls for the blotting. (B) Quantitative analysis of p53 protein levels in hypoxia-treated cardiac myocytes. The data for each time point represent at least three independent determinations. C and D. Representative Western blots of p53 protein expression in cardiac myocytes (C) and fibroblasts (D) treated with 100 nM bafilomycin for the times indicated. E. Quantitative analysis of p53 protein levels in bafilomycin-treated cardiac myocytes (filled bars) and fibroblasts (open bars) as a function of time (three independent determinations each).

To determine whether the increase in p53 expression in isolated neonatal cardiomyocytes was sufficient to cause apoptosis, myocytes were infected with a replication-defective recombinant adenovirus expressing wild-type p53 (AdCMV.p53) under normal oxygen conditions (Figure 7). Recombinant adenoviruses were employed for gene delivery because most neonatal myocytes have withdrawn from the cell cycle at the time of their isolation and are, therefore, relatively refractive to gene transfer by standard transfection techniques. In addition, recombinant adenoviral infection allows transgene expression in almost 100% of the cells in a culture, so apoptosis can be monitored by multiple measures (e.g., DNA laddering, TUNEL, and annexin IV staining), and changes in intracellular protein and mRNA expression, including p53 expression, can be determined. Infection of the myocytes with AdCMV.p53 resulted in a persistent and elevated expression of wild-type p53 in virtually all the cells (8). Myocytes expressing the p53 transgene, but not those infected with control adenoviruses without an inserted transgene (AdCMV.null) showed extensive apoptosis as measured by DNA laddering and TUNEL staining (Figures 7A and B, respectively) (8). In contrast, no evidence for DNA laddering or changes in TUNEL positive cells were detectible in AdCMV.p53 infected- cardiac fibroblasts (Figures 7A and B).

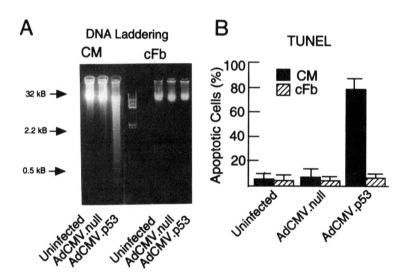

Figure 7 AdCMV.p53 infection induces DNA fragmentation in neonatal cardiomyocytes. **(A)** DNA fragmentation assay. Genomic DNA was isolated from uninfected, AdCMV.null-infected, and AdCMV.p53-infected cardiomyocytes (left panel) or fibroblasts (right panel) 48 h after infection. **(B)** Quantification of the results of TUNEL assay performed 48 h after infection. The data for each condition represent the average of at least four different infections.

The mechanism by which p53 induces apoptosis in cardiomyocytes but not cardiac fibroblasts is still unknown but may have been partially clarified in recent experiments. Infection of adult cardiac myocytes with a recombinant adenovirus expressing wild type p53 leads to significant apoptosis and is accompanied with increased expression of BAX and downregulation of BCL-2 mRNA (35). These two proteins are members of the bcl-2 family and have been shown to have pro-apoptotic and anti-apoptotic actions, respectively, and to be transcriptionally regulated by p53. Expression of p53 in myocytes (and many other cell types, as well) and its regulation of BAX and BCL-2 expression creates a pro-apoptotic environment within the cell. In addition, p53-infected myocytes have elevated levels of both angiotensinogen (AO) and the angiotensin type 1 receptor (AT1). The promoters driving expression of AO and AT1 contain p53-binding sites, although these sites have not yet been shown to be required for promoter activity (35).

Changes in BCL-2/BAX expression alone do not seem to be sufficient to induce apoptosis in cardiomyocytes since incubation of the cells with Losartan, a blocker of the angiotensin receptor type 1 (AT1), prevents apoptosis in the p53-infected myocytes but does not alter the p53-induced changes in bax and BCL-2 expression. It is interesting that not only does expression of p53 lead to increased expression of some components of the renin-angiotensin system, but that angiotensin II (AII) by itself can lead to increased p53 DNA-binding activity and increased expression of BAX. Under some circumstances, AII alone can cause cardiomyocyte apoptosis (37,38), although it is not clear if this process is p53-dependent.

p21/WAF1/CIP1/ IN CARDIOMYOCYTE APOPTOSIS

In addition to BCL-2 and BAX, other downstream targets for p53 sequence-specific transactivation are the cyclin-dependent kinase inhibitor, p21/WAF1/cip1 (39), the p53 binding protein, mdm2 (40), the growth arrest-associated gene, GADD45 (41), cyclin G (42), and the death receptors, FAS (43) and DR5 (44). From this list, the genes with established links to apoptosis are BAX, FAS, and DR5. A possible role for BAX in cardiomyocyte apoptosis was briefly described above. Little is known about the role of DR5 in cardiomyocytes, while increased FAS mRNA expression can be induced in cardiomyocytes by hypoxia (7) and elevated FAS levels are observed in animal models of heart failure (45). Interestingly, while hypoxia increases FAS mRNA in cardiomyocytes, it decreases its expression in cardiac fibroblasts (7).

Less obvious and more controversial is the role that p21/WAF1/cip1 plays in the regulation of apoptosis. It is well-established that p21/WAF1/cip1 is involved in the regulation of cell cycle progression through its ability to inhibit cyclin-dependent kinases (46) and proliferating cell nuclear antigen (PCNA)-dependent DNA replication (47,48). Conflicting evidence exists, however, on its role in apoptosis. Most studies in non-cardiac cells have been unable to demonstrate a direct role for p21/WAF1/cip1 in apoptosis (49), while others have suggested that the ability of p21/WAF1/cip1 to induce growth arrest may actually be important in protecting some cells from apoptosis (50). Nonetheless, forced expression of p21/WAF1/cip1 has been shown to cause apoptosis in at least some cell types. Matsushita et al. (51) reported that forced expression of p21/WAF1/cip1 in vascular smooth muscle cells caused a significant cell loss attributable to apoptosis, while Boudreau and colleagues (52) showed that constitutively expressed p21/WAF1/cip1 caused apoptosis in primary mammary cell cultures that are normally protected from apoptosis by serum.

The induction of apoptosis by bafilomycin or hypoxia in cultured cardiomyocytes and in adult myocytes during the transition from hypertrophy to heart failure in the SHR rat (Figure 1) are all accompanied by elevated expression of the p21/WAF1/cip1 gene. The role that this gene plays in cardiomyocyte apoptosis, however, is unknown. To determine whether forced expression of p21/WAF1/cip1 would have a protective effect on cardiomyocyte apoptosis, cause apoptosis on its own, or have no effect at all, neonatal cardiomyocytes were infected with a replication-defective adenovirus expressing human p21/WAF1/cip1. Whether p21/WAF1/cip1 gene expression in cardiomyocytes in response to hypoxia could be activated in the absence of functionally active p53, as has been shown for other cell types (53,54), was also determined.

Figure 8A shows the DNA laddering profiles that were detected in cardiomyocytes using the LM-PCR assay. Myocytes infected with control virus (AdCMV.null) and maintained under normoxic conditions for 24 hours showed little indication of DNA laddering, while infected cells exposed to hypoxia exhibited a marked increase in DNA nucleosomal fragments.

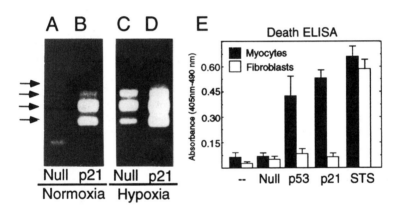

Figure 8 A-D. Forced expression of p21/WAF1/cip1 causes cardiomyocyte apoptosis and potentiates hypoxia-induced apoptosis. LM-PCR DNA ladder assay of neonatal rat cardiomyocytes maintained under normoxic conditions or exposed to hypoxia for 48 hours. Cardiomyocytes were infected either with AdCMV.p21 (AdWAF1) or AdCMV.null immediately prior to exposure to hypoxia. Arrows indicate oligonucleosomal bands indicative of DNA laddering. **E** Quantitation of apoptosis in cardiac myocytes and fibroblasts using the cell death ELISA to detect nucleosomal fragments. Quantitation of apoptosis in mock-infected cells, AdCMV.p53- and AdCMV.p21-infected cells, and cells treated with 100 nM staurosporine for 24 hours. Results are the mean +/- SEM, n = 6.

Infection with AdCMV.p21 potentiated the response of the myocytes to hypoxia and caused a significant increase in DNA fragmentation in myocytes maintained under normoxic conditions. Quantitative analyses of cell death by ELISA and TUNEL staining are shown in Figure 8B and C, respectively. The fold increases in apoptosis resulting from forced p21/WAF1/cip1 expression as measured by both assays were remarkably comparable, showing a 5.3-fold increase in apoptosis measured by TUNEL and a 5.6 fold increase measured by the cell death ELISA.

In contrast to the myocytes, forced expression of human p21/WAF1/cip1 in cardiac fibroblasts did not induce apoptosis as assessed by either conventional DNA laddering (Figure 8A), the cell death ELISA (Figure 8B), or TUNEL staining (data not shown). Infection with the virus, however, did result in growth arrest as assessed by direct cell counting and suppression of serum-stimulated bromodeoxyuridine (BrdU) incorporation (not shown). Although infection with recombinant adenoviruses expressing either wild type p53 or p21/WAF1/cip1 were not able to induce apoptosis in cardiac fibroblasts, apoptosis could be induced in these cells with the nonspecific protein kinase inhibitor, staurosporine (STS, Figure 8E), which causes apoptosis in a variety of cell types through an undefined mechanism.

THE SIGNIFICANCE OF THE p53-SIGNALING PATHWAY FOR CARDIOMYOCYTE APOPTOSIS

Hypoxia is a component of myocardial ischemia. The significance of the p53 signaling pathway to cardiac cell apoptosis in response to ischemia in vivo has been questioned by in vivo experiments using an acute myocardial infarct model in mice in which the p53 gene has been removed from the genome by gene knock-out technology (55). These experiments involved ligation of the left coronary artery in mice that were either wild type (p53+/+) or homozygous knockout (p53 -/-) for the p53 gene. Genomic DNA was then isolated from the hypoperfused areas up to a week after ligation and examined for DNA laddering. DNA laddering in wild type mice (p53 +/+) was detectible within 4 hours of surgery and persisted until sometime between 48 and 72 hours post-ligation. When the same experiments were performed in p53 (-/-) knockout mice, no apparent difference in the extent or kinetics of apoptosis was observed compared to wild type littermates. These results demonstrate that the apoptosis found within the hypoperfused (infarct) area early after surgery does not require p53. They do not, however, exclude a role for p53 in the area outside the infarct in which apoptosis may occur over a longer period of time in response to increased stretching that results from the loss of damaged myocardium in the infarct. In fact, adult cardiac myocytes in cell culture can be seen to undergo apoptosis in response to stretching and the pathway that mediates this response involves angiotensin II release and activation of p53 (56). Because remodeling of the myocardium in response to the loss of muscle mass in the immediate infarct may continue for weeks to months and involve at any one time, a very limited number of cardiomyocytes, it is unlikely to be detected by standard DNA laddering techniques.

The pronounced DNA laddering that can be detected in the hearts of both wild type and p53 knockout mice suggest that a relatively large number of cells are dying early after arterial ligation, a suggestion that is indeed confirmed by perfusion studies which show the size of the infarct to be relatively large (55). These cells are likely to have been present in the infarcted zone and to have died by necrosis as a result of chronic ischemia. In time, chronic ischemia results in multiple insults to the cell, including hypoxia, depletion of metabolizable substrates, and the build-up of toxic products. The lack of oxygen and metabolizable substrates leads to the loss of high energy content within the cells and the likely collapse of the mitochondrial transmembrane potential. This, in turn, results in the release of cytochrome c and other intramembranous components into the cytosol. Cytosolic cytochrome c has been shown to be necessary and sufficient to activate caspase 9 through its binding to Apaf-1. Caspase 9, in turn, can activate the distal executioner caspase 3, the substrates of which include the DNA fragmentation factor (DFF/ICAD) responsible for DNA laddering. Thus, although these cells may die by necrosis, their particular "death actî involves activation of a part of the apoptotic pathway. The activation of this partial pathway may have protective consequences in terms of preventing or minimizing the inflammatory response associated with cell death by necrosis, but it is not the primary mode by which cells die in the infarct. As such, the inhibition of caspases, while possibly preventing the appearance of DNA laddering within the infarct, would be ineffective in preventing cell death in this region. Therefore, analyzing cell death in the hypoperfused region of the mouse heart early after surgery may not provide an adequate test of the necessity or sufficiency of candidate proximal signals for apoptosis..

Another fact to consider in interpreting the results from the p53 knockout mouse is that p53 is now recognized as one member of a growing family of functionally related molecules. Deleting one member of a gene family may leave others to functionally substitute for the loss. For example, a p53-homologue named p73 has been identified (57). The gene product is functionally identical to p53 with respect to gene transactivation(i.e., regulation of p21/WAF/cip1 and bax), but its expression is regulated under conditions and by factors that are different from those that regulate p53 expression and activity. Transactivation-deficient mutants of p53 act as dominant negatives not only for p53-induced but also p73-induced gene expression (58) and would be expected to inhibit this function of other p53-related molecule (59). Because of the redundancy in function between the p53-related molecules, deletion of only one of these genes may be compensated by another family member. Aside from deleting all members of this gene family, transgenic expression of a single dominant negative mutant of either p53 or p73 in the heart may be the most effective way to ablate transactivation resulting from these molecules. Such expression could lead to a different conclusion than that seen with knocking out only a single member of the gene family.

SUMMARY

Figure 9 summarizes the differences in the response of cardiac myocytes and fibroblasts to apoptosis-inducing stimuli. A number of different and possibly interrelated stimuli induce apoptosis in isolated cardiac myocytes, including hypoxia, the vacuolar ATPase inhibitor, bafilomycin A1, overexpression of wild type p53, and overexpression of the inhibitor of cyclin-dependent protein kinases, p21/WAF1/cip1. None of these same stimuli, however, cause cardiac fibroblasts isolated from the same hearts as the myocytes to undergo apoptosis. While the ailure of cardiac fibroblasts to undergo apoptosis in the case of bafilomycin or hypoxia may be due to their inability to activate p53, this cannot explain their lack of response to infection with the recombinant adenoviruses expressing either wild-type p53 or p21/WAF1/cip1.

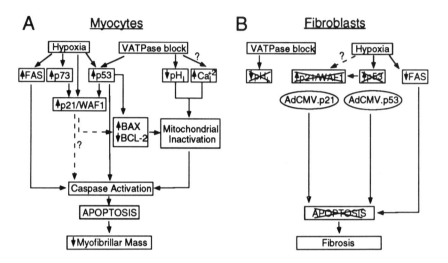

Figure 9 Summary of the effects and potential pathways for apoptosis in cardiac myocytes (A) and fibroblasts (B).

Infection with either virus resulted in elevated levels of transgene expression in both myocytes and fibroblasts. Indeed, elevated expression of p21/WAF1/cip1 in cardiac fibroblasts is functional as well, resulting in growth arrest of the cells. These results demonstrate that neonatal cardiac myocytes are particularly sensitive to apoptosis, whereas fibroblasts are relatively resistant to these same stimuli. It is clear that there are many gaps in our knowledge about the differences in signaling between myocytes and fibroblasts that need to be addressed. Among the more promising approaches to identifying the critical genes regulating this difference in sensitivity would be the differential array analyses of the cDNAs expressed by cardiac myocytes and fibroblasts overexpressing p53.

Differences in the susceptibility of cardiac myocytes and fibroblasts to apoptosis is likely to be an important factor in the progression to heart failure. This progression is likely to begin during the remodeling of the heart as it adapts either to an absolute or relative increase in load as a result of peripheral vessel disease or loss of functional myocardium. One of the important signals for remodeling under these conditions is an increased diastolic load (stretch). Stretching of adult myocytes in culture increases apoptosis through a process that involves angiotensin II release and p53 signaling (56). Stretching of the myocardium may, therefore, lead to selective cell death among myocytes, leaving fibroblasts and the extracellular matrix products secreted by them free to occupy the space once inhabited by contracting myocytes. Because this myocyte loss is irreversible, the replacement of contractile tissue with a stiff and inelastic network of noncontractile cells and extracellular matrix begins the progression to heart failure, a process amplified by the growing mismatch between the functional demands placed on the heart and its dwindling ability to perform.

The functional significance of p53 signaling pathways to cardiomyocyte apoptosis will require additional experiments, preferably in isolated cardiomyocytes exposed to defined apoptotic-inducing stimuli. Cells could be isolated from wild type (p53+/+) or p53-deficient (p53 -/-) mice or infected with adenoviruses carrying dominant negative mutants of p53 or p53-related genes. If the mechanism by which p53 or p53-related genes mediate apoptosis involves transcriptional activation, the approach using dominant negative mutants would be more inclusion of the role of these p53-related genes . The value of in vitro experimentation is cell death can be verified to occur through apoptosis and not necrosis. The presence of DNA ladders or TUNEL staining may not be sufficient for verification. A stringent functional assessment of apoptosis would be to demonstrate that cell death can be blocked by generic caspase inhibitors, such as zVAD-fmk, or by bcl-2 overexpression.

One current perspective on apoptosis recognizes that there is an important link between cell proliferation and cell death (60), with the decision on which pathway is chosen dictated by the presence of survival factors which suppress apoptosis. Although cardiac myocytes are, for the most part, non-renewing and terminally differentiated, myocytes do express proliferation-associated genes, such as PCNA, under circumstances in which myocyte apoptosis is promoted (61), and myocyte apoptosis can be suppressed by the growth factor, IGF-1 (63) and the adrenergic agonist, phenylephrine (64). The mechanism by which such factors rescue myocytes from apoptosis and their link to p53 signaling is unknown and may provide important insights into the mechanism(s) responsible for the differential sensitivity of myocytes and fibroblasts to apoptosis.

References

1. Boluyt M, Lakatta EG. Cardiovascular Aging in Health. In: Advances in Organ Biology. Vol. 4B, p. 257-303, 1998 A-14.
2. Li Z, Bing OL, Long X, Robinson KG, Lakatta EG. Increased cardiomyocyte apoptosis during the transition to heart failure in the spontaneously hypertensive rat. Amer. J. Physiol. H2313-H2319, 1997.
3. Zheng JS, Boluyt MO, O'Neill L, Crow MT, Lakatta EG.. Extracellular ATP induces immediate early gene expression but not cellular hypertrophy in neonatal cardiac myocytes. Circ. Res. 74:1034-1041, 1994.
4. Pfeffer MA, Braunwald E. Ventricular remodeling after myocardial infarction. Circulation 81:1161-1172, 1990.
5. Gottlieb,RA, Burleson KO, Kloner RA, Babior BM, Engler RL. Reperfusion injury induces apoptosis in rabbit cardiomyocytes. J. Clin. Invest. 94:1621-1628, 1994.
6. Kajstura, J, Cheng W, Reiss K, Clark WA, Sonnenblick EH, Krajewski S, Reed JC, Olivetti G, Anversa P. Apoptotic and necrotic myocyte cell deaths are independent contributing variables of infarct size in rats. Lab. Invest. 74:86-107, 1996.
7. Tanaka M, Ito H, Adachi S, Akimoto H, Nishikawa T, Kasajima T, Marumo F, Hiroe H. Hypoxia induces apoptosis with enhanced expression of fas antigen messenger RNA in cultured neonatal rat cardiomyocytes. Circ. Res. 75:426-433, 1994.
8. Long X, Boluyt MO, Zheng JS, O'Neill L, Pirelli C, Lakatta EG, Crow MT. p53 and the hypoxia-induced apoptosis of cultured neonatal rat cardiac myocytes. J. Clin. Invest. 99:2635-2643, 1997.

9. Long X, Boluyt MO, Li X, Crow MT, Lakatta EG. Hypoxia-induced expression of heme-oxygenase gene expression in cultured neonatal rat cardiac myocytes. Circ. Suppl. 92:I693, 1995.
10. Forgac M. Structure and function of vacuolar class of ATP-driven proton pumps. Physiol. Rev. 69:765-796, 1989.
11. Crider BP, Xie X-S, Stone DK. Bafilomycin inhibits proton flow through the H^+-channel of vacuolar proton pumps. J. Biol. Chem. 269:17379-17381, 1994.
12. Gottlieb RA, Giesing HA, Zhu JY, Engler RL, Babior, BM. Cell acidification in apoptosis: granulocyte colony-stimulating factor delays programmed cell death in neutrophils by upregulating the vacuolar H^+-ATPase. Proc. Natl. Acad. Sci. USA 92:5965-5968, 1995.
13. Gottlieb RA, Gruol DL, Zhu YJ, Engler RL. Preconditioning in rabbit cardiomyocytes: role of pH, vacuolar proton ATPase, and apoptosis. J. Clin. Invest. 97:2391-2398, 1996.
14. Nishihara T, Akifusa S, Koseki T, Kato S, Muro M, Hanada N. Specific inhibitors of vacuolar type H^+-ATPases induce apoptosis. Biochem. Biophys. Res. Comm. 212:255-262, 1995.
15. Long X, Crow M, Sollott S, O'Neil L, Menees D, Boluyt MO, Hipolito L, Asai T, Lakatta, EG. Enhanced expression of p53 and apoptosis induced by blockade of vacuolar proton ATPase induces p53-mediated apoptosis in cardiomyocytes. J. Clin. Invest. 101:1453-1461, 1998.
16. Meisenholder GW, Martin SJ, Green DR, Norberg J, Babior BM, Gottlieb, RA. Events in apoptosis: acidification is downstream of protease activation and BCL-2 protection. J. Biol. Chem. 271:16260-16262, 1996.
17. Gottlieb RA, Nordberg J, Skowronski E, Babior BM. Apoptosis induced in Jurkat cells by several agents is preceded by intracellular acidification. Proc. Natl. Acad. Sci. USA 93:654-658, 1995.
18. Li J, Eastman, E. Apoptosis in an interleukin-2-dependent cytotoxic T lymphocyte cell line is associated with intracellular acidification. J. Biol. Chem. 270:3203-3211, 1995.
19. Perez-Sala D. Collado-Escobar D, Mollinedo F. Intracellular alkalinization supressess lovastatin-induced apoptosis in HL-60 cells through the inactivation of a pH-dependent endonuclease. J. Biol. Chem. 270:6235-6242, 1995.
20. Barry MA, Reynolds JE, Eastman A. Etoposide-induced apoptosis in HL-60 cells in associated with intracellular acidification. Cancer Res. 53:2349-2357, 1993.
21. Rebollo A, Gomez J, Martinez-de Aragon A, Lastres P, Silva A, Prerez-Sala D. Apoptosis induced by IL-2 withdrawal is associated with an intracellular acidification. Exp. Cell Res. 218:581-585, 1995.
22. Rajotte D, Haddad P, Haman A, Cragoe, EJ Jr, Hoang T. Role of protein kinase C and the Na^+/H^+ antiporter in suppression of apoptosis by granulocyte macrophage colony-stimulating factor. J. Biol. Chem. 267:9980-9987, 1992.
23. Gottlieb RA, Giesing HA, Engler RL, Babior BM. The acid deoxyribonuclease of neutrophils: a possible participant in apoptosis-associated genome destruction. Blood 86:2414-2418, 1995.
24. Russo CA, Weber TK, Volpe CM, Stoler DL, Petrelli NJ, Rodriguez-Bigas M, Burhans MCW, Anderson GR. An anoxia inducible endonuclease and enhanced DNA breakage as contributors to genomic instability in cancer. Cancer Res. 55:1122-1128, 1995.
25. Ko YJ, Prices C. p53: puzzle and paradigm. Genes Dev. 10:1054-1072, 1996.
26. Grabber EG, Osmanian C, Jacks T, Houseman DE, Koch CJ, Lowe SW, Giacca AJ. Hypoxia-mediated selection of cells with diminished apoptotic potential in solid tumors. Nature 379:88-91, 1996.
27. Donehower LA, Harvey M, Siagle BL, McAurthur MJ, Mongomery JR, Butel JS, Bradley R. Mice deficient for p53 are developmentally normal but susceptible to spontaneous tumors. Nature 356:215-221, 1997.
28. Schwartz JL, Indignities DZ, Zhao S. Molecular and biochemical reprogramming of oncogenes is through the activity of prooxidiants and antioxidants. Ann. NY Acad. Sci. 686:262-278, 1993.
29. Salivanova G, Wilman KG. p53: a cell cycle regulator activated by DNA damage. Adv. Cancer Res. 66:143-180, 1995.
30. Graeber TG, Peterson JF, Tsui M, Monica K, Fournace AJ, Garcia AJ. Hypoxia induces accumulation of p53, but activation of a G1-phase checkpoint by low oxygen conditions is independent of p53 Status. Mol. Cell. biol. 14:6264-6277, 1994.
31. Miyashita T, Reed JC. Tunor suppressor p53 is a direct transcriptional activator of the human bax gene. Cell 80:293-299, 1995.
32. Miyashita T, Harigani M, Hanada M, Reed JC. Identification of a p53-dependent negative response in the bcl-2 gene. Cancer Res. 54:3131-3135, 1994.

33. Yonish-Rouach E, Resnitsky D, Lotem J, Sachs L, Kimchi A, Oren M. Wild-type p53 induces apoptosis of myeloid leukemia cells that is inhibited by interleukin-6. Nature 353:345-347, 1991.

34. Gottleib E, Haffner R, von Rudin T, Wagner EF, Oren M. Down-regulation of wild-type p53 activity interferes with apoptosis of IL3-dependent hematopoietic cells following IL-3 withdrawal. EMBO J 13:1368-1374, 1994.

35. Pierzchalski P, Reiss K, Cheng W, Cirelli C, Kajstura J, Nitahara JA, Rizk M, Capogrossi MC, Anversa P. p53 induces myocytes apoptosis via the activation of the renin-angiotensin system. Exp. Cell. Res. 234:57-65, 1997.

36. Sharov VG, Sabbah NH, Shimoyama H, Goussev AV, Lesch M, Goldstein S. Evidence of cardiomyocyte apoptosis in myocardium of dogs with chronic heart failure. Am. J. Physiol. H2313-H2319, 1997.

37. Kajstura J, Cigola E, Malhotra A, Li P, Cheng W, Meggs LG, Anversa P. Angiotensin II induces apoptosis of adult ventricular myocytes in vitro. J. Mol. Cell. Cardiol. 29:859-870, 1997.

38. Cigola E, Kajstura J, Li B, Meggs LG, Anversa P. Angiotensin II activates programmed myocyte cell death in vitro. Exp. Cell Res. 231:363-371, 1997.

39. El-Diery WS., Tokino T, Velculesco VE, Levy DB, Parsons R, Trent JM, Lin D,Mercer WE, Kinzler KW, Vogelstein B. WAF-1, a potential mediator of p53 tumor suppression. Cell 75:817-825, 1993.

40. Chen C, Oliner JD, Zhan Q, Fornace AJ, Vogelstein B, Kastan MB. Interactions between p53 and MDM2 in a mammalian cell cycle checkpoint pathway. Proc. Natl. Acad. Sci. USA 91:2684-2688, 1994.

41. Kastan MB, Zhan Q, El-Diery WS, Carrier F, Jacks T, Walsh WV, Plunkett WS, Vogelstein B, Fournace AJ. A mammalian cell cycle checkpoint pathway utilizing p53 and GADD45 is defective in ataxia-telangiectasia. Cell 13:587-597, 1992.

42. Okamoto L, Beach D. Cyclin G is a transcriptional target of the p53 tumor suppressor protein. EMBO J. 13:4816-4822, 1994.

43. Owen-Schaub L, Zhang W, Cusack JC, Angelo LS, Santee SM, Fujiwara T, Roth JA,. Diesseroth AB, Zhang WW, Kruzel E, Radinsky R. Wild type p53 and a temperature sensitive mutant induce fas/Apo-1 expression. Mol. Cell. Biol. 15:3032-3040, 1995.

44. Wu GS, Burns TF, MacDonald ERIII, Jiang W, Meng R, Krantz ID, Kao G, Gan D-D, Zhou J-Y, Muschel R, Hamilton SR, Spinner N, Markowitz S, Wu G, El-Diery WS. Killer/DR5 is a DNA damage-inducible p53-regulated death receptor gene. Nature Gen. 17:141-143, 1997.

45. Nishigaki K, Minatoguchi S, Asano K, Noda T, Sano H, Kumada H, Tanaka T, Watanabe S, Seishima M, Fujiwara H. Plasma levels of soluble fas and fas ligand, apoptosis signaling receptor molecules, in patients with congestive heart failure. Circulation 94 (Suppl I):1-32, abstract.

46. Xiong Y, Hannon GJ, Zhang H, Casso D, Kobayashi R, Beach D. p21 is a univeral inhibitor of cyclin kinases. Nature 366:701-704, 1993.

47. Li R, Waga S, Hannon GJ, Beach D, Stillman B. Differential effects by the p21 cdk inhibitor on PCNA-dependent DNA replication and repair. Nature 371:534-537, 1994.

48. Waga S, Hannon GJ, Beach D, Stillman B. The p21 inhibitor of cyclin-dependent kinases controls DNA replication by interaction with PCNA. Nature 369:574-578, 1994.

49. Katayose D, Wersto R, Cowan KH, Seth P. Effects of a recombinant adenovirus expression WAF1/cip1 on cell growth, cell cycle, and apoptosis. Cell Growth Diff. 6:1207-1212, 1995.

50. Canman CE, Gilmer TM, Coutts SB, Kastan MD. Growth factor modulation of p53-mediated growth arrest versus apoptosis. Genes Dev. 9:600-611, 1995.

51. Matsushita H, Morishita R, Kida I, Aoki M, Hayashi SI, Tomita N, Yamamoto K, Moriguchi A, Noda A, Kaneda Y, Higaki J, Ogihara T. Inhibition of human vascular smooth muscle cells by overexpression of p21 gene through induction of apoptosis. Hypertension 31:493-498, 1998.

52. Boudreau N, Werb Z, Bissell MJ. Suppression of apoptosis by basement membrane requires three-dimensional tissue organization and withdrawal from the cell cycle. Proc. Natl. Acad. Sci. USA 93:3509-3513, 1996.

53. Akashi M, Hachiya M, Osawa Y, Spirin K, Suzuki G, Koeffler HP. Irradiation induces WAF1 expression through a p53-independent pathway in KG-1 cells. J. Biol. Chem. 270:19181-19187, 1995.

54. Michieli P, Chedid M, Lin D, Pierce JH, Mercer WE, Givol D. Induction of WAF1/cip1 by a p53-independent pathway. Cancer Res. 54:3391-3395, 1994.

55. Bialik SG, Geenen DL, Sasson IE, Cheng R, Horner JW Evans SM, Lord EM, Koch CJ, Kitsis RL. Myocyte apoptosis during acute myocardial infarction in the mouse localizes to hypoxic regions but occurs independently of p53. J. Clin. Inv. 100:1363-1372, 1997.

56. Leri A, Claudio PP, Li Q, Wang X, Reiss K, Wang S, Malhotra A, Kajstura J, Anversa P. Stretch-mediated release of angiotensin II induces myocyte apoptosis by activating p53 that enhances the local renin-angiotensin system and decreases the bcl2-to-bax protein ration in the cell. J. Clin. Inv. 101:1326-1342, 1998.

57. Kaghad M, Bonnet H, Yang A, Creancier L, Biscan J-C, Valent A, Minty A, Chaon P, Lelias J-M, Dumont X, Ferrara P, McKeon F, Caput D. Monoallelically expressed gene related to p53 a 1p36, a region frequently deleted in neuroblastoma and other human cancers. Cell 90:809-819, 1997

58. Just CA, Marin MC, Kaolin GW. P73 is a human p53-related protein that can induce apoptosis. Nature 389:191-194, 1997.

59. Osawa M, Ohba M, Kawahara C, Ishioka C, Kanamaru R, Katoh I, Ikawa Y, Nimura Y, Nakagawara A, Obinata M, Ikawa S. Cloning and functional analyses of human p51, which structurally and functionally resembles p53. Nat. Med. 4:839-843, 1998.

60. Evan G, Littlewood T. A matter of life and cell death. Science 281:1317-1322, 1998.

61. Reiss K, Cheng W, Giordano A, DeLuca A, Li B, Kajstura J, Anversa P. Myocardial infarction is coupled with activation of cyclin and cyclin-dependent kinases in myocytes. Exp. Cell Res. 225:44-54, 1996.

62. Kim KK, Soonpaa MH, Daud AI, Koh GY, Kim JS, Field YJ. Tumor suppressor gene expression during normal and pathological myocardial growth. J. Biol. Chem 269:22607-22613.

63. Li Q, Li B, Wang X, Leri A, Jana KP, Liu Y, Kajstura J, Baserga R, Anversa P. Overexpression of insulin-like growth factor-1 in mice protects from myocyte death after infarction, attenuating ventricular dilation, wall stress, and cardiac hypertrophy. J. Clin. Invest. 100:1991-1999, 1997.

64. Long X, Lakatta E, O'Neill L, Boluyt M, Seth P, Crow MT. Cardiomyocyte Apoptosis Triggered the Cyclin Kinase Inhibitor, p21/WAF1, is Suppressed by the Adrenergic Agonist, Phenylephrine. AHA 70th Session. Circ Suppl. 96(8): I-553; 1997.

PART THREE:
Apoptosis in cardiac disorders

III.1
Vascular disease

III.1.1
Hypertension as a cardiovascular proliverative disorder

Denis deBlois, Ph.D., Sergei Orlov, Ph.D., and Pavel Hamet, M.D., Ph.D.
University of Montreal Hospital
Montreal, Canada

INTRODUCTION

The balance between growth and apoptosis: a key determinant of cardiovascular structure.

Cardiovascular hypertrophy is an important feature of hypertension (1). However, the mechanisms regulating cardiovascular mass remain poorly defined. Spontaneously hypertensive rats (SHR) are born with elevated cardiovascular mass and DNA content, indicating the influence of genetic factors (2). Hypertrophy also develops secondarily to an increase in mechanical load as in aortic coarctation, or to chronic endocrine stimulation with, e.g., angiotensin II (AngII) (3,4). Hypertrophy which is associated with increased DNA replication is less readily reversible than hypertrophy that is solely due to increased protein synthesis without *de novo* DNA synthesis. Thus, in the vascular wall, DNA content (due to SMC hyperplasia or polyploidy (5)) may be considered as a record of past episodes of vascular growth, contributing to the persistence of the hypertensive disease. The prevention or regression of cardiovascular hypertrophy is now considered a key therapeutic target in the reduction of hypertension-associated morbidity and mortality. Apoptosis is an ubiquitous and highly regulated form of programmed cell death that is involved in tissue morphogenesis and homeostasis as the essential counterpart of cell replication (6,7). In this context, the balance between cell growth and apoptosis is a potential determinant of cardiac structure during development, disease and therapy (8).

Apoptosis is distinct from necrosis (accidental cell death) (9). Cells undergoing necrosis typically swell and show lytic disintegration, triggering an inflammatory response. In contrast, apoptotic cells show cell volume shrinkage, loss of asymmetry of the phospholidid bilayer (exposure of phosphatidylserine outside the cell membrane), margination and fragmentation of the chromatin, and budding of membranes to produce densely packed apoptotic bodies which are phagocytosed by neighboring cells without triggering an inflammatory response. The fact that apoptosis and necrosis are, or at least can be controled by distinct mechanisms in SMC is exemplified by our recent study where we demonstrated that, while necrosis can be prevented significantly by prior induction of tolerance with hsp70 and hsp27 increase, apoptosis induced by serum deprivation or staurosporine remains unmodified (10).

The significance of apoptosis has been acknowledged in various fields of physiopathology, including cancer and degenerative diseases (7). In the field of vascular biology, however, apoptosis is a newly recognized phenomenon, with potentially far reaching implications because the balance between cell replication and apoptosis is likely to be a major determinant of cardiovascular structure, resulting in organ hypertrophy, atrophy or tissue remodeling as a consequence of increased cell turnover (8,11,12). In genetically determined hypertension, we and others have described the heightened proliferative capacity of SMC (13-15) and the elevated neonatal cardiac hyperplasia, a feature which is followed by cardiac hypertrophy in the adult stage (2). Recently, we reported that the increased growth in adult hypertensive organs occurs in parallel to an increase in apoptosis (16,17), suggesting a compensatory balance between cell replication and deletion in maintaining tissue homeostasis. A similar balance between increased SMC growth and apoptosis has been described in lamb arteries showing regression after birth (18) and in intimal lesions formed after vascular injury (reviewed in (8)). Taken together, these observations raise the intriguing possibility that SMC may undergo significant turnover in the arterial wall during the course of life and disease.

COMMON PATHWAYS OF APOPTOSIS

Cell volume shrinkage is one of the most universal early markers of apoptosis. In the immune system, apoptotic cell shrinkage is so impressive that the term "shrinkage-mediated necrosis" was firstly used to describe this mechanism of cell death (6). Recently, we reported that a transient cell volume decrease precedes chromatin cleavage in SMC undergoing apoptosis (19). Interestingly, this step is amplified in SMC from hypertensive animals, suggesting that cell shrinkage could be involved in the abnormal development of the apoptotic program in genetically hypertensive SMC.

Two stages of shrinkage have been revealed in immune system cells undergoing apoptosis. In gamma-irradiated thymocytes, a rapid 24% shrinkage of cell volume was followed by a further gradual 20% decline of volume in the next few hours. The first stage of initial volume decrease is caused by loss of the organic osmolytes and obliged water, whereas the second stage is due to chromatin condensation and intracellular membrane rearrangement (20). The Coulter Counter technique cannot be used for cell volume measurements in adherent SMC undergoing apoptosis, in contrast to non-adherent (e.g., immune) cells. To overcome this problem, we developed a novel approach, i.e. we measured the volume of 14C-urea-available space in the SMC (19). We showed that serum deprivation cause a transient volume decrease that is greater in SMC from SHR, in correlation with a faster progression of apoptosis. Cell shrinkage caused by a hyperosmotic shock stimulated by two- to three-fold the apoptotic response to serum deprivation in SMC. Bortner and Sidowski (21) reported similar results in mouse thymocytes undergoing cycloheximide-dependent apoptosis. These results suggest that the initial volume decrease in SMC is a primary event rather than a consequence of the terminal steps of apoptosis, possibly leading to the condensation of biopolymers and loss of cytoplasmic and membrane components. Our observations are consistent with the reported kinetics of cell shrinkage, internucleosomal chromatin cleavage and cell density alteration in apoptotic thymocytes and T lymphocytes (22-24). Interestingly, partial inhibition of cell shrinkage and apoptosis was obtained in eosinophils treated with K+ channel blockers (25). Taken together, these results suggest that the initial cell volume decrease in SMC undergoing apoptosis is caused by alterations in monovalent ion transporter activity. Furthermore, cell shrinkage may play a central role in the induction and progression of apoptosis in SMC.

The next unifying theme of the apoptosis pathway is the necessary activation of caspases, a family of cysteine proteases that cleave their substrates at specific aspartate-containing sites and that are analogous to the CED-3 death-protein of the nematode. Characterization of caspases as effectors of apoptosis is now a booming issue in biology (26). Members of the mammalian caspase family are analogs of interleukin-1beta-converting enzyme (ICE) and may be grouped in three classes based on the recognition sequence on the substrate. Proteolytic activation of caspases is an early event in apoptosis in response to various death stimuli (27-29), including in SMC. Different caspases can activate each other in a proteolytic cascade converging towards cell death (30). As a consequence, it is likely that different caspases can be used as markers of the activation of apoptosis. Substrates for activated caspases include molecules regulating cell structure (nuclear lamins), cell cycle progression (Rb) and DNA repair (poly (ADP-ribose) polymerase, or PARP). Apoptosis is characterized by heightened specific endonuclease activity, as often evidenced by the degradation of DNA into oligonucleosomal 180-200 base pair integer fragments (appearing as a "ladder" of DNA fragments after conventional agarose gel electrophoresis) (31). The presence of internucleosomal cleavage fragments of DNA is a commonly used marker of apoptosis. It should be noted, however, that oligonucleosomal DNA fragmentation is actually a post-mortem event in the apoptosis pathway. Because of this, caspase activity may provide a more reliable marker in studies of cell population undergoing rapid changes in levels of apoptotic activity (27).

REGULATION OF CARDIOVASCULAR APOPTOSIS BY ANTIHYPERTENSIVE DRUGS

Evidence that specific antihypertensive drugs modulate cardiovascular cell survival in vivo came from studies in SHR treated with specific antihypertensive agents, notably calcium channel blockers and inhibitors of the angiotensin pathway. With losartan treatment, for instance, we showed that SMC apoptosis is transiently increased in the aorta early during reversal of arterial hypertrophy (32). In this model, the induction of arterial apoptosis precedes the inhibition of arterial DNA synthesis and the reduction of DNA content (schematized in Figure 1).

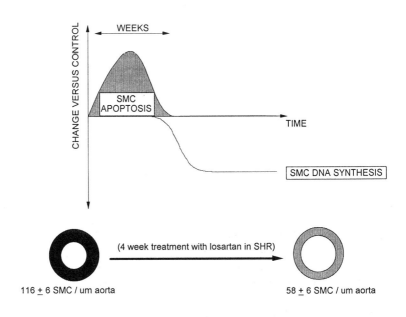

Figure 1   Schematic representation of the time course of apoptosis induction and DNA synthesis inhibition in SMC during the regression of aortic hypertrophy in SHR treated with antihypertensive drugs. Administration of losartan for 4 weeks resulted in a significant decrease in SMC number in the SHR aorta (35c).

Moreover, arterial cell death is not a secondary response to blood pressure reduction because effective antihypertensive treatment with hydralazine does not affect arterial mass, growth or apoptosis. The group of Diez et al (33) also showed that SMC expression of the apoptosis-regulatory proteins BAX and BCL-2 was altered in SHR coronary arteries in a way that favored SMC survival. Moreover, the ratio of BAX to BCL-2 expression was normalized in association with regression of arterial hypertrophy by long term treatment with the ACE inhibitor quinapril, further suggesting a role for apoptosis in the process. Increased SMC apoptosis also occurs in the hypertrophied aorta of DOCA-salt hypertensive rats (34). In this model, an antagonist of the endothelin receptor subtype A further accentuated SMC apoptosis therefore reducing vascular growth.

Studies in SHR also showed that cardiac cell apoptosis is regulated by antihypertensive drugs and these effects appear to follow complex time courses. Aging SHR show increased levels of cardiomyocyte apoptosis compared normotensive controls, a feature that is prevented by long term treatment with an ACE inhibitor (35a). With long term administration of losartan, there is a significant prevention of cardiomyocyte apoptosis and BAX expression in the aging SHR heart (35b). These effects possibly reflect a mechanism for increased myocardial survival. In the short term, however (i.e. within the first 2 weeks after initiation of drug treatment with losartan), there is transient induction of programmed cell death in the heart, possibly reflecting the suppression of fibrosis (35c). The transient increase in apoptosis in response to losartan reaches a maximum around 7 days of treatment, and it is associated with the sustained inhibition of cardiac DNA synthesis and reversal of hypertrophy in the following weeks (35c). Interestingly, we previously observed a transient induction of apoptosis also in rat hearts undergoing cardiac hypertrophy in response to an acute pressure-overload induced by aortic coarctation. In this model, the stimulation of cardiac apoptosis reaches a maximum within the first week of pressure overload (3). Taken together, these observations lead us to suggest that studies of cardiovascular tissue remodeling should take into account the existence of "time windows of apoptosis" during pathogenesis and pharmacotherapy (36). Moreover, these results suggest that the regulation of cardiac apoptosis by inhibitors of the angiotensin II pathway is complex and dependent on the duration of drug administration.

These results implicating ACE and AT1 receptors in the regulation of cardiac cell apoptosis in SHR are consistent with the emerging role of AngII as a key regulator of cardiac mass and structure. Suppressing the angiotensin II pathway prevents or reverses the development of cardiac and vascular hypertrophy and increases survival in patients and animal models (37,38). Tissue activity of the angiotensin system (ACE, AT1 expression) is increased in the overloaded heart (39). Stretching of cardiomyocytes as in pressure overload stimulates a hypertrophic growth response that is partly dependent on the autocrine production of AngII (40). Stretching also induces cardiomyocyte expression of the death mediator Fas in association with increased cardiomyocyte apoptosis (12). Stimulation of AT1 receptors for AngII in cardiomyocytes induces both cellular hypertrophy and apoptotic cell death (41). Cardiomyocyte apoptosis induced by p53 is also AngII-dependent (42). Interestingly, AngII acts as a trigger for programmed cell death in cardiomyocytes primed for apoptosis by a high Bax to Bcl-2 ratio of apoptosis regulatory proteins (42). In contrast to myocytes, cultured fibroblasts respond to AT1 receptor stimulation with increased proliferation (43). Taken together these data suggest that AngII regulates the cell growth / cell death balance in opposite direction in myocytes and non-myocytes in the heart.

Signal transduction pathways triggering apoptosis are not specific to this biological response. SMC apoptosis can be induced in vitro by cAMP, nitric oxide (NO), protein kinase C inhibitors or calcium channel blockers (reviewed in (8)). A well-known method of inducing apoptosis in vitro is growth factor deprivation by serum withdrawal (44). The state of "survival factor deprivation" seen in cultured cells may reflect what happens in the arterial wall undergoing SMC apoptosis and regression in response to antihypertensive drugs targeting L-type calcium channels, angiotensin II AT1 receptors or endothelin A receptors (34,45). These pharmacotherapeutic tools are thus potentially useful in identifying molecular pathways regulating cardiovascular apoptosis in vivo. Dysregulations causing accelerated progression into the cell cycle stimulate apoptosis ("activation-induced apoptosis" (46)). Two major checkpoints exist during cell cycle progression to ensure the fidelity of the genetic information before and after DNA replication, at the G1/S and G2/M transition points, respectively (47). Several lines of evidence suggest that cell cycle checkpoints are altered in SMC from SHR. First, SHR SMC show shortened G1/S and G2/M phases of the cell cycle (48). Second, the heart weight/body weight (HW/BW) ratio in adult recombinant inbred strain (RIS) sets (p=0.006) and in 12 newborns strains which remained in their tercile of low or high heart weight from newborn to adulthood mapped (p=0.0009) to the Acaa locus on the rat chromosome 8 (49). Finally, apoptosis caused by unscheduled progression into the cell cycle has been described in SMC overexpressing c-myc (a growth-related transcription factor) or E1A (an adenoviral functional homologue of c-myc) (50,51).

CANDIDATE GENES INVOLVED IN CARDIOVASCULAR CELL SURVIVAL IN HYPERTENSION

Apoptosis is a cytokine-regulated form of cell death (52). Indirect evidence suggest that TNF is a candidate mediator for abnormalities of apoptosis in hypertension. TNF is a major apoptotic stimulus implicating the ceramide pathway and resulting in the activation of caspases in cardiovascular tissues (53). Hypertensive cells show polymorphism of the TNF gene (63). The two forms of TNF, alpha and ß, are encoded by two genes localized at the boundary of complexes III and I of the major histocompatibility complex (MHC) on chromosome 6 in humans and, in the rat, in the RT1 complex on chromosome 20 which contains gene(s) contributing to hypertension (54). Importantly, conditions resulting in TNF stimulation include serum withdrawal (45,56). Activation of the caspase cascade of proteolysis can be blocked by small heat shock proteins (56). It is worthy to note that under certain conditions, TNF or ceramide can inhibit apoptosis, e.g., in hippocampal neurons stimulated by oxidative insult (56). TNF can also induce the antideath factor bcl-2 (57), further suggesting that TNF is able both to stimulate and inhibit apoptosis (56,58). Consistent with this, we reported that TNF increases apoptosis in cells from normotensive animals while decreasing it in cells obtained from SHR (17). In a recent report, Krown and colleagues demonstrated that TNF induced apoptosis in cardiac myocytes (59). These authors observed a biphasic response to TNF (stimulation, then inhibition of apoptosis as concentrations of TNF were increased). The bivalent potential of TNF in regulating apoptosis may thus be relevant to cardiovascular structure determination in hypertension.

Interestingly, several small heat shock proteins including hsp27, drosophilia D hsp27 and human ß-crystallin are able to inhibit apoptosis induced via the TNF pathway (60,61). The fact that hsp27 functions as an important regulator of TNF-induced apoptosis is relevant to hypertension since we found a single base mutation in the 3' untranslated region. (UTR) of hsp27 gene (62) segregates with blood pressure and increased left ventricular mass in recombinant inbred strains (RIS) and F2 crosses of rats (62). Moreover, hsp27 mutation segregates with left ventricular mass independently of blood pressure and salt intake. It is, therefore, exciting to envision that hsp27 plays a role as an apoptotic inhibitor. Thus, hsp70 and TNF both localized in the RT1 complex of the rat and both are prime candidates for an altered environmental responsiveness underlying high blood pressure (64,65).

In conclusion, the balance between cell growth and apoptosis is emerging as a key determinant of cardiovascular hypertrophy. Studies of pathways and underlying genetic determinants of the balance between cell growth and apoptosis may help reduce cardiovascular morbidity and mortality associated with high blood pressure.

ACKNOWLEDGEMENTS

Supported in part by the Medical Research Council of Canada, Bayer Canada and Merck-Frosst Canada. D.D. is a Scholar of the Fonds de la Recherche en Santé du Québec.

References

1. Folkow, B. 1982. Physiological aspects of primary hypertension. Physiol Rev 62:347-504.
2. Walter, S. V. and P. Hamet. 1986. Enhanced DNA synthesis in heart and kidney of newborn spontaneously hypertensive rats. Hypertension 8:520-525.
3. Teiger, E., T. V. Dam, L. Richard, C. Wisnewsky, B. S. Tea, L. Gaboury, J. Tremblay, K. Schwartz, and P. Hamet. 1996. Apoptosis in pressure overload-induced heart hypertrophy in the rat. J Clin Invest 97:2891-2897.
4. Kim, S., K. Ohta, A. Hamaguchi, T. Yukimura, K. Miura, and H. Iwao. 1995. Angiotensin II induces cardiac phenotypic modulation and remodeling in vivo in rats. Hypertension 25:1252-1259.
5. Owens, G. K. 1989. Control of hypertrophic versus hyperplastic growth of vascular smooth muscle cells. Am J Physiol 257(6Pt2):H1755-H1765.
6. Kerr, J. F. R., A. H. Wyllie, and A. R. Currie. 1972. Apoptosis: a basic biological phenomenon with wide-ranging implications in tissue kinetics. Br J Cancer 26:239-257.
7. Thompson, G. B. 1995. Apoptosis in the pathogenesis and treatment of disease. Science 267:1456-1462.
8. Hamet, P., D. deBlois, T. -V. Dam, L. Richard, E. Teiger, B. -S. Tea, S. N. Orlov, and J. Tremblay. 1996. Apoptosis and vascular wall remodeling in hypertension. Can J of Physiol & Pharmacol 74(7):850-861.
9. Majno, G. and I. Joris. 1995. Apoptosis, oncosis and necrosis. An overview of cell death. Am J Pathol 146:3-15.
10. Champagne, M. -J., P. Dumas, M. R. Bennett, S. N. Orlov, P. Hamet, and J. Tremblay. 1998. HSPs expression selectively protects against heat shock protein-induced growth inhibition and necrosis but not apoptosis in vascular smooth muscle cells. Hypertension 33(3):906-913.
11. Kajstura, J., M. Mansukhani, W. Cheng, K. Reiss, S. Krajewski, J. C. Reed, F. Quaini, E. H. Sonnenblick, and P. Anversa. 1995. Programmed cell death and expression of the protooncogene bcl-2 in myocytes during postnatal maturation of the heart. Exp Cell Res 219:110-121.
12. Cheng, W., B. Li, J. Kajstura, P. Li, M. S. Wolin, E. H. Sonnenblick, T. H. Hintze, G. Olivetti, and P. Anversa. 1995. Stretch-induced programmed myocyte cell death. J Clin Invest 96:2247-2259.
13. Hadrava, V., J. Tremblay, and P. Hamet. 1989. Abnormalities in growth characteristics of aortic smooth muscle cells in spontaneously hypertensive rats. Hypertension 13:589-597.

14. Scott-Burden, T., T. J. Resink, U. Baur, M. Burgin, and F. R. Buhler. 1989. Epidermal growth factor responsiveness in smooth muscle cells from hypertensive and normotensive rats. Hypertension 13:295-304.

15. Paquet, J. L., M. Baudouin-Legros, P. Marche, and P. Meyer. 1989. Enhanced proliferating activity of cultured smooth muscle cells from SHR. Am J Hypertens 2:108-110.

16. Hamet, P. 1995. Proliferation and apoptosis in hypertension. Curr Opin Nephrol Hypertens 4:1-7.

17. Hamet, P., L. Richard, T. -V. Dam, E. Teiger, S. N. Orlov, L. Gaboury, F. Gossard, and J. Tremblay. 1995. Apoptosis in target organs of hypertension. Hypertension 26:642-648.

18. Cho, A., D. W. Courtman, and B. L. Langille. 1995. Apoptosis (programmed cell death) in arteries of the neonatal lamb. Circ Res 76:168-175.

19. Orlov, S. N., T. V. Dam, J. Tremblay, and P. Hamet. 1996. Apoptosis in vascular smooth muscle cells: Role of cell shrinkage. Biochem Biophys Res Commun 221:708-715.

20. Klassen, N. V., P. R. Walker, C. K. Ross, J. Cygler, and B. Lach. 1993. Two-stage cell shrinkage and the OER for radiation-induced apoptosis of rat thymocytes. Intern J Rad Biol 64:571-581.

21. Bortner, C. D. and J. A. Cidlowski. 1996. Absence of volume regulatory mechanisms contributes to the rapid activation of apoptosis in thymocytes. Am J Physiol 271:C950-C961.

22. Wyllie, A. H. and R. G. Morris. 1982. Hormone-induced cell death. Purification ad properties of thymocytes undergoing apoptosis after glucocorticoid treatment. Am J Pathol 109:78-87.

23. Wesselborg, S. and D. Kabelitz. 1993. Activation-driven death of human T cell clones: time course kinetics of the induction of cell shrinkage, DNA fragmentation, and cell death. Cellular Immunology 148:234-241.

24. Thomas, N. and P. A. Bell. 1981. Glucocorticoid-induced cell-size changes and nuclear fragility in rat thymocytes. Mol Cell Endocrinol 22:71-84.

25. Beauvais, F., L. Michel, and L. Dubertret. 1995. Human eosinophils in culture undergo a striking and rapid shrinkage during apoptosis. J Leukocyte Biol 57:851-855.

26. Vaux, D. L., G. Haecker, and A. Strasser. 1994. An evolutionary perspective on apoptosis. Cell 76:777-779.

27. Nicholson, D. W., A. Ali, N. A. Thornberry, J. P. Vaillancourt, C. K. King, M. Gallant, Y. Gareau, P. R. Friffin, M. Labelle, Y. A. Lazebnik, N. A. Munday, S. M. Raju, M. E. Smulson, T. T. Yamin, V. L. Yu, and D. K. Miller. 1995. Identification and inhibition of the ICE/CCED-3 protease necessary for mammalian apoptosis. Nature 376:37-43.

28. Darmon, A. J., D. W. Nicholson, and R. C. Bleackley. 1995. Activation of the apoptotic protease CPP32 by cytotoxic cell-derived granzyme B. Nature 377:446-448.

29. Schlegel, J., I. Peters, S. Orrenius, D. K. Miller, N. A. Thornberry, T. T. Yamin, and D. W. Nicholson. 1996. CPP32 apopain is a key interleukin 1-beta converting enzyme-like protease involved in Fas-mediated apoptosis. J Biol Chem 271:1841-1844.

30. Orth, K., K. O'Rourke, G. S. Salvesen, and V. M. Dixit. 1996. Molecular ordering of apoptotic mammalian CED-3/ICE-like proteases. J Biol Chem 271:20977-20980.

31. Bortner, C. D., N. B. E. Oldenburg, and J. A. Cidlowski. 1995. The role of DNA fragmentation in apoptosis. Trends in Cell Biology 5:21-26.

32. deBlois, D., B. -S. Tea, T. -V. Dam, J. Tremblay, and P. Hamet. 1997. Smooth muscle cell apoptosis during vascular regression in spontaneously hypertensive rats. Hypertension 29:340-349.

33. Diez, J., A. Panizo, M. Hernandez, and J. Pardo. 1997. Is the regulation of apoptosis altered in smooth muscle cells of adult spontaneously hypertensive rats? Hypertension 29:776-780.

34. Sharifi, A. M. and E. L. Schiffrin. 1997. Apoptosis in aorta of deoxycorticosterone acetate-salt hypertensive rats: effect of endothelin receptor antagonism. J Hypertens 15:1441-1448.

35a. Diez, J., A. Panizo, M. Hernandez, F. Vega, I. Sola, M. A. Fortuno, and J. Pardo. 1997. Cardiomyocyte apoptosis and cardiac angiotensin-converting enzyme in spontaneously hypertensive rats. Hypertension 30:1029-1034.

35b. Fortuno, M. A., S. Ravassa, J. C. Etayo, and J. Diez. 1998. Overexpression of Bax protein and enhanced apoptosis in the left ventricle of spontaneously hypertensive rats: effects of AT1 blockade with losartan. Hypertension 32:280-286.

35c. Tea B-S, Dam T-V, Moreau P, Hamet P, deBlois D, 1999. Apoptosis during regression of cardiac hypertrophy in spontaneously hypertensive rats: temporal regulation and spatial heterogeneity. Hypertension (In press)

36. Hamet, P., P. Moreau, T-V. Dam, S. N. Orlov, B-S. Tea, D. deBlois, and J. Tremblay. 1996. The time window of apoptosis: a new component in the therapeutic strategy for cardiovascular remodeling. J Hypertens 14 (Suppl 5):S65-S70.

37. Schiffrin, E. L., L. Y. Deng, and P. Larochelle. 1994. Effects of a beta-blocker or a converting enzyme inhibitor on resistance arteries in essential hypertension. Hypertension 23:83-91.

38. Touyz, R. M., J. Fareh, G. Thibault, and E. L. Schiffrin. 1996. Intracellular Ca2+ modulation by angiotensin II and endothelin-1 in cardiomyocytes and fibroblasts from hypertrophied hearts of spontaneously hypertensive rats. Hypertension 28:797-805.

39. Brooks, W. W., O. H. Bing, K. G. Robinson, M. T. Slawsky, D. M. Chaletsky, and C. H. Conrad. 1997. Effect of angiotensin-converting enzyme inhibition on myocardial fibrosis and function in hypertrophied and failing myocardium from the spontaneously hypertensive rat (see comments). Circulation 96:4002-4010.

40. Li, Z., O. H. Bing, X. Long, K. G. Robinson, and E. G. Lakatta. 1997. Increased cardiomyocyte apoptosis during the transition to heart failure in the spontaneously hypertensive rat. Am J Physiol 272:H2313-H2319.

41. Tomanek, R. J. and M. T. Whitaker. 1990. Compensated function in hypertrophied ventricles of Wistar Kyoto and spontaneously hypertensive rats. Cardiovasc Res 24:204-209.

42. Friberg, P. and M. A. Adams. 1990. Cardiac and vascular structural adaptation in experimental hypertension. Eur Heart J 11 Suppl G:65-71.

43. Conrad, C. H., W. W. Brooks, K. G. Robinson, and O. H. Bing. 1991. Impaired myocardial function in spontaneously hypertensive rats with heart failure. Am J Physiol 260:H136-H145.

44. Bennett, M. R., G. I. Evan, and S. M. Schwartz. 1995. Apoptosis of human vascular smooth muscle cells derived from normal vessels and coronary atherosclerotic plaques. J Clin Invest 95(5):2266-2274.

45. Hannun, Y. A. 1996. Functions of ceramide in coordinating cellular responses to stress. Science 274:1855-1859.

46. Green, D. R., A. Mahboubi, W. Nishoka, F. Echeverri, Y. Shi, J. Glynn, Y. Yang, J. Ashwell, and R. Bissonnette. 1994. Promotion and inhibition og activation-induced apoptosis in T-cell hybridomas by oncogenes and related signals. Immunol Rev 142:321-342.

47. Paulovicj, A. G., D. P. Toczyski, and H. L. Hartwell. 1997. When checkpoints fail. Cell 88:315-322.

48. Hadrava, V., J. Tremblay, R. P. Sekaly, and P. Hamet. 1992. Accelerated entry of aortic smooth muscle cells from spontaneously hypertensive rats into the S phase of the cell cycle. Biochem Cell Biol 70:599-604.

49. Hamet, P., Y. L. Sun, J. Kunes, M. Pravenec, V. Kren, and J. Tremblay. 1997. The persistance of rat neonatal phenotype of heart weight into adulthood is associated with Acaa locus on chromosome 8. Hypertension 30(3):485.(Abstr.)

50. Bennett, M. R., G. I. Evan, and A. C. Newby. 1994. Deregulated expression of the c-myc oncogene abolishes inhibition of proliferation of rat vascular smooth muscle cells by serum reduction, interferon-gamma, heparin, and cyclic nucleotide analogues and induces apoptosis. Circ Res 74:525-536.

51. Bennett, M. R., G. I. Evan, and S. M. Schwartz. 1995. Apoptosis of rat vascular smooth muscle cells is regulated by p53 dependent and independent pathways. Circ Res 77:266-273.

52. Nagata, S. 1997. Apoptosis by death factor. (Review) (85 refs). Cell 88:355-365.

53. Vilcek, J. and T. H. Lee. 1991. Tumor necrosis factor. New insights into the molecular mechanisms of its multiple actions. (Review) (99 refs). J Biol Chem 266:7313-7316.

54. Hamet, P., D. Kong, M. Pravenec, J. Kunes, V. Kren, P. Klir, Y. Sun, and J. Tremblay. 1992. Restriction fragment length polymorphism of hsp70 gene, localized in the RT1 complex, spontaneously hypertensive rats. J Hypertens 19:611-614.

56. Goodman, Y. and M. P. Mattson. 1996. Ceramide protects hippocampal neurons against excitotoxic and oxidative insults, and amyloid beta-peptide toxicity. J Neurochem 66:869-872.

57. Fernandez, A., M. C. Marin, T. McDonnell, and H. N. Ananthaswamy. 1994. Differential sensitivity of normal and Ha-ras-transformed C3H mouse embryo fibroblasts to tumor necrosis factor: induction of bcl-2, c-myc, and manganese superoxide dismutase in resistant cells. Oncogene 9:2009-2017.

58. Park, E., C. I. Kalunta, T. T. Nguyen, C. L. Wang, F. S. Chen, C. K. Lin, J. S. Kaptein, and P. M. Lad. 1996. TNF-alpha inhibits anti-IgM-mediated apoptosis in Ramos cells. Exp Cell Res 226:1-10.

59. Krown, K. A., M. T. Page, C. Nguyen, D. Zechner, V. Gutierrez, K. L. Comstock, C. C. Glembotski, P. J. Quintana, and R. A. Sabbadini. 1996. Tumor necrosis factor alpha-induced apoptosis in cardiac myocytes. Involvement of the sphingolipid signaling cascade in cardiac cell death. J Clin Invest 98:2854-2865.

60. Kim, Y. M., M. E. de Vera, S. C. Watkins, and T. R. Billiar. 1997. Nitric oxide protects cultured rat hepatocytes from tumor necrosis factor-alpha-induced apoptosis by inducing heat shock protein 70 expression. J Biol Chem 272:1402-1411.

61. Mehlen, P., K. Schulze-Osthoff, and A. P. Arrigo. 1996. Small stress proteins as novel regulators of apoptosis. Heat shock protein 27 blocks Fas/APO-1- and staurosporine-induced cell death. J Biol Chem 271:16510-16514.

62. Hamet, P., M. A. Kaiser, Y. Sun, V. Page, M. Vincent, V. Kren, M. Pravenec, J. Kunes, J. Tremblay, and N. J. Samani. 1996. HSP27 locus cosegregates with left ventricular mass independently of blood pressure. Hypertension 28:1112-1117.

63. Pravenec, M., Y. L. Sun, J. Kunes, D. Kong, V. Kren, P. Klir, J. Tremblay, and P. Hamet. 1991. Environmenta suceptibility in hypertension: potential role of HSP70 and TNFalpha genes. J Vasc Med Biol 3:297-302.

64. Hamet P., Pausova Z., Adarichev V., Adaricheva K., Tremblay J. 1996. Hypertension: genes and environment. J Hypertens 1998 Apr;16(4):397-418

65. Pausova Z., Tremblay J. and P. Hamet. 1999. Gene-environment interaction in hypertension. Curr Hypertens Report (In press).

III.1.2
Apoptosis in human atherosclerosis

Gerhard Bauriedel, M.D., Randolph Hutter, M.D.,
Ulrich Welsch, M.D., and Berndt Lüderitz, M.D.
Universität Bonn, Bonn, and Universität München, München, Germany

INTRODUCTION

A better understanding and more effective treatment of acute coronary syndrome and postangioplasty restenosis remain major issues in clinical cardiology. As for acute coronary syndromes, from the pathobiologic perspective, instability of coronary atheroma (e.g. plaque rupture), and subsequent thrombosis may result in myocardial infarction and death, as well as the progression of the arteriosclerotic disease. The underlying factors and mechanisms causing plaque rupture are not completely understood. Recent investigational work on human vulnerable lesions shows a low density of smooth muscle cells (SMCs) and collagen as well as an increased frequency of inflammatory cells, associated with a considerable tissue degrading activity, to be basically implicated in the breakdown of the plaque fibrous cap (1-8). Indeed, elimination of SMCs *via* apoptosis (programmed cell death) may contribute to a weakened plaque texture and to a reduced production and deposition of extracellular matrix proteins, both leading to plaque instability.

Also, restenosis remains a pertinacious limitation of any angioplasty mode including stent application, though novel insights into the process of restenosis, i.e. constrictive remodeling or inadequate compensatory enlargement have been made (9-18). Based on the concept that apoptosis of SMCs plays an important role in vascular wall remodeling, recent studies on human plaque tissue have focussed on apoptosis in different intimal settings, such as saphenous vein grafts (19), early and advanced atherosclerotic lesions (20-22) and, also, restenotic lesions (23). From histo-morphometric evaluation, it is widely accepted that clinically symptomatic, human restenotic lesions show an increased density of SMCs (24-27). Recent experimental work using atherectomy tissue from coronary and peripheral recurrent lesions demonstrates a phenotypic modulation of these cells (25,26) as a prerequisit for their mitogenic stimulation (28). Initiating and constitutive stimuli are believed to be several growth factors and vasoactive peptides, some of which, including PDGF and bFGF, are known to be upregulated in cell-rich restenotic tissue (18,25,29,30). For a long time, enhanced proliferative activity of SMCs has been favoured to explain the high cell density in restenosis (24,31,32). However, recent experimental work on the expression of the proliferation marker PCNA *in situ* is controversial (27,33). A large atherectomy study compared 100 coronary restenotic with 118 primary lesions. More than 70% of all lesions showed no proliferative activity; of the remaining immunoreactive restenoses the majority revealed ≤1% of the cells to be PCNA-positive, thereby exhibiting a similar expression pattern as seen in chronic lesions (33). Notably, the authors postulated that, because the constituent cells of primary and recurrent stenoses replicate at similar rates, a mitigated cell death rate (low apoptosis) may accelerate the growth of restenotic tissue (33).

Based on these concepts, the present contribution reports on the presence and extent of apoptosis in human coronary atherosclerosis with specific regard on acute coronary syndromes and postangioplasty restenosis as clinically important scenarios. Furthermore, we report on different stages and cell-specific attribution of apoptosis by using human coronary tissue samples retrieved by percutaneous atherectomy.

PRESENCE OF APOPTOSIS IN HUMAN ATHEROSCLEROSIS - STAGES OF APOPTOSIS AND DISTINCTION FROM NECROSIS

The ultrastructural morphology of programmed cell death seen in human atherosclerotic lesions is comparable with transmission electron microscopic (TEM) findings previously reported for different tissues of human and animal origin, i.e. epidermis, intestinum, liver, thymus and variable tumors (34-37). Apoptosis of SMCs and macrophages, typically characterized by cell shrinkage, chromatin condensation and membrane budding (34,35) are present in coronary, but also in carotid and femoral plaque tissue (Figures 1 and 2). Consistently, in addition, numerous apoptotic bodies are found in these atheroma. Figure 2b illustrates representative ultrastructural examples. Apoptotic bodies exhibit diameters of 5-20 μm, are round and predominantly reveal granular or fragmented contents. Furthermore, a surrounding membrane of about 5 nm thickness is detectable (Figure 2b). Systematic analysis demonstrates apoptotic bodies to be either encircled by extracellular matrix fields or to be membrane-bound to adjacent SMCs or macrophages; others are located within the cytoplasm. Extracellular matrix fields contiguous to apoptotic bodies commonly reveal a normal texture without focal desintegration. Importantly, a clear differentiation of apoptosis from necrosis can be easily accomplished by TEM analysis. Findings typical for necrosis are an intracellular decompartimentation, loss of an intact cell membrane, accompanied by the dispersion of cytoplasmic organelles in pericellular areas as well as degraded extracellular matrix (Figure 2c).

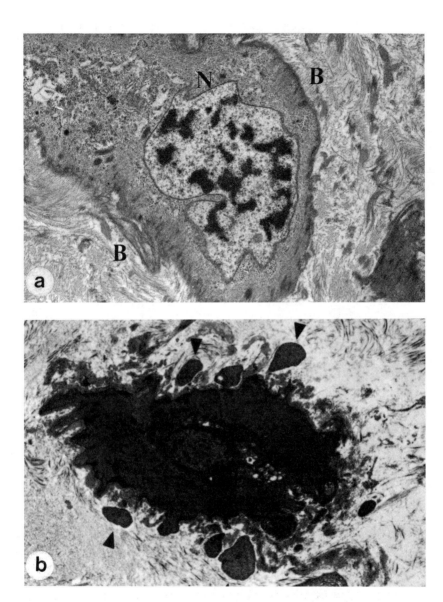

Figure 1 TEM of primary coronary lesions illustrating ultrastructural features of viable compared with apoptotic SMC. (a) Viable SMC of beginning intermediate phenotype, surrounded by a distinct basement membrane (B). The nucleus is intact with a granular pattern of chromatin organization (N); x6,700. (b) High-power magnification of a small apoptotic SMC in an UA lesion. Characteristic signs of SMC apoptosis are the dark, electron dense appearance indicative of cross-linking events of cytoplasmic proteins leading to SMC shrinkage, the condensed clumped chromatin lining the nuclear envelope, and the increased activity and outpouching of membrane segments (arrowheads); x8,200.

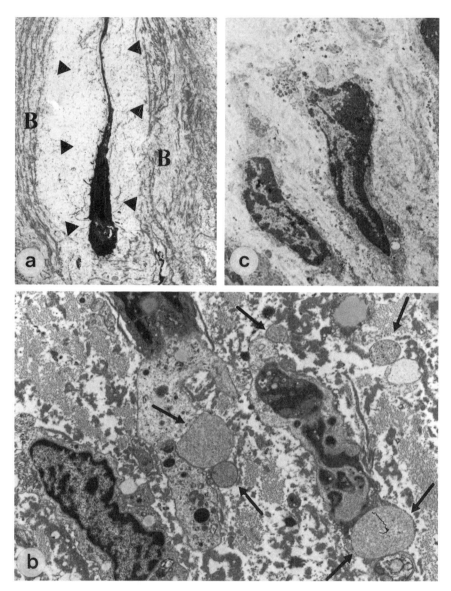

Figure 2 TEM of coronary primary lesions. (a) Shrinkage of an apoptotic SMC and detached anchorage from surrounding extracellular matrix are indicated by its condensed cytoplasm and a *de novo* pericellular territory (arrowheads), known as anoikis phenomenon. The multi-lamellated basal laminae (B) encircling the apoptotic SMC suggest repetitive loss of SMC/matrix adhesion and reconstitution of B synthesis; x7,600. (b) Ultrastructural features of apoptotic remnants (apoptotic bodies) found in different intra- and extracellular locations (arrows). The variable, often speckled appearance of these vesicles is due to gradual differences in the organization and the electron density pattern of their content, and suggests ongoing degradation processes; x6,000. (c) Two necrotic cells in an UA lesion. Typical findings are almost lost cell membranes, dispersed cytoplasmic organelles and degraded pericellular matrix; x7,000.

Frequently, in the neighborhood of necrosis, macrophages can be seen, signalling local inflammatory events. Our findings complement previous reports from us (25,26,38) and from other groups (21,32) which demonstrate TEM to be a valuable method for obtaining important information about texture, composition, and identity of extra- and intracellular structures found in the arterial intima. Also, TUNEL (terminal deoxynucleotidyl transferase-mediated dUTP nick-end labeling) testing (32,39,40) indicates apoptosis by the detection of fragmented DNA. Importantly, any overestimation of intimal apoptosis by this immunohistochemical test that may occur due to methodical problems can be largely excluded, when tissue slices are systematically preincubated in citric acid. By this pretreatment step, unspecific binding on matrix vesicles and apoptotic bodies *via* biotin- or digoxigenin-conjugated nucleotides is prohibited, thereby significantly increasing the specifity of the TUNEL test to detect apoptotic nuclei (41). Indeed, important work by Kockx *et al.* on human carotid plaques has revealed that additional citric acid or EDTA incubation leads to a more than 50% loss of TUNEL signals in areas full of non-nuclear calcified structures (41). Recent studies in our laboratory could confirm this experience and, in addition, showed that there is a strong correlation by use of either TUNEL labeling or TEM analysis to detect and quantitate intimal apoptosis (23). Figure 3 illustrates a histology of a coronary restenosis, demonstrating typically high cellularity and sparse TUNEL signals.

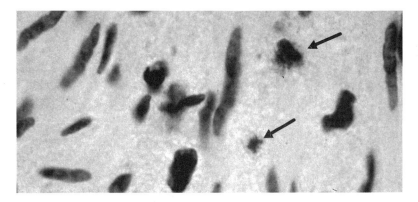

Figure 3 Photomicrograph of *in situ* detection of DNA fragmentation by (TUNEL) testing. Cell-rich restenotic tissue illustrates TUNEL-signals of only a few cells associated with nuclear shrinkage and fragmentation (arrows). Adjacent unlabeled nuclei fail to bear these typical light microscopic signs of apoptosis; x650.

APOPTOSIS IN SPECIFIC TYPES OF HUMAN ATHEROSCLEROSIS - RELATION TO INTIMAL CELL COMPOSITION

Acute coronary syndrome *versus* stable angina primary atheroma

Background. Plaque rupture and subsequent thrombosis are key events in the onset of acute coronary syndromes and in the progression of the underlying arteriosclerotic disease (1,2,5). Therefore, a better understanding of the mechanisms and factors that allow the fibrous cap to become vulnerable is of outstanding importance. However, our knowledge of the underlying pathogenic elements that (i) predispose to or (ii) elicit the rupture of coronary atheroma is still incomplete. A body of intense work on human vulnerable lesions demonstrates that a sparse density of SMCs and collagen, as well as an increased frequency of inflammatory cells, associated with a considerable tissue degrading activity, are basically implicated in the breakdown of the plaque fibrous cap (1-8). Based on the concept that SMC apoptosis plays an important role in the remodeling of atheromatous tissue, recent studies have focussed on apoptosis in early and advanced atherosclerotic lesions (20-22). Indeed, apoptotic self-elimination of SMCs may represent a beneficial adaptive response with the ultimate result of less obstructive vascular lesions. However, SMC apoptosis may also contribute to a weakened intimal plaque texture and to the reduced elaboration and deposition of extracellular matrix proteins, both leading to plaque instability.

Cell composition. Specifically, tissue specimens of primary coronary origin from 50 patients presenting unstable angina (UA) and stable angina (SA) were compared with regard to cell density, cell type and frequency of cell death, specifically SMC apoptosis and necrosis. Cellular composition of SMCs and inflammatory cells, such as macrophages and lymphocytes, is different in both plaque groups (Figure 4). As a key finding, the cell pool of UA lesions contains significantly less SMCs compared to that of SA lesions ($75\pm23\%$ *vs.* $90\pm13\%$, $P<0.01$). Also, macrophages and lymphocytes are more frequently found in plaques associated with unstable *vs.* stable angina ($25\pm19\%$ *vs.* $10\pm9\%$, $P<0.01$), whereas the average cellularity of both plaque types is similar (about 300 cells/mm^2). As expected, macrophages and lymphocytes that indicate inflammatory events encompass a larger portion in UA compared to SA plaques. These data are confirmed by several *ex vivo* and *post mortem* studies that show the prevalence of macrophages in vulnerable lesions with focal localization in ruptured and eroded zones, irrespective of the dominant plaque architecture (2-8).

Apoptosis. Sparse SMC density represents another key finding associated with vulnerable coronary lesions. In UA atheroma, importantly, morphometric evaluation demonstrates a 2-fold ($P<0.01$) higher proportion of SMCs undergoing apoptosis compared to SA lesions, whereas the proportion of viable SMCs is significantly lower ($P=0.001$) in UA *vs.* SA lesions (Figure 4). Also, macrophages that undergo apoptosis are more frequently seen in UA *vs.* SA atheroma (4% *vs.* 1% of the intimal cell pool, $P=0.01$). Importantly, our finding of increased percentages of SMCs and macrophages that undergo apoptosis with the onset of unstable angina (Figure 4) is accompanied by an increased frequency of apoptotic remnants (Figure 5).

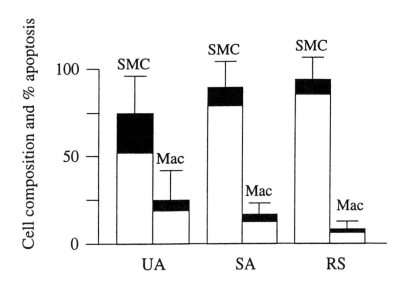

Figure 4 Cell composition and % cell type-attributed apoptosis. UA=unstable angina; SA=stable angina; RS=restenotic. ☐ denotes viable cells; ■ apoptotic cells. SMC=smooth muscle cells; Mac=macrophages.

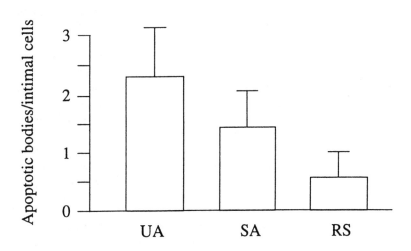

Figure 5 Density of apoptotic bodies (compare Figure 4).

Therefore, apoptosis could principally explain the loss of viable SMCs. Also, necrotic cells, whose morphology did not allow a classification of their previous cell type, are frequently seen adjacent to macrophages, indicating local inflammation. Quantitatively, necrosis is more frequent in lesions associated with UA *vs.* SA angina (19 ± 16 *vs.* 10 ± 11 necrotic cells/total cells, $P<0.05$).

When we analyze these data on apoptosis in more detail, apoptotic SMCs encompass a markedly higher proportion in unstable *versus* stable angina plaque tissue with 24% and 12%, related to the total intimal cell pool, respectively (Figure 4). These findings are confirmed by recent reports using immunohistochemical TUNEL labeling that described an apoptotic index between 10% and 46% for human coronary and peripheral plaque tissue (20,21). Interestingly, Han and co-workers (21) found maximal apoptosis in macrophage-rich areas, however, did not differentiate between arteriosclerotic lesions associated with unstable and stable angina. Although we observed high, yet different levels of apoptosis for each lesion type, mean cell density remained similar, and self-elimination or regression of the atheroma that may be anticipated as a consequence, was not documented. Also, proliferation of SMCs in coronary plaques is known to be low (33,42). Therefore, one may speculate that apoptosis, particularly that of SMCs, may be reversible at early stages or reveal an incomplete late course, as recently reported for dermal tissue cells (20). Indeed, our data give evidence for this hypothesis by the ultrastructural scenario specifically observed for apoptotic SMCs (Figure 2a). These cells reveal typical features of apoptosis and, notably, an intense loss of pericellular adhesion, a phenomenon called anoikis ("homelessness") (43). Most interestingly, this discriminant pattern of SMC apoptosis frequently found in human coronary plaque tissue is accompanied by the presence of surrounding multi-layered, basal lamina cages (Figure 2a), suggesting repetitive alternating episodes of cellular recovery, including basal lamina synthesis, and apoptosis, indicated by the loss of cell adhesion. Also, apoptosis of macrophages can be observed in 1% to 4% of the intimal cell pool, the more with acute coronary syndromes. This finding coincidences with a higher frequency of macrophages in vulnerable coronary lesions, pointing to an increased intimal turn-over of macrophages with the onset of unstable angina. In this context, recent work on human carotid plaques demonstrated proliferative activity to be largely restricted to macrophages, but not to SMCs (44).

Apoptotic bodies. Membrane-bound remnants of apoptotic cells, or matrix vesicles, reflective of final stages of apoptosis (22,37) were consistently seen in all lesions. These apoptotic remnants were present in extracellular matrix areas, isolated or in membrane contact to SMCs and macrophages, respectively, as well as in the cytoplasm of both cell types. Quantitatively, their density was markedly higher ($P<0.001$) in UA *vs.* SA lesions (Figure 5), supporting the higher level of apoptosis in primary coronary lesions with UA *vs.* SA. Also, as illustrated in Figure 2b, neighboring cells were engaged in binding and internalizing the apoptotic remnants. These findings have several implications. Apparently, intimal SMCs bear a similarly developed capacity to engulf apoptotic debris as macrophages that are prototypes of phagozytosing cells. Indeed, SMCs found in human arteriosclerotic lesions express specific integrins (Bauriedel *et al.*, in preparation) such as the vitronectin receptor ($\alpha_v\beta_3$) and the thrombospondin receptor (CD36) that are adequate binding structures for apoptotic bodies as known from experimental work with human peritoneal macrophages (40,45,46). As a consequence, competition for the cellular binding sites between apoptotic debris and other potential ligands, such as the proliferation-promoting thrombospondin, the extracellular matrix components fibronectin, vitronectin, tenascin, osteopontin or other proteins with RGD sequences (46,47), may impede with SMC/matrix interactions and, thereby, modify intimal tissue texture. Though the engulfment phase of apoptotic structures is completed within hours (34,35,37) and mediated in part by exposure of phosphatidylserine (46,48), as recently shown by *in vitro* work, we still lack information about the further cytoplasmic pathway of apoptotic debris and its degraded products in human plaque SMCs. Several questions are still unanswered that concern the identity of the enzymes degrading apoptotic bodies, the effect of phagozytosed structures on the cytoskeleton architecture and the differentiation degree of SMCs, and the SMC engulfment capacity that may become exhausted at a definite threshold, thus possibly leading to tissue destabilization. Though UA lesions compared to SA lesions contain more macrophages (Figure 4) as "professional" phagocytes, the present study demonstrates a larger pool of apoptotic endstage products in these lesions (Figure 5). The residual, smaller portion of viable SMCs that was detectable in unstable angina lesions (Figure 4) is apparently not capable to compensate or even to eliminate the accumulated output of the apoptosis machinery. In summary, high apoptosis and necrosis in human coronary primary lesions, clinically associated with acute coronary syndromes, indicate the presence of one or more intimal factors that induce intimal cell death. Therefore, implications of our findings point to the identification of these factors and to the modulation of endogeneous apoptosis to increase the regional density of viable SMCs with the ultimate goal to prevent plaque rupture.

Stable angina primary atheroma *versus* postangioplasty restenosis

Cell composition. TEM analysis reveals that restenotic chronic lesions (n=20) contain a lower number of macrophages and lymphocytes than primary atheroma (Figure 4). About 95% of the intimal cells were SMCs, 5% were macrophages and lymphocytes (Figure 4).

Apoptosis and apoptotic bodies. Recent investigational work by our group (23,38) shows that both TEM analysis and TUNEL labeling indicate restenotic lesions to contain fewer apoptotic cells compared with primary atheroma (3% *vs.* 12%; $P<0.01$). With regard to cell type, the lower frequency of apoptosis observed in restenotic tissue is attributable to both SMCs and macrophages (Figure 4). Furthermore, the number of apoptotic bodies is significantly reduced in restenotic compared to primary stenotic tissue (Figure 5), whereas the frequency of necrosis is similar in both lesion groups. As expected, at the same time, intimal cell density was found to be increased by the factor 2 to 3 in hyperplastic restenosis (23,26). Intimal cell density and the frequency of apoptosis and apoptotic bodies, respectively, show inverse correlations. Herein, our data are consistent with the concept that downregulation of SMC apoptosis permits an elongated life span of these cells and thereby leads to their continuous accumulation in the intimal space, histologically characterized as hyperplastic restenosis. In analogy, the chronic lesions reveal an increased density of apoptotic bodies, coincident with a smaller number of SMCs that are qualitatively more differentiated (25,26,38) and whose growth is only modestly influenced by growth factors (28). Previous cell culture studies have demonstated atherectomy samples from primary stenoses to show poor results when transfered to cell culture, and that even when cell cultivation is successful, these cells are characterized by a largely lost passage capacity. In addition, unlike cells of restenotic origin, these cells show a weak response to serum and growth factors (49,50). More recent experimental work has shown that human SMCs isolated from chronic arteriosclerotic lesions and transfected with the protooncogene BCL-2 were easier to grow in culture, particularly after the reduction of growth factor concentrations or in low serum conditions (51,52).

APOPTOSIS AND INTIMAL MICROECOLOGY - PATHOGENIC IMPLICATIONS

Cross-talk between apoptosis and necrosis - evidence from *in situ* data

An important, not yet answered question, in particular in plaque rupture, addresses to a possible cross-talk between apoptosis and necrosis (as the accidental form of cell death). Indeed, a significant correlation can be found (i) between the frequency of apoptotic cells and that of necrosis ($r=0.41$, $P=0.04$), and (ii) between the frequency of apoptotic remnants and that of necrosis ($r=0.63$, $P=0.001$). Most interestingly, this correlation is only apparent for lesions associated with UA, but not for the SA group. Thus, increased necrosis that goes parallel with increased levels of apoptotic cells and apoptotic remnants in unstable angina may explain the loss of (viable) SMCs as a characteristic feature in coronary atheroma complicated by plaque rupture. Additional important findings of the present report concern the normal pattern of the extracellular matrix and the paucity of cell debris adjacent to apoptotic structures. This suggests an effective sealing of the putative caustic contents of apoptotic structures (53), as commonly defined for apoptosis *versus* inflammatory necrosis. However, importantly, this also implies a focal destructive activity in case of a lost integrity of the membrane surrounding the apoptotic cell or its cytoplasmic remnants. Based on the concept of a cross-talk between apoptosis and necrosis, plaque areas rich in apoptotic structures may reflect a focally labile tissue architecture and, therefore, should be considered to predispose to plaque fissures and rupture. Conversely, locally effective proteinases, such as interstitial collagenase, 92-kD gelatinase, stromelysin or matrilysin (2,4,54-56), may not only induce the degradation of specific extracellular matrix components, but also digest the membranes of nearby apoptotic structures with the ultimate result of non-selective "boostering" of tissue degradation processes.

Regulation of apoptosis - preliminary aspects

Apoptosis and plaque rupture. Our recent work on human atheroma has sought to quantify the extent of all apoptosis events implicated, in particular in acute coronary syndromes. By necessity, this is a momentaneous and not a sequential insight into the lesional composition. Therefore, these data do not allow to conclude for the rate or the spatiotemporal pattern of intimal apoptosis. Also, this work does not specifically focus on the pathways and mechanisms of apoptosis. However, with regard to the different extent of SMC apoptosis (24% *vs.* 12%) observed in UA compared to SA lesions, one may question, whether there are two (or even more) different pathways of apoptosis. Basically, one pathway may specifically regulate intimal cell density in chronic arteriosclerosis, apparently by a complex framework of protooncogenes (BCL-2, BCL-X$_L$, BAX), cell cycle regulators (E2F1, RB, p53) and growth factors (PDGF, IGF), as shown by recent reports (22,52,57-62). In addition to this pathway that is responsible for the basal extent of apoptosis found in primary coronary lesions, a second or even more pathways of apoptosis are postulated leading to plaque vulnerability and rupture, as demonstrated by the present study. Specific cytokines, such as interferon-γ (IFN-γ) and tumor necrosis factor-α (TNF-α) and/or interleukin-1β (IL-1β) that are produced by activated macrophages (2) have recently been shown to lead to a severe loss of cellular integrity and, finally, to predispose to apoptosis *in vitro* (63).

Hypercellular Restenosis. There is a striking similarity observed between postangio-plasty restenosis and keloid wound healing. Recently, Desmoulière *et al.* (64) demonstrated that apoptosis plays a role in the decrease in cellularity which occurs as granulation tissue evolves into a scar. Their data revealed that apoptosis of granulation tissue cells takes place essentially after wound closure and affects target cells consecutively rather than producing a single wave of cell disappearance. Indeed, the authors speculated that a lack of apoptosis could result in the establishment of a hypertrophic scar or keloid, both characterized by a high degree of cellularity (64). If our concept of low SMC apoptosis in the remodeling restenotic intima is valid, the development of anti-restenotic approaches to enhance apoptosis may be possible. Since numerous agents have been reported to promote the occurence of apoptosis, including NO (65) and cytostatic agents such as protein kinase C inhibitors (40), local delivery of these agents may have a positive influence on early remodeling processes. In addition, local somatic gene therapy using tumor suppressor genes, such as p53, or blockade of protooncogenes may have beneficial effects (40,65,66). Recently, the use of catheter-based radiotherapy has been shown to inhibit restenosis in patients (67,68). Based on knowledge of radiation-induced apoptosis (69) and on recent work from animal models in which neointimal formation and cellularity were markedly suppressed by a ß-particle emitting stent (70), beneficial therapeutic effects of intracoronary radiation could be explained by an additional pro-apoptotic action. However, induction of apoptosis may also increase the higher basal levels of apoptosis in adjacent primary lesions. Most importantly, as demonstrated in the present contribution, this may lead to a pronounced SMC loss in vulnerable regions of the atheroma and result into plaque rupture and thrombosis.

References

1. Davies MJ. Stability and instability: Two faces of coronary atherosclerosis. Circulation 1996;94:2013-20.
2. Libby P. Molecular bases of acute coronary syndromes. Circulation 1995;91:2844-50.
3. Moreno PR, Falk E, Palacios IF, Newell JB, Fuster V, Fallon JT. Macrophage infiltration in acute coronary syndroms - implications for plaque rupture. Circulation 1994;90:775-78.
4. Shah PK, Falk E, Badimon JJ, Fernandez-Ortiz A, Mailhac A, Villareal-Levy G, Fallon JT, Regnstrom J, Fuster V. Human monocyte-derived macrophages induce collagen breakdown in fibrous caps of atherosclerotic plaques - potential role of matrix degrading metalloproteinases and implications for plaque rupture. Circulation 1995;92:1565-69.
5. Falk E, Shah PK, Fuster V. Coronary plaque disruption. Circulation 1995;92:657-71.
6. Kovanen PT, Kaartinen M, Paavonen T. Infiltrates of activated mast cells at the site of coronary atheromatous erosion or rupture in myocardial infarction. Circulation 1995;92:1084-88.
7. Arbustini E, De Servi S, Bramucci E, Porcu E, Costante AM, Grasso M, Diegoli M, Fasani R, Morbini P, Angoli L, Boscarini M, Repetto S, Danzi G, Niccoli L, Campolo L, Lucreziotti S, Specchia G. Comparison of coronary lesions obtained by directional coronary atherectomy in unstable angina, stable angina and restenosis after either atherectomy or angioplasty. Am J Cardiol 1995;75:675-82.
8. Van der Wal AC, Becker AE, V d Loos CM, Das PK. Site of intimal rupture or erosion of thrombosed coronary atherosclerotic plaques is characterized by an inflammatory process irrespective of the dominant plaque morphology. Circulation 1994;89:36-44.
9. Gibbons GH, Dzau VJ. The emerging concept of vascular remodeling. N Engl J Med 1994;330:1431-38.
10. Andersen HR, Maeng M, Thorwest M, Falk E. Remodeling rather than neointimal formation explains luminal narrowing after deep vessel wall injury. Circulation 1996;93:1716-24.
11. Gertz SD, Banai S, Perez LS, Gimple LW, Ragosta M, Powers ER, Sarembock IJ, Roberts WC. Remodeling after PTCA: from shrinkage to compensatory enlargement. Circulation 1995;91:2002-03.
12. Gordon PC, Gibson CM, Cohen DJ, Carrozza JP, Kuntz RE, Baim DS. Mechanisms of restenosis and redilation within coronary stents - quantitative angiographic assessment. J Am Coll Cardiol 1993;21:1166-74.
13. Kuntz RE, Baim DS. Defining coronary restenosis - newer clinical and angiographic paradigms. Circulation 1993;88:1310-23.
14. Mintz GS, Pichard AD, Kent KM, Satler LF, Popma JJ, Leon MB. Intravascular ultrasound comparison of restenotic and de novo coronary artery narrowings. Am J Cardiol 1994;74:1278-80.
15. Nishioka T, Luo H, Eigler NL, Berglund H, Kim CJ, Siegel RJ. Contribution of inadequate compensatory enlargement to development of human coronary artery stenosis: An in vivo intravascular ultrasound study. J Am Coll Cardiol 1996;27:1571-76.
16. Pasterkamp G, Wensing PJW, Post MJ, Hillen B, Mali WP, Borst C. Paradoxical arterial wall shrinkage may contribute to luminal narrowing of human atherosclerotic femoral arteries. Circulation 1995;91:1444-49.
17. Post MJ, Kuntz RE, Borst C. Remodeling after PTCA: From shrinkage to compensatory enlargement. Circulation 1995;91:2002
18. Ross R. The pathogenesis of atherosclerosis: A perspective for the 1990s. Nature 1993;362:801-09.
19. Kockx MM, De Meyer GR, Bortier H, de Meyere N, Muhring J, Bakker A, Jacob W, v Vaeck L, Herman AG. Luminal foam cell accumulation is associated with smooth muscle cell death in the intimal thickening of human saphenous vein grafts. Circulation 1996;94:1255-62.
20. Geng YJ, Libby P. Evidence for apoptosis in advanced human atheroma. Colocalization with interleukin-1β-converting enzyme. Am J Pathol 1995;147:251-66.
21. Han DKM, Haudenschild CC, Hong MK, Tinkle BT, Leon MB, Liau G. Evidence for apoptosis in human atherogenesis and in a rat vascular injury model. Am J Pathol 1995; 47:267-77.
22. Kockx MM, De Meyer GR, Muhring J, Jacob W, Bult H, Herman AG. Apoptosis and related proteins in different stages of human atherosclerotic plaques. Circulation 1998;97:2307-15.
23. Bauriedel G, Schluckebier S, Hutter R, Welsch U, Kandolf R, Lüderitz B, Forney Prescott M. Apoptosis in restenosis versus stable angina atherosclerosis. Implications for the pathogenesis of restenosis. Arterioscler Thromb Vasc Biol 1998;18:1132-39.

24. Austin GE, Ratliff NB, Hollman J, Tabei S, Phillips DF. Intimal proliferation of smooth muscle cells as an explanation for recurrent coronary artery stenosis after percutaneous transluminal coronary angioplasty. J Am Coll Cardiol 1985;6:369-75.

25. Bauriedel G, Kandolf R, Welsch U, Höfling B. Mechanismen der Re-Stenosierung nach Angioplastie. Z Kardiol 1994;83(suppl 4):31-41.

26. Bauriedel G, Kandolf R, Schluckebier S, Welsch U. Ultrastructural characteristics of human atherectomy tissue from coronary and lower extremity arterial stenoses. Am J Cardiol 1996;77:468-74.

27. Pickering JG, Weir L, Jekanowski J, Kearney MA, Isner JM. Proliferative activity in peripheral and coronary atherosclerotic plaque among patients undergoing percutaneous revascularization. J Clin Invest 1993;91:1469-80.

28. Thyberg J, Hedin U, Sjölund M, Palmberg L, Bottger BA. Regulation of differentiated properties and proliferation of arterial smooth muscle cells. Arteriosclerosis 1990;10:966-90.

29. Bauriedel G, Heidemann P, Heimerl J, Kandolf R, Höfling B. Detection of PDGF mRNA in human restenotic plaque tissue by in situ hybridization: Implication for novel therapeutic approaches. J Am Coll Cardiol 1994;23:124A.

30. Flugelman MY, Virmani R, Correa R, Yu ZX, Farb A, Leon MB, Elami A, Fu YM, Casscells W, Epstein SE. Smooth muscle cell abundance and fibroblast growth factor in coronary lesions with nonfatal unstable angina. Circulation 1993;88:2493-2500.

31. Isner JM. Vascular remodeling. Circulation 1994;89:2937-41.

32. Isner JM, Kearney M, Bortman S, Passeri J. Apoptosis in human atherosclerosis and restenosis. Circulation 1995;91:2703-11.

33. O'Brien ER, Alpers CE, Stewart DK, Ferguson M, Tran N, Gordon D, Benditt EP, Hinohara T, Simpson JB, Schwartz SM. Proliferation in primary and restenotic coronary atherectomy tissue: implications for antiproliferative therapy. Circ Res 1993;73:223-31.

34. Kerr IFR, Harmon BV. "Definition and Incidence of Apoptosis: An Historical Perspective." In *Apoptosis: The Molecular Basis of Cell Death,* ed. Tomei LD and Cope FO: New York, Cold Springs Harbor Laboratory Press, pp 5-29, 1991.

35. Kerr JF, Winterford CM, Harmon BV. Apoptosis. Its significance in cancer and cancer therapy. Cancer 1994;73:2013-26.

36. Majno G, Joris I. Apoptosis, oncosis, and necrosis. An overview of cell death. Am J Pathol 1995;146:3-15.

37. Wyllie AH, Kerr JFR, Currie AR. Cell death: The significance of apoptosis. Int Rev Cytol 1980; 68:251-306.

38. Bauriedel G, Schluckebier S, Welsch U, Höfling B, Kandolf B. Evidence of apoptosis in human arteriosclerosis. Circulation 1995;92:I-500.

39. Wijsman JH, Jonker RR, Kreijzer R, DeVelde CJH, Cornelisse CJ, v Dierendonck JH. A new method to detect apoptosis in paraffin sections: *In situ* end-labeling of fragmented DNA. J Histochem Cytochem 1993;41:7-12.

40. Savill J. Apoptosis in disease. Eur J Clin Invest 1994;24:715-23.

41. Kockx MM, Muhring J, Bortier H, De Meyer GR, Jacob W. Biotin- or digoxigenin-conjugated nucleotides bind to matrix vesicles in atherosclerotic plaques. Am J Pathol 1996;148:1771-77.

42. Gordon D, Reidy M, Benditt EP, Schwartz S. Cell proliferation in human coronary arteries. Proc Natl Acad Sci USA 1990;87:4600-06.

43. Ruoslahti E, Reed JC. Anchorage dependence, integrins, and apoptosis. Cell 1994;77:477-78.

44. Brandl R, Richter T, Haug K, Wilhelm MG, Maurer PC, Nathrath W. Topographic analysis of proliferative activity in carotid andarterectomy specimens by immunocytochemical detection of the cell cycle-related antigen Ki-67. Circulation 1997;96:3360-68.

45. Savill J, Dransfield I, Hogg N, Haslett C. Vitronectin receptor-mediated phagocytosis of cells undergoing apoptosis. Nature 1990;343:170-73.

46. Savill J, Fadok V, Henson P, Haslett C. Phagocyte recognition of cells undergoing apoptosis. Immunol Today 1993;14:582-90.

47. Hynes RO. Integrins: Versatility, modulation, and signaling in cell adhesion. Cell 1992;69:11-25.

48. Bennett MR, Gibson DF, Schwartz SM, Tait JF. Binding and phagocytosis of apoptotic vascular smooth muscle cells is mediated in part by exposure of phosphatidylserine. Circ Res 1995;77:1136-42.

49. Bauriedel G, Windstetter U, DeMaio SJ, Kandolf R, Höfling B. Migratory activity of human smooth muscle cells cultivated from coronary and peripheral primary and restenotic lesions removed by percutaneous atherectomy. Circulation 1992;85:554-64.

50. Dartsch P, Voisard R, Bauriedel G, Höfling B, Betz E. Growth characteristics and cytoskeletal organization of cultured smooth muscle cells from human primary stenosing and restenosing lesions. Arteriosclerosis 1990;10:62-75.

51. Bennett MR, Evan GI, Newby AC. Deregulated expression of the c-*myc* oncogene abolishes inhibition of proliferation of rat vascular smooth muscle cells by serum reduction, interferon-γ, heparin, and cyclic nucleotide analogues and induces apoptosis. Circ Res 1994;74:525-36.

52. Bennett MR, Evan GI, Schwartz SM. Apoptosis of human vascular smooth muscle cells derived from normal vessels and coronary atherosclerotic plaques. J Clin Invest 1995;95:2266-74.

53. Cohen JJ. Apoptosis. Immunol Today 1993;14:126-30.

54. Brown DL, Hibbs MS, Kearney M, Loushin C, Isner JM. Identification of a 92-kD gelatinase in human coronary atherosclerotic lesions - association of active enzyme synthesis with unstable angina. Circulation 1995;91:2125-31.

55. Halpert I, Sires UI, Roby JD, Potter-Perigo S, Wight TN, Shapiro SD, Welgus HG, Wickline SA, Parks WC. Matrilysin is expressed by lipid-laden macrophages at sites of potential rupture in atherosclerotic lesions and localizes to areas of versican deposition, a proteoglycan substrate for the enzyme. Proc Natl Acad Sci USA 1996;93:9748-53.

56. Henney AM, Wakely PR, Davies MJ, Foster K, Hembry R, Murphy G, Humphries S. Localization of stromelysin gene expression in atherosclerotic plaques by in situ hybridization. Proc Natl Acad Sci USA 1991;88:8154-58.

57. Bennett MR, Evan GI, Schwartz SM. Apoptosis of rat vascular smooth muscle cells is regulated by p53-dependent and -independent pathways. Circ Res 1995;77:266-73.

58. Bennett MR, Macdonald K, Chan SW, Boyle JJ, Weissberg PL. Cooperative interactions between RB and p53 regulate cell proliferation, cell senescence, and apoptosis in human vascular smooth muscle cells from atherosclerotic plaques. Circ Res 1998;82:704-12.

59. Cai WJ, Devaux B, Schaper W, Schaper J. The role of Fas/APO 1 and apoptosis in the development of human atherosclerotic lesions. Atherosclerosis 1997;131:177-86.

60. Jacobson MD, Burne J, Raff MC. Programmed cell death and bcl-2 protection in the absence of a nucleus. EMBO J 1994;13:1899-1910.

61. Pollman MJ, Hall JL, Mann MJ, Zhang L, Gibbons GH. Inhibition of neointimal cell bcl-x expression induces apoptosis and regression of vascular disease. Nature Medicine 1998;4:222-27.

62. Schwartz SM, Bennett MR. Death by any other name. Am J Pathol 1995;147:229-34.

63. Geng YJ, Wu Q, Muszynski M, Hansson GK, Libby P. Apoptosis of vascular smooth muscle cells induced by in vitro stimulation with interferon-γ, tumor necrosis factor-α, and interleukin-1β. Arterioscler Thromb Vasc Biol 1996;16:19-27.

64. Desmoulière A, Redard M, Darby I, Gabbiani G. Apoptosis mediates the decrease in cellularity during the transition between granulation tissue and scar. Am J Pathol 1995;146:56-66.

65. Meßmer UK, Ankarcrona M, Nicotera P, Brüne B. p53 expression in nitric oxide-induced apoptosis. FEBS Letters 1994;355:23-26.

66. Symonds H, Krall L, Remington L, Saenz-Robles M, Lowe S, Jacks T, v Dyke T. p53-dependent apoptosis suppresses tumor growth and progression in vivo. Cell 1994;78:703-11.

67. Condado JA, Waksman R, Gurdiel O, Espinosa R, Gonzalez J, Burger B, Villoria G, Acquatella H, Crocker IR, Seung KB, Liprie SF. Long-term angiographic and clinical outcome after percutaneous transluminal coronary angioplasty and intracoronary radiation therapy in humans. Circulation 1997;96:727-32.

68. Teirstein PS, Massullo V, Jani S, Popma JJ, Mintz GS, Russo RJ, Schatz RA, Guarneri EM, Steuterman S, Morris NB, Leon MB, Tripuraneni P. Catheter-based radiotherapy to inhibit restenosis after coronary stenting. N Engl J Med. 1997;336:1697-1703.

69. Thompson CB. Apoptosis in the pathogenesis and treatment of disease. Science 1995;267:1456-62.

70. Hehrlein C, Gollan C, Dönges K, Metz J, Riessen R, Fehsenfeld P, v Hodenberg E, Kübler W. Low dose radioactive stents inhibit smooth muscle cell proliferation and neointimal thickening in rabbits. Circulation 1995;92:1570-75.

III.2
Cardiac disease

III.2.1
Apoptosis in myocardial infarction

Andreas V. Sigel, M.D., and Günter A.J. Riegger, M.D.
Universität Regensburg, Regensburg, Germany

INTRODUCTION

Accumulating evidence suggests that programmed cell death plays an important role in myocardial infarction. The occurrence of programmed cell death has clearly been shown in several clinical (1,2,3) and experimental settings involving myocardial injury. Experimental data in vivo and in vitro suggest that cardiomyocytes are able to undergo apoptosis during hypoxia (4,5), hypoxia-reoxygenation (6,7), myocardial infarction (8,9), ischemia-reperfusion (10,11), and heart failure (12,13). Based on these studies the present concept of myocardial injury attributes the major portion of cell loss during cardiac ischemia and reperfusion to primary necrosis (14,15). However, based on the observation that apoptosis can be the early and predominant form of cell death in infarcted human myocardium, the possibility of apoptosis as inducer of secondary necrosis has already been raised (9,16). Thus, investigating the role of programmed cell death in myocardial infarction as well as documenting its underlying mechanisms may lead to new therapeutic strategies to prevent serious cell loss following ischemia and reperfusion.

Furthermore, the induction of cardiomyocyte apoptosis in the border zone (17) and the surviving myocardium (1) after infarction has been observed. These studies provide evidence that in addition to overt necrosis, a subset of myocytes undergo apoptosis after acute myocardial infarction in patients with patent infarct-related arteries and, thus, may initiate progressive congestive heart failure (17). Because apoptosis represents a potentially preventable form of cell death owing to its active nature, these findings may also have important clinical implications as new cardioprotective strategies for the treatment of congestive heart failure are being developed (18).

Despite these controversies whether programmed cell death represents an important feature in the onset and progression of myocardial infarction and ventricular dysfunction, programmed cell death constitutes a major challenge for future research in the field of ischemia-reperfusion and congestive heart failure (18,19).

EVIDENCE FOR APOPTOSIS IN MYOCARDIAL INFARCTION

Evidence that death of cardiomyocytes during ischemia and reperfusion might occur, at least in part, by apoptosis has accumulated rapidly over the last 4 to 5 years. Initial hallmark studies demonstrated programmed cell death in tissue samples of human subjects post myocardial infarction (2,13,16,20). In these studies, apoptosis appeared to be predominantly localized in the hypoperfused border zone between the central infarct area and noncompromised myocardial tissue (3,17).

Table 1 Hallmark studies and key findings on apoptosis following myocardial infarction. *Abbreviations*: R = reference.

Species	Model	Key findings	Author	R
In vivo *Human*	Myocardial infarction	Apoptosis	Itoh G, 1994	3
	Myocardial infarction	Early apoptosis	Bardales RH, 1996	20
	Myocardial infarction	Apoptosis and Bax expression	Misao J, 1996	53
	Ischemic cardiomyopathy	Apoptosis	Narula J, 1996	13
	Myocardial infarction	Apoptosis in the surviving myocardium	Olivetti G, 1996	2
	Ischemia / reperfusion	Apoptosis in the borderzone	Saraste A, 1997	17
	Myocardial infarction	Early apoptosis	Veinot JP, 1997	16
Rabbit	Ischemia / reperfusion	Apoptosis solely in reperfusion	Gottlieb RA, 1994	10
	Myocardial infarction	Apoptosis and iNOS expression	Wildhirt SM, 1995	70
	Myocardial infarction	Apoptosis and iNOS expression	Bing RJ, 1996	21
	Myocardial infarction	Apoptosis and iNOS expression	Suzuki H, 1996	63
	Ischemia / reperfusion	Apoptosis and Fas expression	Yue TL, 1998	11
Rat	Myocardial infarction	Early apoptosis and Fas expression	Kajstura J, 1996	8
	Ischemia / reperfusion	Early apoptosis and acceleration	Fliss H, 1996	9
	Ischemia / reperfusion	Late apoptosis and p38 MAP kinase	Yin T, 1997	23
	Ischemia / reperfusion	Apoptosis and complement activation	Vakeva AP, 1998	71
	Myocardial infarction	Apoptosis and JNK activation	Li WG, 1998	48
	Myocardial infarction	Earlier apoptosis in old hearts	Liu L, 1998	72
Mouse	Myocardial infarction	Apoptosis independent of p53 expression	Bialik S, 1997	55
Ex vivo *Rat*	Ischemia / reperfusion	Apoptosis solely in reperfusion	Maulik N, 1998	15
In vitro *Rat*	Hypoxia	Apoptosis and Fas expression	Tanaka M, 1994	4
	Hypoxia	Apoptosis and p53 expression	Long X, 1997	5
	Hypoxia / reoxygenation	Apoptosis solely after reperfusion	Laderoute KR, 1997	6
	Hypoxia / reoxygenation	Apoptosis and ERK expression	Aikawa R, 1997	7
	Ischemia / reperfusion	Apoptosis solely after reperfusion	Bielawska AE,1997	24

In addition to various animal models of ischemia-reperfusion (10,21) the occurrence of apoptosis and its underlying mechanisms have been documented by studies using apoptosis preventing therapies, thus, inhibiting cardiomyocyte death (11,22). The pathophysiological context in which cardiac muscle apoptosis has been documented now also include several animal models of acute myocardial infarction as well as in-vitro studies on hypoxia and reoxygenation (table 1). These studies showed both the occurrence of early apoptosis as predominant form of cell death (8) as well as apoptosis as contributing cause for delayed myocyte loss after myocardial infarction (23).

However, based on limited and inconsistent data, at present, it is impossible to answer the question whether apoptosis is a critical etiological factor in the onset and progression of myocardial infarction. Maulik (14), Gottlieb (10) and Yue (11) reported apoptotic cells only in reperfused myocardium, whereas continuous ischemia provoked no evidence of apoptosis (figure 1). In addition, in a left coronary artery occlusion model, ischemia with subsequent reperfusion, but not ischemia alone, induced apoptosis in myocardial cells (24). By contrast, Fliss and Gattinger (9) showed that rats subjected to continuous coronary artery occlusion display characteristic signs of apoptosis solely in the ischemic myocardium after about 2 hours of ischemia. However, reperfusion after a 45-minute occlusion accelerated this process, with apoptosis becoming evident in the reperfused myocardium after only 1 hour of reperfusion. This observation was confirmed by other groups (4,5,6).

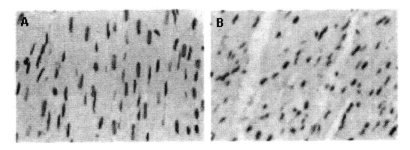

Figure 1   Apoptotic cell death in reperfused myocardium using the TUNEL method. *A*: normoxic cardiac myocytes, *B*: apoptotic cardiac myocytes after ischemia/reperfusion injury. (Reprinted with permission of Tian-Li Yue, M.D.).

The onset of apoptosis was also examined in human studies: Veinot et al. examined the time of appearance and extent of apoptosis in human acute myocardial infarction and compared these with necrotic cell death (16). In autopsied tissue from cases of acute myocardial infarct there was widespread apoptosis even in infarcts only a few hours in age before the appearance of coagulative necrosis. During the next 1 to 2 days, programmed cell death remained extensive but increasingly appeared in cells with morphological features of coagulative necrosis. In addition, in older infarcts, the incidence of apoptosis declined in myocytes, but increased in invading inflammatory cells. These data suggest that apoptosis may be the early and predominant form of cell death in infarcted human myocardium, and that its appearance is accelerated in reperfused myocardium.

In summary, observations in both clinical as well as experimental settings of myocardial infarction have confirmed the contribution of apoptosis to cardiomyocyte death. At present, the relative importance of apoptotic cell death in both the acute and chronic phases of myocardial infarction is not known. Therefore, there is a variety of controversies on the role of apoptosis in cardiac damage (table 2).

Table 2 Controversies and common features of apoptosis in myocardial infarction.

Large variation in onset of induction and duration
Large variation in prevalence and distribution
No clear dissociation between apoptosis and necrosis

Apoptosis but not necrosis occurs at sites remote to the core ischemic region
Apoptosis in both cardiomyocytes and nonmyocytes
Association with specific gene expression

However, there is increasing evidence that ischemia-induced apoptosis preceeds necrosis, suggesting the possibility to inhibit substantial myocye death by inhibiting apoptosis.

REPERFUSION AS ACCELERATOR OF APOPTOSIS

Reperfusion of the infarct-related coronary artery is a central therapeutical goal in patients with acute myocardial infarction. However, cardiomyocytes continue to die during reperfusion (figure 2).

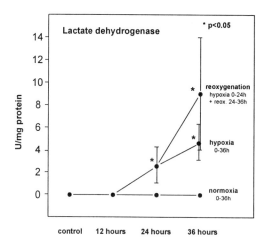

Figure 2 Differential effects of hypoxia (0-36h) and hypoxia (0-24h) and reoxygenation (24-36h) in cultured neonatal rat cardiac myocytes. LDH activity in the medium increases to higher levels with reoxygenation suggesting more extensive cellular damage.

The mechanisms of cell death during this phase of infarction have already been subject to debate (25). Therefore, the role of apoptosis following reperfusion has been addressed in various animal models. These studies showed both the occurrence of apoptosis during ischemia alone, as well as acceleration of apoptotic cell death in cardiomyocytes after reperfusion (3,6,9,10,14). In order to document the impact of reoxygenation on myocyte injury we established a reliable cell culture model of apoptosis and linked morphological findings to biochemical parameters of necrosis and apoptosis (26). For this purpose neonatal rat myocytes were cultured in 2% oxygen for 24 hours to produce hypoxic conditions and then exposed to 20% oxygen for additional 12 hours to simulate reoxygenation. Hypoxia led to a 10-fold increase in LDH leakage ($p<0.05$) and an almost complete loss in myocyte creatine kinase (CK) activity ($p<0.05$). This pattern of severe necrosis further increased during additional reoxygenation (figure 2). In addition, reoxygenation was followed by nucleosomal DNA fragmentation that was detectable by gel electrophoresis (DNA ladder) (figure 3) as well as significant induction of Fas receptor protein, cytochrome c release and caspase-3 activation, mediators of apoptotic cell death. Interestingly, the expression of Fas receptor occurred as early as 12 hours after hypoxia, much earlier than the occurence of necrosis parameters. Taken together, these results suggest that reoxygenation augments hypoxia-induced cell death in cardiac myocytes and that induction of Fas receptor, cytochrome c release and caspase-3 activation may set the stage for this process.

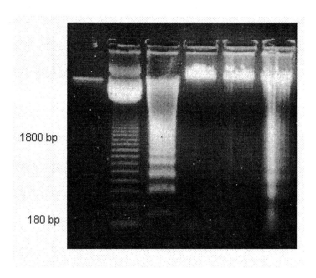

Figure 3 Effect of hypoxia and reoxygenation on apoptosis in cardiac myocytes using DNA laddering. *lane 1*: high molecular weight DNA control, *lane 2*: 123 ladder, *lane 3*: thymus cell DNA positive apoptosis control, *lane 4*: normoxic myocyte DNA, *lane 5*: myocyte DNA after 36h of hypoxia, *lane 6*: apoptotic myocyte DNA after 24h of hypoxia followed by 12 hours of reoxygenation. Significant DNA fragmentation only occurs in reoxygenated cardiac myocytes.

Albeit the consecutive occurrence of indicators of apoptosis (DNA laddering), and necrosis (CK and LDH activities) there is no proof for apoptosis-induced secondary necrosis following myocardial infarction. The early induction of mediators of programmed cell death (induction of Fas receptor, cytochrome c release and caspase-3 activation) may substantiate the hypothesis that apoptosis is an early form of cardiomyocyte death in this setting. Less clear is, however, as to whether these cellular alterations increase the amount of cells that subsequently undergo necrosis. By contrast, there is no doubt that reoxygenation augments programmed cell death, thus contributing substantially to myocardial injury.

MECHANISMS OF APOPTOSIS IN MYOCARDIAL INFARCTION

Although increasing descriptive evidence suggests that apoptosis occurs in myocardial infarction, it is less clear what the relevant pathophysiological triggers might be. However, it has been documented that control of programmed cell death in the myocardium depends on a balance between inducers and inhibitors of apoptosis. Oxidative stress, calcium overload, mitochondrial defects, stimulation of proapoptotic factors, or loss of cardiac myocyte survival factors each could, theoretically, result in apoptosis (27) (table 3).

Table 3   Possible therapeutical strategies to inhibit apoptosis based on the underlying mechanisms. *Abbreviations*: R = reference.

Species	Model	Key findings	Author	R
In vivo *Human*	No studies			
Rabbit	Ischemia / reperfusion	Cardioprotection of antioxidants	Yue TL, 1998	11
Rat	Ischemia / reperfusion	Cardioprotection of IGF-1	Buerke M, 1995	73
	Ischemia / reperfusion	Cardioprotection of FGF-1	Cuevas P, 1997	62
Mouse	Myocardial infarction	Cardioprotection of IGF-1	Li Q, 1997	45
Ex vivo *Rat*	Ischemia / reperfusion	Cardioprotection of NHE inhibition	Chakrabarti S, 1997	50
In vitro *Rat*	Hydrogen peroxide	Cardioprotection of ERK inhibition	Aikawa R, 1997	7
	Staurosporine	Cardioprotection of caspase-3 inhibition	Yue TL, 1998	59
	Metabolic inhibition	Cardioprotection of VPATPase activation	Karwatowska E,1998	22
	Hypoxia/reoxygenation	Cardioprotection of antioxidants	Sigel AV, 1998	26

Importance of oxidative stress and *Mitogen-Activated Protein Kinases*

Reactive oxygen intermediates

Many studies have suggested that both neutrophils and reactive oxygen intermediates (ROI) play important roles in ischemia-reperfusion-induced cardiac abnormalities (11,14,28). It is widely accepted knowledge that low levels of ROI are regularly produced during a process of physiological metabolism, and every cell contains several enzymes such as catalase, glutathione peroxidase, and superoxide dismutase, which scavenge ROI from the cell. High levels of ROI are generated from a variety of sources such as the xanthine oxidase system, the leakage of electrons from mitochondria (29), the cyclooxygenase pathway of arachidonic acid metabolism (30), and the respiratory burst of phagocyte cells (31). In the heart, it has been reported recently that ROI evoke a variety of abnormalities including cytotoxicity (32), cardiac stunning (33), and arrhythmia (34). In addition, administration of oxygen free-radical scavengers such as superoxide dismutase and catalase results in a significant decrease in infarct size (35). Furthermore, Horwitz et al. showed that N-(2-mercaptopropionyl)-glycine, an endogenous antioxidant, markedly reduced cytotoxicity caused by hydrogen peroxide in cultured cardiac myocytes (36). Although, the molecular mechanism by which ROI induce cardiac injuries remains largely unknown, it has been suggested that the mitogen-activated protein kinase family may trigger some of the effects.

Oxidative stress is a condition in which oxidant metabolites exert toxic effects because of their increased production or an altered cellular mechanism of protection (28). Because the formation of oxygen radicals has been implicated as one of the pathomechanisms for tissue injury during reperfusion, the finding that oxidative stress induces apoptosis may provide an important mechanistic link between reperfusion and cardiomyocyte injury (37,7). Extracellular signal-regulated kinases (ERKs) have been reported to play pivotal roles in many aspects of cell functions and to be activated by oxidative stress. ERKs are transiently and concentration-dependently activated by hydogen peroxide (H_2O_2) in cardiac myocytes in conjunction with programmed cell death and activation of caspase-3. A specific tyrosine kinase inhibitor, genistein, suppressed H_2O_2-induced ERK activation.

In addition, the presence of apoptotic cells and DNA fragmentation were abolished by reperfusing the hearts in the presence of the antioxidant ebselen. These results clearly demonstrate that oxidative stress developed in the ischemic reperfused myocardium induces apoptosis. In addition, in 45 autopsy cases histological disassociation between CuZn-SOD expression and apoptosis suggests the possibility of a cytoprotective role played by endogenous CuZn-SOD against free radical generation in the human heart (38). Furthermore, data from our own group clearly document the importance of ROI production during hypoxia and reoxygenation on myocyte death (figure 4 left). Interstingly, we could show that ROI production significantly contributes to acidification during hypoxia under myocyte cell culture conditions (figure 4 right).

Mitogen-Activated Protein Kinases

The mitogen-activated protein kinases (MAPKs) are serine/threonine protein kinases, which play pivotal roles in a variety of cell functions in many cell types. Three subfamilies of MAPKs consisting of extracellular signal-regulated kinase (ERK), c-Jun NH2-terminal protein kinase (JNK) and p38-MAPK, which are regulated by three distinctive signal transduction pathways and show different functions (39).

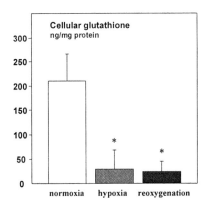
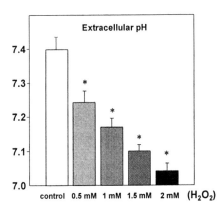

Figure 4 Effect of hypoxia and reoxygenation on glutathione loss (left), effect of ROI on extracellular pH (right).

In cardiac myocytes, the activation of ERKs has been reported to be critical for the development of the morphological feature of hypertrophy and specific gene expression (40). Stimulation of receptor tyrosine kinases often activates the Raf-1-MAPK/ERK kinase (MEK)-ERK cascade through Ras (41). Activation of Src family tyrosine kinases and Ras is required for activation of ERKs in smooth muscle cells (42), however, in cardiac myocytes protein kinase C (PKC) (7). Therefore, the signal transduction pathways leading to activation of ERKs may be different among cell types. In cardiac myocytes, JNK is activated by ischemia-reperfusion (43) and mechanical stretch (44). While activation of ERKs functions to protect cells from a variety of cellular stresses, activation of JNK and p38MAPK induce apoptosis (44) (figure 5).

It could be shown that oxygen-derived free radicals induce activation of ERKs and p38MAPK in cultured cardiac myocytes and that Src family tyrosine kinases and Ras are essential for H_2O_2-induced ERK activation. In addition, H_2O_2 induces apoptotic death of cardiac myocytes, and selective inhibition of ERK activation further increases the number of apoptotic cells. Yue et al. documented that myocardial ischemia-reperfusion leads to a rapid activation of stress-activated protein kinase (SAPK) in the ischemic area but not in nonischemic regions. In addition, SAPK activity was increased four-fold after 30 minutes of of ischemia followed by 20 minutes of reperfusion (11).

Laderoute et al. demonstrated that reoxygenation, but not hypoxia alone, caused sustained increases in phosphorylation of the amino-terminal domain of the c-Jun transcription factor (6). The activation correlated with hypoxia-mediated depression of intracellular glutathione, indicating significant production of oxygen radicals. Reoxygenation-induced c-Jun kinase activation was reduced by preincubating myocytes during the hypoxia period with the spin-trap agent alpha-phenyl N-tert-butylnitrone or N-acetylcystein, potent ROI scavengers.

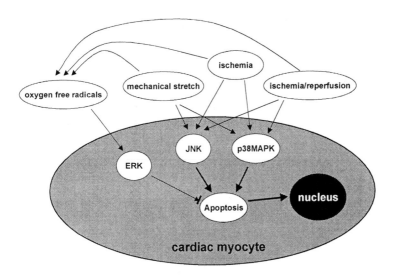

Figure 5 Effect of pathophysiological stimulation of MAPkinases during hypoxia and reoxygenation. *Abbreviations*: ERK: extracellular signal-regulated kinase, *JNK*: c-Jun NH2-terminal protein kinase, *p38-MAPK*: p38 MAP kinase.

In addition, kinase activity was also inhibited by the tyrosine kinase inhibitor genistein but not by other protein kinase inhibitors. These results implicate unquenched reactive oxygen intermediates as the stimulus that initiates a kinase pathway involving the stress-activated protein kinases (JNKs/SAPKs) in reoxygenated cardiac myocytes.

In addition, it could be shown that there is an almost 4-fold increase in JNK phosphorylation within the remote myocardium, in conjunction with a 52% increase in TBARS suggesting increased lipid peroxidation (45,48). Furthermore there is a significant increase in myocyte apoptosis within the remote myocardium.

Furthermore, the molecular mechanisms that contribute to tissue damage following ischemia and ischemia coupled with reperfusion (ischemia/reperfusion) were studied in the rat heart (23). The investigators observed the activation of three stress-inducible mitogen-activated protein (MAP) kinases in the rat heart: p38 MAP kinase and the 46- and 55-kDa isoforms of Jun N-terminal kinase (JNK46 and JNK55). During ischemia alone only p38 MAP kinase was activated. However, additional reperfusion led to activation of p38 MAP and JNK55 kinase. In addition, c-Jun and ATF3, two stress-response genes, were induced by ischemia and ischemia/reperfusion. A close correlation was found between DNA laddering, indicating apoptosis, and the pattern of kinase activation, supporting a link between stress kinase activation and apoptotic cell death in the heart.

Role of pH

Intracellular acidification is a general feature of the ischemic myocardium and develops as a result of anaerobic metabolism, hydrolysis of ATP, and CO_2 retention (46). In addition, interventions that limit myocardial ischemia, also attenuate intracellular acidosis suggesting a harmful effect of acidosis on the ischemic myocardium (10,47). Furthermore, there is growing evidence that acidification is a common characteristic of apoptotic cells (10). Major mechanisms by which the heart adapts to and recovers from intracellular acidosis during ischemia and reperfusion include the sodium-hydrogen exchanger (NHE) and the vacuolar proton ATPase (VPATPase).

Sodium-hydrogen exchanger

There are at least 5 NHE isoforms identified with the NHE-1 subtype representing the major one found in the mammalian myocardium (49). Extensive studies using NHE inhibitors like amiloride, HOE 694 or HOE 642 have consistently shown protective effects against ischemia- and reperfusion-induced apoptosis in a large variety of experimental models and animal species particularly in terms of attenuating contractile function. This observation was confirmed by Chakrabarti et al. in a rabbit model of ischemia-reperfusion where they documented the anti-apoptotic effect of HOE 642 (cariporide) (50).

Vacuolar proton ATPase

The vacuolar proton ATPase (VPATPase) operates in cardiomyocytes as a complementary proton-extruding mechanism, with increased activity by preconditioning resulting in attenuation of intracellular acidification during ischemia (22). VPATPase inhibition increased the amount of apoptosis and abrogated the protective effect of inhibition of N+-H+ exchange by amiloride indicating an important accessory role in cardiomyocyte protection by reducing acidosis and Na+-H+ exchange-induced Ca2+ overload.

Classical Pathway

Fas

The Fas-Fas ligand (Fas-L) system is one of the representative systems of apoptosis signaling molecules. Fas (CD95) is a cell surface protein belonging to the nerve growth factor/TNF receptor family (51). Human soluble Fas-L is predominantly expressed in activated T cells (52). Binding of Fas-L or agonistic anti-Fas antibodies to Fas induce apoptosis (52). The so called death receptor Fas is markedly upregulated in cardiomyocytes during ischemia and reperfusion, and cardiomyocytes may thus become susceptible to programmed cell death by interaction with Fas ligand (figure 6). Whereas under control conditions less than 1% of cardiomyocytes express the Fas receptor, Fas is detectable in more than 50%

of myocytes within a few hours of ischemia and reperfusion (8,11) in conjunction with cardiomyocyte apoptosis.

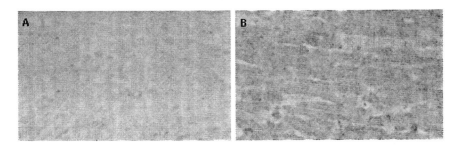

Figure 6 Effect of hypoxia and reoxygenation on Fas receptor expression in cardiac myocytes. *A*: normoxic cardiac myocytes, *B*: cardiac myocytes after ischemia/reperfugion injury. (reprinted with permission of Tian-Li Yue, M.D.).

Furthermore, Fas mRNA levels show a close correlation with apoptotic myocyte death during hypoxia alone (4). In addition, Nishigaki et al. documented elevated levels of sFas in patients with chronic congestive heart failure, suggesting an important role in the pathophysiologic mechanisms of congestive heart failure (52).

Bcl-2 and Bax

Bcl-2 is localized to the outer mitochondrial and nuclear membranes. The ratio of Bcl-2, an inhibitor of apoptosis, and bax protein, an inducer of apoptosis, determines survival or death after an apoptotic stimulus (53). Bcl-2 protein is induced in the salvaged myocytes at the acute stage of infarction, but bax protein is overexpressed at the chronic stage. Cheng et al. reported a decrease in the expression of Bcl-2 and an increase in the expression of Bax after myocardial infarction, an imbalance that favours apoptosis (54). Thus, the expression of bcl-2 and the overexpression of bax may play an important pathophysiological role in the protection or acceleration of the apoptosis of human myocytes after ischemia and/or reperfusion.

p53

Exposure of cardiac myocytes to hypoxia results in increased p53 transactivating activity and protein accumulation (5). Expression of p21/WAF-1/CIP-1, a well-characterized target of p53 transactivation, also increases in response to hypoxia. To determine whether the increase in p53 expression in myocytes is sufficient to induce apoptosis, normoxic cultures were infected with a replicon-defective adenovirus expressing wild-type human p53. Infected cells expressed high intracellular levels of p53 protein and exhibited morphological changes and genomic DNA fragmentation characteristic of apoptosis, suggesting that the intracellular signaling pathways activated by p53 might play a critical role in the regulation of hypoxia-induced apoptosis in cardiomyocytes. However, this hypothesis could not be confirmed by Bialik ct al., who studied the necessity of p53 for myocyte apoptosis in the hearts of mice nullizygous for p53 (55). Myocyte apoptosis following myocardial infarction occurred as readily in the hearts of mice nullizygous for p53 as in wild-type littermates. These data may demonstrate the existence of a p53-independent pathway that mediates myocyte apoptosis during myocardial infarction.

Caspase 3

Like in other tissues, a key phenomenon of apoptotic cell death in the myocardium is the activation of a unique class of aspartate-specific proteases with at least 10 members, termed caspases, which are responsible for internucleosomal DNA fragmentation (56). For activation, the caspase proform has to be cleaved into a large subunit and a small subunit that finally reassociate to form a complex comprising 2 small and 2 large subunits (19). Initiation of apoptosis following ischemia and reperfusion involves the binding of extracellular death signal proteins, such as TNF-alpha or Fas-L to their myocyte surface receptors, thus, activating caspase-3 (CPP32). In addition, recent studies identified the mature heme-containing form of cytochrome c that is located in the mitochondrial intermembranous space as activator of caspase-3 (57).

Target proteins for caspases comprise a plethora of different proteins, including nuclear proteins, proteins involved in signal transduction, and cytoskeletal targets (56). In order to investigate the specific role of caspases in ischemia-induced cardiomyocyte death Sprague-Dawley rats were subjected to 30 minutes coronary occlusion followed by 24 hours reperfusion (58). Intravenous administration of Z-Val-Ala-Asp(OMe)-CH2F (ZVAD-fmk), a tripeptide inhibitor of the caspase family, significantly reduced programmed cell death and cardiomyocyte death in conjunction with an improvement of left ventricular function. To further determine whether caspase-3 and stress-activated protein kinase (SAP/JNK) are involved in cardiac apoptosis, neonatal cardiac myocytes were treated with staurosporin (59). Staurosporine induced caspase activity in cardiac myocytes by five- to eight-fold, peaking at 4-8 hours after stimulation. Based upon substrate specific analysis, the major component of caspases activated in myocytes was consistent with caspase-3. The results of Yaoita et al. were confirmed by the observation that apoptosis was reduced by administration of ZVAD-fmk.

Growth factors and cytokines

Growth factors can profoundly affect many aspects of cell death and production of extracellular matrix proteins, thus leading to cardiac remodeling. In the heart, myocytes, fibroblasts and endothelial cells are major endogenous sources of growth factors. In addition, growth factors are also synthesized by inflammatory cells such as macrophages. Accordingly, studying the role of growth factors in myocardial infarction, may not only lead to mechanisms of apoptotic cell death but may also document pathways responsible for cardiac remodeling and congestive heart failure (figure 7).

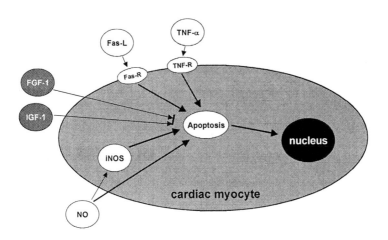

Figure 7 Effect of growth factors on programmed cell death in cardiac myocytes. *Abbreviations: Fas-L*: Fas ligand, *Fas-R*: Fas receptor, *NO*: nitric oxide, *iNos*: inducible nitric oxide synthase, *TNF-R*: TNF receptor, *FGF-1*: fibroblast growth factor 1, *IGF-1*: insulin like growth factor 1.

Fibroblast Growth Factor

Fibroblast growth factor is widely distributed in developing and mature heart tissue (60) and stimulates mitosis in several types of cells (61). The effect of native (FGF-1) and non-mitogenic fibroblast growth factor-1 (m FGF-1) on apoptosis was assessed in a rat model of 20 minutes regional myocardial ischemia and 24 hours of reperfusion (62). When given as a systemic bolus immediately after myocardial ischemia, both FGF-1 and mFGF-1 significantly attenuate apoptosis, suggesting that this cardioprotection does not depend on the mitogenic properties of this protein.

Insulin-like Growth Factor 1

To determine whether insulin like growth factor 1 (IGF-1) opposes the stimulation of myocyte death in the surviving myocardium after infarction, transgenic mice overexpressing human IGF-1B in myocytes (FVB.IgF+/-) and wild-type littermates were subjected to coronary ligation (45). Myocardial infarction involved an average 50% of the left ventricle and produced cardiac failure. In the region proximate to infarction, myocyte apoptosis and necrosis were increased in wild-type animals. By contrast, the changes in wall thickness, chamber diameter, and cavitary volume were significantly smaller in FVB.IgF+/-. The differential response to infarction of FVB.IgF+/- mice resulted in an attenuated increase in diastolic wall stress, cardiac weight, and left and right ventricular weight-to-body weight ratio.

Nitric Oxide

Activated macrophages produce nitric oxide through the inducible form of nitric oxide synthase (iNOS) (63). Previously a significant increase of iNOS activity in macrophaged in infarcted rabbit heart tissue was observed. The peak activity of iNOS was found on day 3 postinfarction, which corresponded with the induction of apoptosis. In another study, Bing et al. documented that iNOS was significantly increased in the infarcted area beginning on the third day following ligation of a coronary artery, with primarily induction in macrophages (21). The specific inhibitor of iNOS, S-methylisothiourea (SMT) prevented apoptosis with the greatest effect occurring in the normal non-affected area of the heart.

Tumor Necrosis Factor

The heart is a tumor necrosis factor (TNF) producing organ (64). Both myocardial macrophages and cardiac myocytes themselves synthesize TNF. Locally produced TNF contributes to postischemic myocardial dysfunction via direct depression of contractility and induction of apoptosis. Lipopolysaccharide or ischemia-reperfusion activates myocardial p38 mitogen-activated protein (MAP) kinase and nuclear factor kappa B, which lead to TNF production. TNF activation of TNF receptor 1 or Fas may induce apoptosis. In addition, endogenous anti-inflammatory ligands, which trigger the gp signaling cascade, heat shock proteins, and TNF-binding proteins, also control TNF production and activity.

Furthermore, Krown et al. have been shown that physiological relevant levels of the proinflammatory cytokine TNF-alpha induced apoptosis in rat cardiomyocytes in conjunction with stimulated production of the endogenous second messenger, sphingosine, suggesting sphingolipid involvement in TNF-alpha-mediated cardiomyocyte apoptosis (65). Consistent with this hypothesis, sphingosine strongly induced cardiomyocyte apoptosis. Taken together, these findings suggest that the elevated TNF-alpha levels seen in a variety of clinical conditions, including sepsis and ischemic myocardial infarction, may contribute to TNF-alpha-induced cardiac cell death.

IMPACT ON THE SURVIVING MYOCARDIUM

Myocardial ischemia and acute myocardial infarction are the major etiological causes of congestive heart failure in western society (figure 8). Myocardial ischemia may acutely result in myocardial dysfunction, or chronically affect the heart when recovery is delayed (stunning), perfusion is chronically at an insufficient level (hibernation) or ischemia results in apoptosis or necrosis, thus, contributing to myocardial cell loss and congestive heart failure. Despite preliminary data on the occcurence of programmed cell death in hibernating myocardium and congestive heart failure the question remains whether apoptosis is a critical event in both entities.

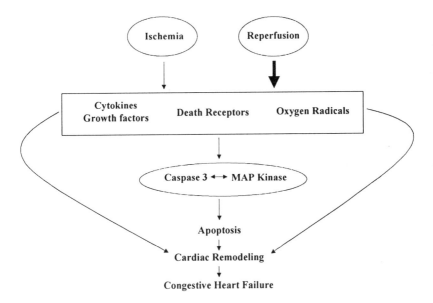

Figure 8 Molecular mechanisms of ischemia-reperfusion-induced apoptosis and possible link to congestive heart failure.

The hibernating myocardium

The term „hibernating myocardium" refers to the presence of persistently impaired LV function at rest, due to a reduced coronary blood flow that can partially or completely be restored to normal after revascularization (66). To test the hypothesis that hibernating myocardium represents an incomplete adaption to a reduced myocardial oxygen supply, biopsies taken in 38 patients with areas of hibernating myocardium showed structural degeneration in addition to an increased amount of extracellular matrix proteins resulting in a significant degree of reparative tissue fibrosis (67,68). The occurrence of apoptotic myocytes was clearly shown using TUNEL and electronmicroscopy.

In addition, Chen et al. observed apoptotic myocytes in the hibernating myocardial regions of all animals after coronary artery stenosis for 24 hours (69). The severity of myocyte apoptosis correlated significantly with regional coronary blood flow reduction. Both studies demonstrate that there is ongoing myocyte death through myocyte apoptosis in hypoperfused hibernating myocardium. Accordingly, cellular degeneration rather than adaption is present in hibernating myocardium. Therefore, the consequence is progressive diminution of the chance for complete structural and functional recovery after restoration of blood flow. However, the practical consequence from these studies should be early vascularization in conjunction with anti-apoptotic therapy in patients showing areas of hibernating myocardium.

Initiation of congestive heart failure

At present, there is a variety of hypothesis available to explain the progressive functional deterioration and cardiac remodeling that characterize end-stage heart failure. Left ventricular dysfunction, once established as a consequence of acute myocardial infarction, can continue to worsen over months or years, despite the absence of clinically apparent intercurrent adverse effects. Electron microscopic studies using myocardial specimen obtained from hypertrophied and failed human hearts (13) and hearts of dogs with experimentally induced chronic failure (12) have clearly established the existence of cardiomyocyte degeneration. In addition, recent studies from Sabbah et al. of dogs with heart failure have shown that cardiomyocyte death through apoptosis occurs in end-stage heart failure.

On this basis, a new hypothesis is presented that apoptotic myocyte death may occur in the surviving portion of the heart following coronary artery disease or myocardial infarction (figure 9). In order to substantiate this hypothesis, myocardial samples were obtained from the region adjacent to and remote from infarction in patients who died within 10 days from the initial clinical symptoms. Apoptosis was observed in all infarcted hearts in both the regions bordering on and distant from the necrotic myocardium. However, the number of apoptotic nuclei was greater in the peri-infarcted region than in that away from infarction. Thus, apoptosis appears to be a significant complicating factor of acute myocardial infarction increasing the magnitude of myocyte cell death associated with coronary artery occlusion.

Olivetti et al. studied the magnitude of apoptosis in patients suffering from end-stage congestive heart failure (2). Heart failure was characterized by a more than 200-fold increase in myocyte apoptosis. In conclusion, programmed cell death of myocytes occured in the decompensated human heart in spite of the enhanced expression of BCL-2, thus, may contributing to the progression of cardiac function.

Table 4 Evidence for apoptosis in congestive heart failure following myocardial infarction. *Abbreviations*: R = reference.

Species		Model	Key findings	Author	R
In vivo	*Human*	End-stage heart failure	Apoptosis in LV tissue	Narula J, 1996	13
		End-stage heart failure	Apoptosis in LV tissue	Olivetti G, 1996	2
		End-stage heart failure	Apoptosis in LV tissue	Nishigaki K, 1996	52
	Dog	Myocardial infarction	Apoptosis in LV tissue	Sabbah HN, 1998	12

In addition, it has been recently reported that apoptotic cell death occurs in myocytes of dogs with congestive heart failure (12). Furthermore, in order to examine plasma levels of soluble Fas/APO-1 receptor (sFas), an inhibitor of apoptosis, and soluble Fas ligand (sFas-L), an inducer of apoptosis, and their relation to other clinical variables, 70 patients with chronic congestive heart failure mostly due to coronary artery disease were studied (52).

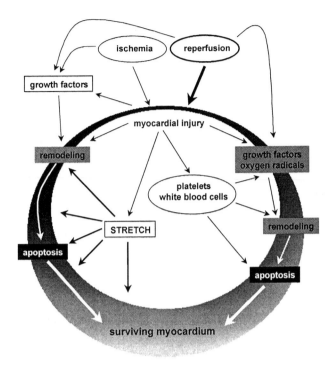

Figure 9 Summary of events involved in ischemia/reperfusion, apoptosis and the surviving portion of the myocardium.

sFas levels increased with the severity of functional classification in conjunction with elevated pulmonary artery wedge pressure and decreased cardiac index. In addition, plasma levels of sFas tended to decrease in patients with clinical improvement.

However, these results do not prove that the degree of cell death is the cause of the terminal outcome of the disease. In addition, at present, little is known concerning the duration of the apoptotic process in myocytes in vivo thus limiting the estimation of the rate of apoptosis in the human heart. Moreover, the lack of information regarding the relationship between ongoing cell death and ventricular dimension and function further complicates the full understanding of the role of apoptosis in the failing heart.

SUMMARY

Accumulating evidence documents that programmed cell death represents an important feature in myocardial infarction. Although apoptosis has been verified in several clinical as well as experimental in vivo and in vitro settings, the role of apoptosis in the pathogenesis of ischemia-reperfusion injury requires substantiation. In this respect, it is important to determine whether programmed cell death represents one of the early causes rather than a terminal event that is associated with the end stage of these entities. In addition, given the fact that apoptosis may be a very short process on the one side, the detection of apoptotic patterns, however, very time consuming and sometimes nonspecific on the other, it is difficult to determine the true incidence of apoptosis. By contrast, increasing data on the underlying mechanisms already helped to define targets for therapeutical inhibition of apoptosis. Preliminary data on the effect of growth factor therapy, the use of specific caspase-inhibitors and antioxidants have already been shown to prevent ischemia-induced myocardial cell loss by preventing programmed cell death. However, the ultimate fate of the „rescued" myocyte, that has already initiated the apoptosis pathway, may simply be a delayed death.

Despite these problems and questions, programmed cell death constitutes a major challenge for future research in the field of ischemia-reperfusion and congestive heart failure. In addition, apoptosis may represent an exciting target for the development of new therapeutical stratagies.

References

1.   Olivetti G, Quaini F, Sala R, Lagraste C, Corradi D, Bonacina E, Gambert SR, Cigola E, Anversa P. Acute myocardial infarction in humans is associated with activation of programmed myocyte cell death in the surviving portion of the heart. J Mol Cell Cardiol 1997; 28: 2005-2016.
2.   Olivetti G, Abbi R, Quaini F, Kajstura J, Cheng W, Nitahara JA, Quaini E, Loreto C, Beltrami CA, Krajewski S, Reed JC, Anversa P. Apoptosis in the failing human heart. N Engl J Med 1997; 336: 1131-1141.
3.   Itoh G, Tamura J, Suzuki M, Suzuki Y, Ikeda H, Koike M, Nomura M, Jie T, Ito K. DNA fragmentation of human infarcted myocardial cells demonstrated by the nick end labeling method and DNA agarose gel electrophoresis. Am J Pathol 1995; 146: 1325-1331.
4.   Tanaka M, Itoh H, Adachi S, Akimoto H, Nishikawa T, Kasajima T, Marumo F, Hiroe M. Hypoxia induces apoptosis with enhanced expression of Fas antigen messenger RNA in cultured neonatal rat cardiomyocytes. Circ Res 1994; 75: 426-433.
5.   Long X, Boluyt MO, Hipolito ML, Lundberg MS, Zheng JS, O'Neill L, Cirelli C, Lakatta EG, Crow MT. p53 and the hypoxia-induced apoptosis of cultured neonatal rat cardiac myocytes. J Clin Invest 1997; 99: 2635-2643.
6.   Laderoute KR, Webster KA. Hypoxia/reoxygenation stimulates Jun kinase activity through redox signaling in cardiac myocytes. Circ Res 1997; 80: 336-340.
7.   Aikawa R, Komuro I, Yamazaki T, Zou Y, Kudoh S, Tanaka M, Shiojima I, Hiroi Y, Yazaki Y. Oxidative stress activates extracellular signal-regulated kinases through Src and Ras in cultured cardiac myocytes of neonatal rats. J Clin Invest 1997; 100: 1813-1821.
8.   Kajstura J, Cheng W, Reiss K, Clark WA, Sonnenblick EH, Krajewski S, Reed JC, Olivetti G, Anversa P. Apoptotic and necrotic myocyte cell deaths are independent contributing variables of infarct size in rats. Lab Invest 1996; 74: 86-107.
9.   Fliss H, Gattinger D. Apoptosis in ischemic and reperfused rat heart myocardium. Circ Res 1996; 79: 949-956.
10.   Gottlieb RA, Gruol DL, Zhu JY, Engler RL. Preconditioning rabbit cardiomyocytes: role of pH, vacuolar proton ATPase, and apoptosis. J Clin Invest 1996; 97: 2391-2398.
11.   Yue TL, Ma XL, Wang X, Romanic AM, Liu GL, Louden C, Gu JL, Kumar S, Poste G, Ruffolo RR Jr, Feuerstein GZ. Possible involvement of stress-activated protein kinase signaling pathway and Fas receptor expression in prevention of ischemia/reperfusion-induced cardiomyocyte apoptosis by carvedilol. Circ Res 1998; 82: 166-174.
12.   Sabbah HN, Sharov VG. Apoptosis in heart failure. Prog Cardiovasc Dis 1998; 40: 549-562.
13.   Narula J, Haider N, Virmani R, DiSalvo TG, Kolodgie FD, Hajjar RJ, Schmidt U, Semigran MJ, Dec GW, Khaw BA. Apoptosis in myocytes in end-stage heart failure. N Engl J Med 1996; 335: 1182-1189.

14. Maulik N, Yoshida T, Das DK. Oxidative stress developed during the reperfusion of ischemic myocardium induces apoptosis. Free Radic Biol Med 1998; 24: 869-875.
15. Maulik N, Kagan VE, Tyurin VA, Das DK. Redistribution of phosphatidylethanolamine and phosphatidylserine precedes reperfusion-induced apoptosis. Am J Physiol 1998; 274: H242-H248.
16. Veinot JP, Gattinger DA, Fliss H. Early apoptosis in human myocardial infarction. Hum Pathol 1997; 28: 485-492.
17. Saraste A, Pulkki K, Kallajoki M, Hendriksen K, Parvinen M, Voipio-Pulkki LM. Apoptosis in human acute myocardial infarction. Circulation 1997; 95: 320-323.
18. Dzau VJ, Gibbons GH, Mann M, Braun-Dullaeus R. Future horizons in cardiovascular molecular therapeutics. Am J Cardiol 1997; 80: 331-391.
19. Haunstetter A, Izumo S. Apoptosis. Basic mechanisms and implications for cardiovascular disease. Circ Res 1998; 82: 1111-1129.
20. Bardales RH, Hailey LS, Xie SS, Schaefer RF, Hsu SM. In situ apoptosis assay for the detection of early acute myocardial infarction. Am J Pathol 1996; 149: 821-829.
21. Bing RJ, Suzuki H. Myocardial infarction and nitric oxide. Mol Cell Biochem 1997; 160-161: 303-306.
22. Karwatowska-Prokopczuk JA, Nordberg JA, Li HL, Engler RL, Gottlieb RA. Effect of vacuolar proteon ATPases on pHi, Ca2+, and apoptosis in neonatal cardiomyocytes during metabolic inhibition/recovery. Circ Res 1998; 82: 1139-1144.
23. Yin T, Sandhu G, Wolfgang CD, Burrier A, Webb RL, Rigel DF, Hai T, Whelan J. Tissue-specific pattern of stress kinase activation in ischemic/reperfused heart and kidney. J Biol Chem 1997; 272: 19943-19950.
24. Bielawska AE, Shapiro JP, Jiang L, Melkonyan HS, Piot C, Wolfe CL, Tomei LD, Hannun YA, Umansy SR. Ceramide is involved in triggering of cardiomyocyte apoptosis induced by ischemia and reperfusion. Am J Pathol 1997; 151: 1257-1263.
25. Kloner RA. Does reperfusion injury exist in humans ? J Am Coll Cardiol 1993; 21: 537-545.
26. Sigel AV, Romanic AM, Peng CF, Schunkert H, Feuerstein G, Riegger GAJ and Yue TL. Hypoxia and reoxygenation related injuries in cardiac myocytes are enhanced by programmed cell death: Differential protective effects of beta-adrenergic receptor blockers. Circulation 1998; 19: 742A.
27. MacLellan WR, Schneider MD. Death by design. Programmed cell death in cardiovascular biology and disease. Circ Res 1997; 81: 137-144.
28. Ferrari R, Agnoletti L, Comini L, Bachetti T, Cargnoni A, Ceconi C, Curello S, Visioli O. Oxidative stress during myocardial ischemia and heart failure. Eur Heart J 1998; 19 Suppl B: B2-B11.
29. Turner MJ, Evermann DB, Ellington SP, Fields CE. Detection of free radicals during the cellular metabolism of adriamycin. Free Radic Biol Med 1990; 9: 415-421.
30. Plaza V, Prat J, Rosello J, Ballester E, Ramis I, Mullol J, Gelpi E, Vives-Corrons JL, Picado C. In vitro release of arachidonic acid metabolites, glutathione peroxidase, and oxygen-free radicals from platelets of asthmatic patients with and without aspirin intolerance. Thorax 1995; 50: 490-496.
31. McCord JM. Superoxide radical: controversies, contradiction, and paradoxes. Proc Soc Exp Biol Med 1995; 209: 112-117.
32. Hiraishi H, Terano A, Ota S, Mutoh H, Sugimoto T, Harada T, Razandi M, Ivey KJ. Protection of cultured rat gastric cells against oxidant-induced damage by exogenous glutathione. Gastroenterology 1194; 106: 1199-1207.
33. Gross GJ. Do ATP-sensitive potassium channels play a role in myocardial stunning ? Basic Res Cardiol 1995; 90: 266-268.
34. Priori SG, Barhanin J, Hauer RN, Haverkamp W, Jongsma HJ, Kleber AG, McKenna WJ, Roden DM, Rudy J, Schwartz K, Schwartz PJ, Towbin JA, Wilde AM. Genetic and molecular basis of cardiac arrhythmias: impact on clinical management. Circulation 1999; 99: 674-681.
35. Baker K, Marcus CB, Huffman K, Kruk H, Malfroy B, Doctrow SR. Synthetic combined superoxide dismutase/catalase mimetics are protective as a delayed treatment in a rat stroke model: a key role for reactive oxygen species in ischemic brain injury. J Pharmacol Exp Ther 1998; 284: 215-221.
36. Horwitz LD, Wallner JS, Decker DE, Buxser SE. Efficacy of lipid soluble, membrane-protective agents against hydrogen peroxide cytotoxicity in cardiac myocytes. Free Radic Biol Med 1996; 21: 743-753.

37. Jeroudi MO, Hartley CJ, Bolli R. Myocardial reperfusion injury: role of oxygen radicals and potential therapy with antioxidants. Am J Cardiol 1994; 73: 2B-7B.

38. Kashima K, Yokayama S, Daa T, Nakayama I, Iwaki T. Immunohistochemical study on tissue transglutaminase and copper-zinc superoxide dismutase in human myocardium: its relevance to apoptosis detected by the nick end labelling method. Virchows Arch 1997; 430: 333-338.

39. Hazzalin CA, Cuenda A, Cano E, Cohen P, Mahadevan LC. Effects of the inhibition of p38/RK MAP kinase on induction of five fos and jun genes by diverse stimuli. Oncogene 1997; 15: 2321-2331.

40. Yamazaki T, Komuro I, Yazaki Y. Signalling pathways for cardiac hypertrophy. Cell Signal 1998; 10: 693-698.

41. Rozakis-Adcock M, van der Geer P, Mbamalu G, Pawson T. MAP kinase phosphorylation of mSos1 promotes dissociation of mSos1-Shc and mSos1-EGF receptor complexes. Oncogene 1995; 11: 1417-1426.

42. Marrero MB, Schieffer R, Li B, Sun J, Harp JB, Ling BN. Role of Janus kinase/signal transducer and activator of transcription and mitogen-activated protein kinase cascades in angiotensin II- and platelet-derived growth factor-induced vascular smooth muscle cell proliferation. J Biol Chem 1997; 272: 24684-24690.

43. Force T, Pombo CM, Avruch JA, Bonventre JV, Kyriakis JM. Stress-activated protein kinases in cardiovascular disease. Circ Res 1996; 78: 947-953.

44. Komuro I, Kudo S, Yamazaki T, Zou Y, Shiojima I, Yazaki Y. Mechanical stretch activates the stress-activated protein kinases in cardiac myocytes. FASEB 1996; 10: 631-636.

45. Li Q, Li B, Wang X, Leri A, Jana KP, Liu Y, Kajstura J, Baserga R, Anversa P. Overexpression of insulin-like growth factor-1 in mice protects from myocyte death after infarction, attenuating ventricular dilation, wall stress, and cardiac hypertrophy. J Clin Invest 1997; 100: 1991-1999.

46. Dennis SC, Gevers W, Opie LH. Protons in ischemia: where do they come from; where do they go? J Mol Cell Cardiol 1991; 23: 1077-1086.

47. Chen SJ, Bradley ME, Lee TC. Chemical hypoxia triggers apoptosis of cultured neonatal rat cardiac myocytes: modulation by calcium-regulated proteases and protein kinases. Mol Cell Biochem 1998; 178: 141-149.

48. Li WG, Zaheer A, Coppey L, Oskarsson HJ. Activation of JNK in the remote myocardium after large myocardial infarction in rats. Biochem Biophys Res Commun 1998; 246: 816-820.

49. Hayashi M, Yoshida T, Monkawa T, Yamaji Y, Sato S, Saruta T. Na+/H+ -exchanger-3 activity and its gene in the sponaneously hypertensive rat kidney. J Hypertens 1997; 15: 43-48.

50. Chakrabarti S, Hoque AN, Karmazyn M. A rapid ischemia-induced apoptosis in isolated rat hearts and its attenuation by the sodium-hydrogen exchanger inhibitor HOE 642 (cariprotide). J Mol Cell Cardiol 1997; 29: 3169-3174.

51. Senju S, Negishi I, Motoyama N, Wang F, Nakayama KI, Nakayama K, Lucas PJ, Hatakeyama S, Zhang Q, Yonehara S, Loh DY. Functional significance of the Fas molecule in native lymphocytes. Int Immunol 1996; 8: 423-431.

52. Nishigaki K, Minatoguchi S, Seishima M, Asano K, Noda T, Yasuda N, Sano H, Kumada H, Takemura H, Noma A, Tanaka T, Watanabe S, Fujiwara H. Plasma Fas ligand, an inducer of apoptosis, and plasma soluble Fas, an inhibitor of apoptosis in patients with chronic congestive heart failure. J Am Coll Cardiol 1997; 29: 1214-1220.

53. Misao J, Hayakawa Y, Ohno M, Kato S, Fujiwara T, Fujiwara H. Expression of bcl-2 protein, an inhibitor of apoptosis, and Bax, an accellerator of apoptosis, in ventricular myocytes of human hearts with myocardial infarction. Circulation 1996; 94: 1506-1512.

54. Cheng W, Kajstura J, Nitahara JA, Li B, Reiss K, Liu Y, Clark WA, Krajewski S, Reed JC, Olivetti G, Anversa P. Programmed myocyte cell death affects the viable myocardium after infarction in rats. Exp Cell Res 1996; 22: 316-327.

55. Bialik S, Geenen DL, Sasson IE, Cheng R, Horner JW, Evans SM, Lord EM, Koch CJ, Kitsis RN. Myocyte apoptosis during acute myocardial infarction in the mouse localizes to hypoxic regions but occurs independently of p53. J Clin Invest 1997; 100: 1363-1372.

56. Nicholson DW, Thornberry NA. Caspases: killer proteases. Trends Biochem Sci 1997; 22: 299-306.

57. Yang J, Liu X, Bhalla K, Kim CN, Ibrado AM, Cai J, Peng TI, Jones DP, Wang X. Prevention of apoptosis by Bcl-2: release of cytochrome c from mitochondria blocked. Science 1997; 275: 1129-1132.

258

58. Yaoita H, Ogawa K, Maehara K, Maruyama Y. Attenuation of ischemia/reperfusion injury in rats by a caspase inhibitor. Circulation 1998; 97: 276-281.
59. Yue TL, Wang C, Romanic AM, Kikly K, Keller P, DeWolf WE Jr, Hart TK, Thomas HC, Storer B, Gu JL, Wang X, Feuerstein GZ. Staurosporine-induced apoptosis in cardiomyocytes: a potential role of caspase-3. J Mol Cell Cardiol 1998; 30: 495-507.
60. Engelmann GL, Dionne CA, Jaye MC. Acidic fibroblast growth factor and heart development. Role in myocyte proliferation and capillary angiogenesis. Circ Res 1993; 72: 7-19.
61. Basilico C, Ambrosetti D, Fraidenraich D, Dailey L. Regulatory mechanisms governing FGF-4 gene expression during mouse development. J Cell Physiol 1997; 173: 227-232.
62. Cuevas P, Reimers D, Carceller F, Martinez-Coso V, Redondo-Horcajo M, Saenz-de-Tejada I, Gimenez-Gallego G. Fibroblast growth factor 1 prevents myocardial apoptosis triggered by ischemia reperfusion injury. Eur J Med Res 1997; 2: 465-468.
63. Suzuki H, Wildhirt SM, Dudek RR, Narayan KS, Bailey AH, Bing RJ. Induction of apoptosis in myocardial infarction and its possible relationship to nitric oxide synthase in macrophages. Tissue Cell 1997; 89-97.
64. Meldrum DR. Tumor necrosis factor in the heart. Am J Physiol 1998; 274: R577-R595.
65. Krown KA, Page MT, Nguyen C, Zechner D, Gutierrez V, Comstock KL, Glembotski CC, Quintana PJ, Sabbadini RA. Tumo necrosis factor alpha-induced apoptosis in cardiac myocytes. Involvement of the sphingolipid signaling cascade in cardiac death. J Clin Invest 1996; 98: 2854-2865.
66. Ferrari R, Ferrari F, Benigno M, Pepi P, Visioli O. Hibernating myocardium: its pathophysiology and clinical role. Mol Cell Biochem 1998; 186: 195-199.
67. Elsasser A, Schlepper M, Klovekorn WP, Cai WJ, Zimmermann R, Muller KD, Strasser R, Kostin S, Gagel C, Munkel B, Schaper W, Schaper J. Hibernating myocardium: an incomplete adaption to ischemia. Circulation 1997; 96: 2920-2931.
68. Gil VM, Hibernating myocardium. An incomplete adaption to ischemia. Rev Port Cardiol 1998; 17: 293-294.
69. Chen C, Ma L, Linfert DR, Lai T, Fallon JT, Gillam LD, Waters DD, Tsongalia GJ. Myocardial cell death and apoptosis in hibernating myocardium. J Am Coll Cardiol 1997; 30: 1407-1412.
70. Wildhirt SM, Dudek RR, Suzuki H, Bing RJ. Involvement of inducible nitric oxide synthase in the inflammatory process of myocardial infarction. Int J Cardiol 1995; 50: 253-261.
71. Vakeva AP, Agah A, Rollins SA, Matis LA, Li L, Stahl GL. Myocardial infarction and apoptosis after myocardial ischemia and reperfusion: role of the terminal complement components and inhibition by anti-C5 therapy. Circulation 1998; 97: 2259-2267.
72. Liu L, Azhar G, Gao W, Zhang X. Bcl-2 and Bax expression in adult rats after coronary occlusion: age associated differences. Am J Physiol 1998, 275: R315-R322.
73. Buerke M, Murohara T, Skurk C, Nuss C, Tomaselli K, Lefer AM. Cardioprotective effect of insulin-like growth factor 1 in myocardial ischemia followed by reperfusion. Proc Natl Acad Sci USA 1995; 92: 8031-8035.

III.2.2
Pro-inflammatory and pro-apoptotic factors in heart failure

Laura Agnoletti, M.D., Laura Comini, M.D., Giuseppina Gaia, M.D., Salvatore Curello, M.D., and Roberto Ferrari, M.D.

Salvatore Maugeri Foundation, Brescia, and University of Ferrara, Italy

INTRODUCTION

Congestive heart failure (CHF) is a final common pathway of different etiologies that results in a compensatory hypertrophy of myocytes which increase their size and the expression of contractile and other proteins normally expressed only during foetal development (1).

During the 20th century the "concept" of heart failure has been greatly modified. Initially, it was considered to be an oedematous disorder resulting from fluid and salt retention due to renal blood flow impairment. Thereafter, the idea of the cardio-circulatory model was proposed.

Until a decade ago, attention was focused on neuroendocrine activation as a major trigger of cardiovascular reactions. Recently, both in animals and in humans, it has become more and more evident that an altered immune function can promote the cardiac disease. This assumption is based on the observation that an over-expression of vasoconstrictory and pro-inflammatory members of the cytokine family worsens heart failure both locally by favouring cardiodepression and apoptosis, and systemically by triggering inflammation, cachexia and important metabolic alterations.

The compensatory responses that are initiated by left ventricular dysfunction are responsible for a "vicious cycle" that occurs in this disorder and which leads to further progression of cardiac failure, to subsequent multiple organ failure, and finally, to death (Figure 1) (2).

In the present article we will concentrate on the immunological alterations occuring in heart failure which could have a specific role in the induction of apoptosis.

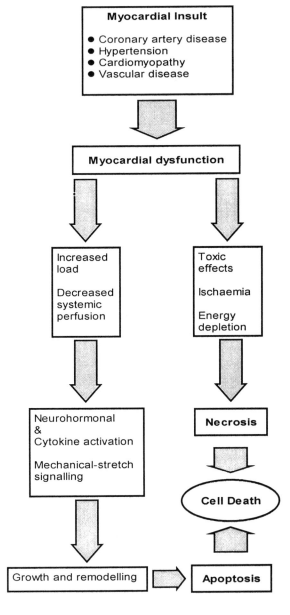

Figure 1 Central signalling pathways in production of adverse biological effects that induce the end fate of the cells.

IMMUNOLOGICAL ACTIVATION

The elevated rate of activity of the nervous sympathetic system is a primary factor in heart failure. Although an enhanced adrenergic drive helps to maintain the perfusion pressure despite a decreased plasma volume, prolonged sympathetic activation may ultimately contribute to the deterioration of cardiac function. The clinical setting of heart failure is so peculiar that humoral and cellular immunity should be considered for its evaluation.

In humoral immunity, the major mechanism of cell injury is complement activation which occurs when factor C1 attaches to an antigen/antibody complex on the surface of the target cell. A cascade of reactions is initiated resulting in the formation of the membrane attack complex which is arranged into a plasma membrane pore (3).

Cellular immunity also plays a role in the mechanism underlying cardiac dysfunction. Cellular immunity is initiated by the recognition of an immunogenic epitope by antigen-specific T lymphocytes. This activation is exerted by helper T cells and requires the presence of histocompatible antigen presenting cells. In dilated cardiomyopathy and myocarditis, abnormalities in cell-mediated immunity have been clinically demonstrated by the findings of a) cytokine production, b) autoantibody elaboration and autoreactive T cell activation and c) subset lymphocyte alteration (4). Moreover, the inappropriate expression of the major histocompatibility complex on cardiac tissue and expression of adhesion molecules on cardiac myocytes are known to occur (Table 1).

Table 1   Alteration in cellular immunity occurring in heart failure.

REFERENCES	ABNORMALITY IN CELLULAR IMMUNITY
• Andreassen at al 1998 (5)	Up-regulation of adhesion molecules and low-grade inflammation
• Toyozaki at al 1993 (6)	Expression of ICAM-1 on cardiac myocytes
• Eckstein at al 1982 (7)	Reduced suppressor T cell activity
• Anderson at al 1985 (8)	Deficient natural killer cell activity
• Hwang at al 1985 (9)	High percentage of helper T cells and high helper/suppressor ratio
• Ronnblom at al 1991(10)	Increased HLA-DR positive T cells
• Caforio at al 1990 (11)	Inappropriate expression of MHC class II molecule
• Koike at al 1989 (12)	Enhanced IL-2 production and reduced expression of IL-2 receptor of lymphocytes
• Limas at al 1995 (13)	Elevate soluble IL-2 receptor levels

The role of cellular and humoral immunity in the pathogenesis of myocyte injury in heart failure, however, is not well understood.

Cytokine production

Cachexia is a prominent feature in patients with end-stage heart failure. Although several theories have been proposed to describe the pathogenesis of cachexia (14,15) the cause of the severe weight loss and anorexia in these patients remains unclear. Reduction in calories intake or malabsorption of nutrients as well as enhanced secretion of endogenous hormones with anti-anabolic and catabolic activities may be related to the weight loss. In the 90's, Levine and Packer discovered that high levels of tumor necrosis factor-alpha (TNF-α) are related to the presence of cachexia (16), this finding encouraged the research on the involvement and role of cytokines in heart failure (Table 2).

Table 2   Proinflammatory cytokines involved in heart failure.

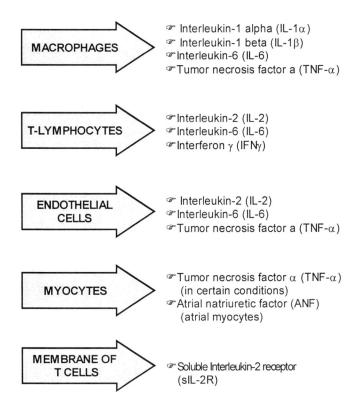

TNF-α is a pleiotropic cytokine with several biological actions. It was originally identified as a systemic mediator of different pathophysiological situations, involving endotoxemic shock, cachexia and tumor regression. Actually, we recognise that TNF-α is a member of a larger family of signalling proteins. These act in a paracrine manner, and they are not only involved in tissue inflammation and injury, but also regulate both cell proliferation and activation of programmed cell death (17,18). This latter function occurs during normal growth and development, but may also result from pathological conditions due to locally and systemically increased cytokine production (19).

TNF-α is a homotrimeric protein and can exist either as a membrane-bound form or as a truncated soluble form (20). TNF-α signalling occurs with high affinity, *in vitro* and *in vivo,* through two distinct receptors, TNF-RI (p55) and TNF-RII (p75). These receptors share extensive homology in their extra-cellular domains but have unrelated cytoplasmatic domains suggesting that they activate differing intracellular pathways. Expression of the two receptors also appears to be differentially regulated and exhibits tissue specificity. Extracellular portions can also exist in soluble forms (sTNF-RI and sTNF-RII) which capture and stabilise the free TNF-α, as well as neutralise and stabilise its biological activity.

As a mediator of general inflammation (21), TNF-α, together with interleukin-1 (IL-1), induces fever by the stimulation of hypothalamic prostaglandin-E2 (PGE2) production. It also activates the synthesis of IL-6 and IL-8 as well as of several other pro-inflammatory mediators. TNF-α, together with IL-1, promotes the expression of adhesive molecules such as integrins on leukocytes and the corresponding ligand, the intracellular adhesion molecule 1, on the endothelial cells. This mechanism is important because it initiates the recruitment of leukocytes to the site of infection. Together with interferon-γ, TNF-α upregulates the expression of the major histocompatibility complex (HLA) class II molecules on monocytes and macrophages (22).

The question arises as to whether cytokines and inflammatory molecules are involved in the pathogenesis of CHF or, conversely, CHF itself causes immune activation. Several scientists are in favour of this latter hypothesis as TNF-α increases in the blood of patients with end-stage heart failure (even in the absence of cachexia) and is associated with a shift from asymptomatic to symptomatic left ventricular dysfunction. Moreover, TNF soluble receptors are also increased in CHF patients and correlate with increased mortality (23). In the SOLVD study, IL-6 plasma levels were increased in CHF patients and correlated with TNF-α (24) values and were inversely associated with the prognosis (25).

Other studies support the pathological potential of inflammatory cytokine since transgenic mice over-expressing TNF-α in the heart develop dilated cardiomyopathy associated to myocyte apoptosis, transmural myocarditis and biventricular fibrosis (26,27) Likewise, in rats, chronic infusion of TNF-α resulted in left ventricular dysfunction and dilatation (28). TNF-α is thought to be dangerous for the heart since 1) it has intrinsic negative inotropic effects, 2) it plays an important role in the regulation of nitric oxide (NO) pathway stimulating the induction of a calcium-independent, macrophage-like nitric oxide synthase (iNOS) in smooth muscle and endothelial cells, as well as in myocytes and 3) it induces apoptosis in cardiac myocytes (29,30). In this context, we studied the induction of monocytic iNOS level and its relation with TNF-α system in patients with CHF. Interestingly, we found that iNOS presence was correlated to the activation of the TNF-α pathway (antigenic TNF and its soluble receptors) and strictly associated with the New York Heart Association (NYHA) functional class (31). This finding suggests that inflammatory cytokines have a central role in the development of the NO-mediated CHF.

Beside the heart, the vascular endothelium is also an important target of TNF-α and undergoes a number of morphological and functional changes at the molecular level including the surface expression of cellular adhesion molecules and the elaboration of other cytokines and chemokines. TNF-α also induces apoptosis in these cells. To evaluate its potential role in endothelial dysfunction occurring during heart failure, we studied the protein expression of endothelial NOS (eNOS) and the rate of apoptosis of human umbilical vein endothelial cells (HUVECs) after incubation with serum from NYHA class IV patients. Our data show that serum from these patients down-regulates eNOS expression and increases apoptosis, indirectly suggesting endothelial dysfunction. The addition of the anti-human TNF-α antibody to the serum from CHF patients reduced but did not counteract this effect suggesting that TNF-α is likely to play a role, but may not be the only responsible factor in the progression of the disease (Figure 2) (32).

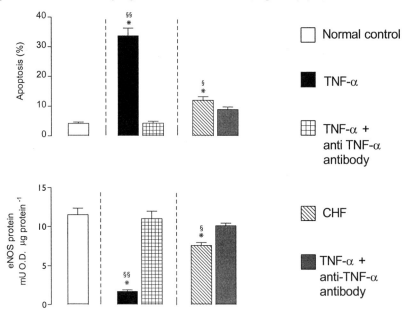

Figure 2 Apoptosis rate and eNOS expression of HUVECs after incubation with serum from healthy subjects and CHF patients. *p<0.001 vs normal control; §p<0.05 and §§p<0.001 vs treatment with antibody.

Another member of the TNF family is the Fas antigen, a cell-surface protein expressed in cardiomyocytes and involved in the signalling of apoptosis. On the cell membrane, Fas induces apoptosis when it binds Fas ligand (Fas-L) or soluble Fas-L (sFas-L) and also TNF-α. However, plasma sFas, a molecule without trans-membrane domain of Fas, blocks apoptosis by inhibiting binding between Fas and Fas-L or sFas-L on the cell membrane (Figure 3).

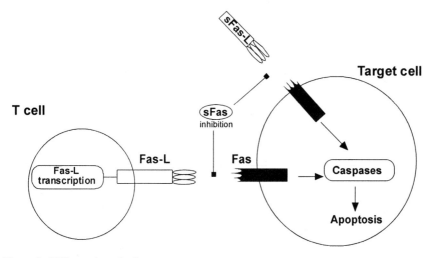

Figure 3 Killing pathway by Fas system.

At present, Fas is an attractive candidate as mediator of apoptosis in heart failure but its role in human myocardium is not well known. It has been recently demonstrated that hypoxia in advanced CHF can stimulate Fas receptor to induce apoptosis in cultured myocytes (33). Moreover, plasma levels of soluble Fas receptor have been studied in CHF patients in relation to TNF-α, IL-6 and NYHA class (34). The authors showed increase levels of TNF-α and IL-6 without significant difference in sFas-L between normal subjects and patients, independently from NYHA class. However, sFas increased with the severity of the functional class underlying an important role of sFas in the pathophysiological mechanisms of the disease.

Future efforts are needed to address the role of other cytokines (such as IL-1 and IL-6, their soluble receptors and receptor antagonists) that are also increased in heart failure. Studies in animals have shown that, as TNF-α, IL-6 and IL-2 inhibit the contractility of papillary muscle in a concentration-dependent reversible manner and that the administration of IL-1 promotes *coxsachievirus* B3 myocarditis in genetically resistant mice (35). Studies in humans demonstrated that patients with acute myocardial infarction had elevated levels of soluble IL-2 receptor (IL-2-R) and IL-1, especially in presence of heart failure and low ejection fraction (36). Munger et al. did not find statistical differences among IL-1β, sIL-2-R and TNF-α concentrations between CHF patients with mild-moderate heart failure and healthy subjects. However, sIL-2-R concentrations correlated with the functional class and were negatively associated with exercise tolerance (37), IL-6 levels were also significantly elevated. Marriot et al. measured serum concentrations of IL-2, IL-4, IL-10 and IL-12 in patients with idiopathic dilated cardiomyopathy (DCM), in their relatives with left ventricular enlargement (LVE), in patients with ischemic heart failure and in healthy subjects. They found IL-2 in DCM and LVE groups, and IL-10 abnormal concentrations in DCM, while IL-12 and IL-4 were not increased in any group, supporting the hypothesis of the immune pathogenesis of the disease (38).

Auto-antibody elaboration

Myocarditis, idiopathic dilated cardiomyopathy and post-myocardial infarction syndrome can be accompanied by the deposition of antibodies within myocardium. These antibodies can be directed against different antigens such as cardiac myosin, β-adrenergic receptor, M2 muscarinic, adenine nucleotide translocator (ANT) and others. Auto-antibodies directed against cell surface proteins are able to cause damage to cells. Antibodies directed against the ANT cause damage to the energetic metabolism *in vitro* and *in vivo* (39). Auto-antibodies directed against intracellular auto-antigen are unlikely to be pathogenic unless the cell membrane is already leaking or auto-antibodies cross-react with other surface molecules. It is expected that patients with more severe cardiac dysfunction have higher antibody titers if the antibody plays a causative role in the disease process. Actually, Limas and colleagues observed a rough correlation between the degree of left ventricular dysfunction and auto-antibody titers (40). Podlowski et al. show that after longer-term treatment with the anti-β_1-adrenergic receptor auto-antibodies, the rat cardiomyocytes showed a down-regulation of the β-adrenergic receptors similar to that observed in failings heart from patients with dilated cardiomyopathy suggesting, for these antibodies, a negative role in the cardiac function (41). On the other hand, Matsui and Fu did not report a significant correlation between the titers of anti-β_1-adrenoceptor and anti M2 muscarinic receptor antibodies and the clinical severity of the patients (42). However, the pathogenetic role of auto-antibodies in myocardial injury, associated with myocarditis and/or cardiomyopathy is not well established. Indeed, it may be that circulating auto-antibodies are a marker for, rather than the cause of, myocardial damage. It is interesting to note that ejection fraction improved in the surviving patients after enhanced immunosuppressive therapy by using corticosteroids and plasmapheresis (43).

Furthermore, genetic studies, showing that patients with dilated cardiomyopathy had an increased frequency of some HLA class II phenotypes, supported the hypothesis that some subjects may be predisposed to an immunoregulatory dysfunction (44).

Subset lymphocyte alteration

Different studies report an alteration of the circulating lymphocyte subsets in patients with congestive heart failure. However, these observations are not homogeneous. Several authors found a decreased $T_{suppressor}$-cell function (45,7), others a decreased natural killer-cell activity (8), while Hwang and co-workers (9) found an important reduction in the number of circulating lymphocytes and a decreased number of natural killer and $T_{suppressor/cytotoxic}$, as well as an increase in the $T_{helper/suppressor}$ ratio in a large group of heart failure patients. The same authors observed that these alterations were not related to the cause of the disease but rather to its severity, thus suggesting that elevated norepinephrine levels could play a role in the abnormal T-cell distribution, synergically with a reduced cardiac output or elevations of other stress hormones, also increased in heart failure. This pathological activation initiates the auto-immune reaction, which leads to destruction of myocardial tissue evolving in myocyte fibrosis and necrosis and in up to contractility depression.

References

1. Chien KR, Zhu H, Knowlton KU et al. Transcriptional regulation during cardiac growth and development. *Annu Rev Phisiol* 1993;55,77-95.
2. Katz AM. The cardiomyopathy of overload: an unnatural growth response in the hypertrophied heart. *Ann Intern Med* 1994;121:363-71.
3. Barry WH. Mechanisms of immune-mediated myocyte injury. *Circulation* 1994;89:2421-32.
4. Limas C. Autoimmunity in dilated cardiomyopathy and the major histocompatibility complex. *Int J Cardiol* 1996;54:113-6.
5. Andreassen AH, Nordoy I, Siminsens S, Ueland T, Muller F, Froland SS, Gullestad L, Aukrust P. Levels of circulating adeshion molecules in congestive heart failure and after heart transplantation. *Am J Cardiol* 1998;81(5):604-8.
6. Toyozaki T, Saito T, Takano H, et al. Expression of intracellular adhesion molecule-1 on cardiac myocyte for myocarditis before and during immuno-suppresive therapy. *Am J Cardiol* 1993;72:441-4.
7. Eckstein R, Mempel W, Bolte HD. Reduced suppressor cell activity in congestive cardiomyopathy and in myocarditis. *Circulation* 1982;65:1224-9.
8. Anderson JL, Carlquist JF, Hammond EH. Deficient natural killer cell activity in patients with idiopathic dilated cardiomyopathy. *Am J Cardiol* 1985;55:755-8.
9. Hwang S, Harris TJ, Wilson NW, Maisel AS. Immune function in patients with chronic stable congestive heart failure. *Am Heart J* 1993;125:1651-8.
10. Rönnblom LE, Forsberg H, Evrin P. Increased level of HLA-DR-expressing T lymphocytes in peripheral blood from patient with idiopathic dilated cardiomyopathy. *Cardiology* 1991;78:161-7.
11. Caforio ALP, Stewart JT, Bonifacio E et al. Inappropriate major histocompatibility complex expression on cardiac tissue in dilated cardiomyopathy. Relative for autoimmunity? *J Autoimmun* 1990;3:187-200.
12. Koike S. Immunological disorders in patients with dilated cardiomyopathy. *Jpn Heart J* 1989;30:799-807.
13. Limas CJ, Goldemberg IF, Limas C. Soluble interleukine-2 receptor levels in patients with dilated cardiomyopathy. *Circulation* 1995;91:631-43.
14. Friedberg CK. *Diseases of the heart.* Philadelphia, PA: Saunders, 1996, p 233.
15. Pittman JC, Cohen P. The pathogenesis of cardiac cachexia. *N Engl J Med* 1964;271:453-60.
16. Levine B, Kalman J, Mayer L, Fillit HM, Packer M. Elevated circulating levels of necrosis factor in severe chronic heart failure. *N Engl J Med* 1990;323:236-41.
17. Ware CF, VanArsdale TL. Apoptosis mediated by the TNF-related cytokine and receptor families. *J Cell Biochem* 1996;60:47-55.
18. Wang CY, Mayo MW, Baldwin ASJ. TNF-α and cancer therapy-induced apoptosis: potentiation by inhibition of NFkB [see comments]. *Science* 1996;274:784-7.
19. Sharov VG, Sabbah HN, Shimoyama H, Goussev AV, Lesch M, Goldstein S. Evidence of cardiocyte apoptosis in myocardium of dogs with chronic heart failure. *Am J Pathol* 1996;148:141-9.
20. Baker SJ, Reddy EP. Transducers of life and death: TNF receptor superfamily and associated proteins. *Oncogene* 1996;12(1):1-9.
21. Tracey KJ. The acute and chronic pathophysiological effects of TNF: mediation of septic shock and wasting. In: Beutler B, editor. Tumor necrosis factors: the molecules and their emerging role in medicine. New York, NY: Raven, 1992:255-73.
22. Van Deuren M, Dofferhoff ASM, Van der Meer JW. Cytokines and the response to infection. *J Pathol* 1992;168:349-56.

APOPTOSIS IN CARDIAC BIOLOGY

23.	Ferrari R, Bachetti T, Confortini R et al. Tumor necrosis factor soluble receptors in patients with various degrees of congestive failure. *Circulation* 1995;92:1479-86.
24.	Torre-Amione G, Kapadia S, Benedict C, Oral H, Young JB, Mann DL. Proinflammatory cytokine levels in patients with depressed left ventricular ejection fraction: a report from the studies of left ventricular dysfunction (SOLVD). *J Am Coll Cardiol* 1996;27:1201-6.
25.	Tsutamoto T, Hisanaga T Wada A, Maeda Y, Fukai D. Plasma concentration of interleukin-6 as a marker of prognosis in patients with chronic congestive heart failure (Abstr). *Circulation* 1994;90:I-381.
26.	Kubota T, McTiernan CF, Frye CS et al. Dilated cardiomyopathy in transgenic mice with cardiac-specific overexpression of tumor necrosis factor-alpha. *Cir Res* 1997;81:627-35.
27.	Bryant D, Becker L, Richardson J et al. Cardiac failure in transgenic mice with myocardial expression of tumor necrosis factor-alpha. *Circulation* 1998;97:1375-81.
28.	Bozkurt B, Kribbs SB, Clubb FJ et al. Pathophysiologiaclly relevant concentrations of tumor necrosis factor-alpha promote progressive left ventricular dysfunction and remodeling in rats. *Circulation* 1998;97:1382-91.
29.	Pinsky DJ, Cai B, Yang X, Rodriguez C, Sciacca RR, Cannon PJ. The lethal effects of cytokine-induced nitric oxide on cardiac myocytes are blocked by nitric oxide synthase antagonism or transforming growth factor beta. *J Clin Invest* 1995;95:677-85.
30.	Krown KA, Page MT, Nguyen C et al. Tumor necrosis factor alpha-induced apoptosis in cardiac myocytes. *J Clin Invest* 1996;98:2854-65.
31.	Comini L, Bachetti T, Agnoletti L, Gaia G, Curello S, Milanesi B, Volterrani M, Parrinello G, Ceconi C, Giordano A, Corti A, Ferrari R. Induction of functional inducible nitric oxide sinthase in monocyte of patients with congestive heart failure: link with tumor necrosis factor-α. *European Heart J*, in press.
32.	Agnoletti L, Curello S, Bachetti T, Malacarne F, Gaia G, Comini L, Volterrani M, Bonetti P, Parrinello G, Cadei M, Grigolato PG, Ferrari R. Serum from patients with severe heart failure down-regulate eNOS and is proapoptotic: role of the tumor necrosis factor-α. *Circulation*, in press.
33.	Tanaka M, Ito H, Adachi S et al. Ipoxia induces apoptosis with enhanced expression of Fas antigen messenger RNA in cultured neonatal rad cardiomyocytes. *Circ Res* 1994;75:426-33.
34.	Nishigaki K, Minatoguchi S, Seishima M, asano K, Noda T, Yasuda N, Sano H, Kumada H, Takemura M, Noma A, Tanaka T, Watanabe S, Fujiwara H. Plasma Fas ligand, an inducer of apoptosis and plasma soluble Fas, an inhibitor of apoptosis in patients with chronic congestive heart failure. *J Am Coll Cardiol* 1997;29(6):1214-20.
35.	Lane JR, Neumann DA, Lafond-Walker A, Herskowitz A Rose NR. Interleukin-1 or tumor necrosis factor can promote coxsackie B3-induced myocarditis in resistant B10.A mice. *J Exp Med* 1992;175:1123-9.
36.	Blum A, Scarovsky S, Rehavia E, Shohat B. Levels of T-lymphocyte subpopulations, interleukin-1 beta, and soluble interleukin-2 receptor in acute myocardial infarction. *Am Heart J* 1994;127:1226-30.
37.	Munger MA, Johnson B, Amber IJ, Callahan KS, Gilbert EM. Circulating concentrations of proinflammatory cytokines in mild or moderate heart failure secondary to ischemic or idiopathic dilated cardiomyopathy. *Am J Cardiol* 1996;77:723-7.
38.	Marriott JB, Goldman JH, Keeling PJ, Baig M K, Dalgleish AG, McKenna WJ. Abnormal cytokine profiles in patients with idiopathic dilated cardiomyopathy and their asymptomatic relatives. *Heart* 1996;75:287-90.
39.	Schulze K, Becker BF, Schauer R, Schultheiss HP. antibodies to ADP-ATP carries – an auto-antigen in myocarditis and dilated cardiomyopathy –impair cardiac function. *Circulation* 1990;81:959-69.
40.	Limas CJ, Limas C. Immune-mediated modulation of b-adrenoceptor function in human dilated cardiomyopathy. *Clin Immunopathol* 1993;68:204-7.
41.	Podlowski S, Luther HP, Morwinski R, Müller J, Wallukat G. Agonistic anti-β1-adrenergic receptor autoantibodies from cardiomyopathy patients reduce the β1-adrenergic receptor expression in neonatal rat cardiomyocytes. *Circulation* 1998;98:2470-6.
42.	Matsui S, Fu M. Characteristic distribution of circulating auto-antibodies against G-protein coupled cardiovascular receptors in patients with idiopathic dilated and hypertrophic cardiomyopathy. *Int J Cardiol* 1996;54:143-7.

270

43. McNamara D, Di-Salvo T, Mathier M, Keck S, Semigran M, Dec GW. Left ventricular dysfunction after heart transplantation: incidence and role of enhanced immunosoppression. *J Heart Lung Transplant* 1996;15:506-15.
44. Carlquist JF, Menlove RL, Murray MB et al.HLA class II (DR and DQ) antigen associations in idiopathic dilated cardiomyopathy. *Circulation* 1991;83:515-22.
45. Fowles RE, Bieber CP, Stinson EB. Defective in vitro suppressor cell function in idiopathic congestive cardiomyopathy. *Circulation* 1979;59:483-91.

III.2.3
Molecular mechanisms of cardiac myocardial remodeling during aging. Role of apoptosis

Ziad Mallat, M.D., and Bernard Swynghedauw, M.D.
U141 and U127-INSERM, Lariboisière Hospital, Paris, France

INTRODUCTION

Studies on myocardial senescence are far from being academic for several reasons. Epidemiological studies have shown that diseases of the heart are one of the major causes of mortality among overall population and the main cause of death in people after 65 years of age (1). Therefore, it is of major importance to determine the physiological structure and function of the heart in healthy aged persons and to assess the limits of normality in all age groups. The clinical problem is far from being simple because obviously the basic process of senescence is intimately associated with an increased incidence of arterial hypertension, atheroclerosis, cancer, and also with several modifications in physical activity and nutritional status which all may seriously modify the myocardial structure. It is possible to carefully select aged people who have normal blood pressure and no clinical history of coronary disease, but anatomical studies have demonstrated the high incidence of occult coronary stenosis in people who die from all causes (2). Therefore, it would be very difficult to eliminate such a disease only on the basis of clinical criteria. It is also ethically difficult to organize a large epidemiological study on aging which would include routine coronarography (reviewed in 2-5). The advent of non invasive imaging techniques such as electron-beam computed tomography (6) may prove to be of value in this setting. From a pure economical point of view, it is quite important to know whether aged myocardium behaves like myocardium of adult persons in their responses to various stimuli and drugs, and whether it would be more suitable to perform the first screening of new therapies in senescent animal models.

From a structural point of view, cardiac remodeling not only occurs during diseased conditions, but also during the normal process of senescence (7). The aged heart is indeed not only enlarged but also different in terms of molecular structures including renin-angiotensin system, receptor densities, myosin content, and capacity to hypertrophy. Myocardial fibrosis also increases with age, and plays a crucial role as a determinant of arrhythmias and changes in ventricular compliance. Finally, myocardial cell loss occurs with aging, and it has been suggested that this may be the result of incresaed cell death (necrosis and apoptosis). Cardiac apoptosis has been repeatedly reported in various diseased conditions which are described in other chapters of this book, nevertheless, studies on cell death in undiseased senescent hearts are extremely rare and provide contradictory results.

PHYSIOLOGICAL AND ANATOMICAL BACKGROUND

Cardiac hypertrophy

The Heart Weight/Body Weight ratio is unchanged during aging, except in very old animals (rats > 27 months) and in humans above 85 years (8). It is not clear whether such hypertrophy may relate to changes intrinsic to the heart or relate to the fact that aged persons or animals do not feed normally depending of various environmental conditions.

Table 1   Effects of aging on cardiovascular structure and function in healthy elderly subjects (2, 3).

Anatomical data
Increased left ventricular mass, normal heart weight/body weight ratio
Dilatation of the aortic orifice and the great vessels
Dilatation of arterioles and diminished capillary density
Myocyte hypertrophy
Fibrosis (interstitial and perivascular)
Cell loss

Functional data
Normal cardiac output at rest and during exercise
Increased characteristic aortic impedance and arterial stiffness
Decreased ventricular early diastolic filling rate
Increased atrial contribution to ventricular filling
Adaptation to exercise with more Frank-Starling mechanism than tachycardia
Exercise-induced increase in cardiac output is normal
Decreased cardiovascular response to catecholamines
Arrhythmias and attenuation of the heart rate variability

In addition, when the results were not normalized for the body weight, the degree of hypertrophy, in g, is always more pronounced on the left side than on the right one, and the Left/Right Ventricular Weight ratio is usually slightly augmented with aging. Such an asymetry has also been confirmed using the tibia length instead of the body weight (Table 1) (9).

Energetics

The senescent heart is in many respects comparable to left ventricular overload. Contraction energetics of papillary muscle was calculated from mechanical parameters, force and velocity. During senescence, the peak power output was significantly depressed and the curvature G of the force /velocity curve was increased, which indicates that each contraction was more economical (Tables 2 and 3) (10). An interesting finding, made in man, is that the force-time integral of the individual myosin cross-bridge cycle is correlated with the age of the patient with nonfailing myocardium, suggesting that, even in man, aging is also associated with an improved contraction economy (Table 2) (11). The blunted response of the autonomous nervous system to exercising is also well-documented (2, 12).

Table 2   Papillary muscle energetics during senescence in rat heart (recalculated from 10, 11).

	3 mo	22-24 mo
Isotonic contraction and relaxation		
Maximum shortening velocity,		
V_{cmax}, in L_{max}/s:	2.38±0.06	1.99±0.08**
Maximum unloaded shortening		
velocity, V_{max}, in L_{max}/s:	3.20±0.06	2.81±0.10**
Maximum lengthening velocity,		
V_{rmax}, in L_{max}/s:	3.25±0.1	2.75±0.09**
Isometric contraction		
Active force per surface area,		
mN/mm^2:	55±2	45±2*
Energetics		
Curvature of the Hill's hyperbola, G:	1.6±0.07	1.93±0.13*
Peak power output, E_{max},		
in $mN . L_{max} . s^{-1} . mm^{-2}$:	30±1	20±1**

* $p < 0.05$, ** $p < 0.01$

Systolic and diastolic function at rest

The Baltimore study has clearly demonstrated that cardiac output, ejection fraction, shortening fraction and velocity of circunferential fiber shortening are not altered with aging (2). The afterload of the left ventricle is represented by aortic impedance.

Aortic impedance is increased with aging mainly because of an increased aortic stiffness and a dilatation of big vessels.

During senescence the global diastolic function remains unchanged despite a pronounced impairment of the early ventricular filling because the contribution of atrial systole to ventricular filling is increased (2). The impairment in early ventricular filling and the diminution of the E wave was shown by EchoDoppler results suggesting both a prolonged active isovolumic relaxation and an increased myocardial stiffness.

Studies on contractility on papillary muscle were complicated by the fact that the senescent papillary muscle is both thicker and stiffer than the young muscles which both impairs the oxygenation of the preparation and limits the accuracy of the measurements of active force. Nevertheless, it has been shown that isometric as well as isotonic contraction is prolonged in every species studied and both the maximum velocity of shortening and the maximum unloaded shortening velocity were depressed. Both the relaxation velocity and the peak of negative force derivative normalized per cross-sectional area were depressed (Table 2) (10, 13).

The cardiovascular response to exercise

One of the most consistent findings in gerontologic research is the age-related decline in VO_2 max, although cardiac output does not decline with age. At least part of the decline in VO_2 max appears to be due to a decrease in maximal arteriovenous oxygen difference. The exercise - induced increase in cardiac output is unchanged during aging, nevertheless in normal young adults such an increase is mainly due to tachycardia while, during senescence, the heart rate is unchanged by exercising and the increase in cardiac output is caused by an increased ejection fraction. The cardiovascular effects of an adrenergic stimulation which is obtained by exercising or isoproterenol infusion, are attenuated (2, 3, 12).

Arrhythmias

Clinical studies demonstrate a prevalence of supraventricular and ventricular ectopic beats. In humans, time domain analysis revealed an age-related diminution of the heart rate variability. In the senescent heart, arrhythmias result from both fibrosis and changes in the structure and concentration of the various membrane proteins which are directly or indirectly responsible for the intracellular calcium movements (14, 15).

PHENOTYPIC MODIFICATIONS OF CARDIOCYTES

Calcium movements

The modifications of the membrane proteins occur at several different levels including the Ca^{2+}ATPase of the sarcoplasmic reticulum, SR, and also the adrenergic and vagal receptors, the calcium channels, the Na^+/Ca^{2+} exchange and the (Na^+, K^+)-ATPase (16-21). This phenoconversion of membrane proteins is directly responsible for the slowing of the intracellular calcium transient as measured with fluorescent probes specific for calcium (22) and can take into account the decrease in V max. In addition, we know that the duration of the action potential is prolonged (23), and that this is likely to be the consequence of a change in the potassium channels and currents. The activity of this exchanger was attenuated in the aged myocardium as in cardiac hypertrophy of mechanical origin. In vitro, the activity of the Na^+/Ca^{2+} exchanger is progressively reduced from 4 to 27 months in the senescent rat ventricle as the capacity of SR to pump calcium (24).

Table 3   Renin-angiotensin-aldosterone system and atrial natriuretic factor in senescent rats.

	Young	Senescent
Circulating RAAS and plasma hormones concentrations		
Renin activity, (ng AngI/mL/h)	38±5	6±1***
Angiotensin I (ng/mL)	6±1	1.7±0.2***
Aldosterone (fmol/mL):	844±99	715±85
Cortisol (nmol/mL)	42±3	68±9*
Free T4 (pg/mL)	29±2	12±2***
Free T3 (pg/mL)	3.1±0.2	2.6±0.2
Plasma ANF (pmol/L)	21±6	52±8*
Ventricular content in mRNAs of RAAS and ANF		
Left Ventricle		
Angiotensinogen (fg mRNA/mgRNA)	18±2	92±29**
ACE (fg mRNA/mgRNA)	50±5	120±21**
ANF (Densitometric score)	2±0.5	23±5***
Right Ventricle		
Angiotensinogen (in fg mRNA/mgRNA)	215±53	181±41
ACE (fg mRNA/mgRNA)	1.9±0.2	2.0±0.2
ANF (Densitometric score)	2.5±0.7	2.0±0.4

$p<0.05 **p<0.01 ***p<0.001
ACE: *A*ngiotensin-I-*C*onverting-*E*nzyme; ANF: *A*trial-*N*atriuretic-*F*actor; RAAS: *R*enin-*A*ngiotensin-*A*ldosterone-*S*ystem; (reprinted from 26 and 28).

Cardiac hormones

Aging also modifies the endocrine system and is associated with an increased plasma level of cortisol and atrial natriuretic factor and low plasma levels of free T4 (but T3 is unchanged), angiotensin I and II, renin activity and angiotensinogen[25-27], which is clearly different from the situation observed in pressure overload.

However, both the myocardial renin-angiotensin system and the angiotensin II subtype 1 receptor density are upregulated (26-27) during aging (Table 3). This upregulation is restricted to the left ventricle and does not occur in the right ventricle suggesting that the trigger for activation is the left ventricular mechanical overload. Since cardiac failure is a disease of the elderly, most patients have a negligible plasma level of angiotensin II. It might therefore be of interest to know how angiotensin converting enzyme inhibitors work in such a setting? The answer is most likely to be found in the various tissue systems, at least the ones located in the myocardium (Tables 3 and 4).

Table 4 Senescent heart versus overloaded heart. Renin-angiotensin system, atrial natriuretic factor and autonomous nervous system receptors.

	Overload	Senescence
Renin-Angiotensin-System		
Circulating:	⇑	⇓⇓•
Myocardial:	⇑	⇑
Aldosterone:	= or ⇑	=
Atrial Natriuretic Factor		
Plasma ANF:	⇑	⇓•
Ventricular mRNA:	⇑	⇑
Autonomous Nervous System		
Heart Rate Variability:	⇓	⇓⇓
Sensitivity to Isoproterenol:	⇓	⇓
β-Adrenergic Receptor Density:	⇓	⇓
mRNA:	⇓	⇓⇓⇓•
Muscarinic Receptor Density:	⇓	⇓⇓⇓•
mRNA:	⇓	⇑⇑⇑•
$G_{\alpha s}$ mRNA:	=	⇓•
$G_{\alpha i2}$ mRNA:	=	=

⇓: decreased. ⇑: increased. =: unchanged. +: pronounced. +++: extremely important. •Indicates significant differences between Senescence and Overload.

In vitro, the basal ANF secretory rate was greater in atria from aged animals, and also the secretory response to phenylephrine, but not to stretch, suggesting that an increased secretory response to adrenergic stimulation may contribute to the enhanced ANF plasma levels. Molecular biological determinations of the relative levels of mRNA coding for ANF showed a strong activation in the left, but not in the right ventricle (26, 28).

Autonomous nervous system

In the senescent Wistar rat heart, the density of both the total β-adrenergic and muscarinic receptors are diminished but the drop in muscarinic receptor density is greater than that in total β-adrenergic receptors (29-31). Several findings suggest that in fact the receptors were not the only component of the myocardial autonomous system to be modified during aging (Table 4). A diminution of the $G_{\alpha s}$ mRNA was also observed and the adenylate cyclase is also modified (32). Aging, as mechanical overload, is accompanied by several modifications of the autonomous myocardial system which are likely to be located "down the road", as initially suggested by E. Lakatta (2).

Table 5 Senescent heart versus overloaded heart. Fibrosis, arrhythmias and mechanics (from 5, 10, 14)

	Overload	Senescence
Fibrosis:	+ or 0	+++ •
Arrhythmias:	+	+++ •
Mechanics of papillary muscle:		
Max. Shortening Velocity:	⇓	⇓
Max. Relengthening Velocity:	⇓	⇓
Active Force per mm²:	⇓	⇓ or =
Energetics:		
Curvature G of the F/V curve:	⇑	⇑
Contractile and Membrane Proteins:		
Action Potential Duration:	⇑	⇑
Calcium Transient Duration:	⇑	⇑
Isomyosin Shift to V3:	+	+
Ca^{2+} ATPase of SR:	⇓	
Na^+/Ca^{2+} Exchanger:	⇓	⇓
Na^+, K^+ ATPase, Shift to A3:	+	+

⇓: decreased. ⇑: increased. =: unchanged. +: pronounced. +++: extremely important. •Indicates significant differences between senescence and overload.

Contractile proteins

The ventricles of a two month old rat contain 100% V1, and this percentage declines in proportion to aging, so the content in V1 is nearly a mean to determine age in this animal species. This shift of the isomyosins, which also occurs during cardiac overload, results in a decreased ATPase activity which parallels the decline in the unloaded shortening velocity and, at least in rats, is likely to constitute the main determinant of the adaptational process (Table 5) (33, 34). Correlation analysis demonstrated a strong positive correlation between shortening velocity and both the content in slow isomyosin and Ca^{2+} ATPase of SR, nevertheless partial correlation analysis showed that the relaxation parameters depended more on the isoforms of myosin than on Ca^{2+} ATPase density of SR. This which outlines the strong dependency of active relaxation, relative to contraction (33), upon the aging process.

Protein turnover, capacity to hypertrophy

The modifications that occur in both protein synthesis and degradation, and in mRNA content during aging would suggest that the senescent heart may also be unable to adapt to an increased load or to further hypertrophy in response to a mechanical stress. This question has more than an academic interest since the main causes of cardiac hypertrophy are indeed much more frequent after 65 years than before (1). Recent studies showed that both the yield in total RNA and the total amount of cardiac polyA containing RNAs relative to ribosomal RNA remained unchanged, and the general opinion is that the capacity of the senescent heart to hypertrophy is unchanged, although the process may be slower (9, 10, 33).

CHANGES IN EXTRACELLULAR MATRIX

Myocardial fibrosis is a constant finding in healthy senescent hearts both in rats and humans (10, 14, 33, 35-37). Cardiac fibrosis in this condition is certainly, at least in part, a reparative process related to myocyte loss and predominates in the subendocardium (Table 5). The concentration of the two main components of fibrosis, namely collagen I and fibronectin, increases during aging. The increased collagen concentration has been evidenced both biochemically by quantitating the tissue content in hydroxyproline (the tissue concentration in this amino acid is doubled by aging) and histologically by quantitative morphometry. By contrast, both type I and type III procollagen mRNA levels were reduced in the senescent rat heart (-63% and -51% as compared to 3 month old animals at the age of 16 and 24 month old animals respectively) showing that changes in myocardial collagen mRNA and protein were not synchronous and suggesting that during senescence collagen concentration is not transcriptionally regulated.

Nevertheless, the regulation of myocardial concentration in collagen during ageing is a complex phenomenon. Two different studies have provided converging results and have shown a paradoxically inverse relationship between the protein and mRNA content of collagen in aging hearts, the lower the mRNA concentration, the higher the protein levels, which is in contrast with the situation observed with fibronectin (33, 36). In addition, a 40-45% decrease in both collagenase (matrix metalloproteinases, MMPs) 2 and MMP 1 has recently been evidenced in 22-24 month old rats, suggesting that collagen accumulation is, at least in part, regulated at the level of the degradative pathway(38). This does not seem to be the case in the overloaded heart which shows increased levels of MMPs mRNAs and activities (39).

CELL DEATH (NECROSIS AND APOPTOSIS)

Clinical and experimental studies had revealed that in the aged heart, loss of myocytes and fibrosis are associated with myocyte hypertrophy which is more significant in the left ventricle (60%) than in the right ventricle (10% to 20%). It was commonly admitted that, after birth, the cardiac cells have lost their capacity to undergo DNA synthesis, cytokinesis and mitosis (35).

A study from Anversa et al. (35) using 3 and 21 month old male Sprague Dawley rats showed a significant degree of cardiac hypotrophy. Such a hypotrophy is a consequence of a pronounced loss in the cardiocytes located mostly in the endocardium of the left ventricle. Such a loss is only partly compensated by an enhanced myocyte volume (from 15 to 31.10^{-3} mm^3), cardiocyte hypertrophy is a constant finding during senescence and is much more pronounced in the left ventricle than in the right ventricle.

The aged heart contains less myocytes than younger hearts. Based on autopsy findings, it has been suggested that the process is gender-specific and does not occur in women (40). The cause of death includes both ischemic necrosis due to the aged-related reduction in coronary reserve and apoptosis which is temporally and spatially unrelated to necrosis. In aged Fischer rat hearts as compared to young hearts, necrosis (which was quantitated with injection with myosin monoclonal antibody) is the predominant cause of cell death. Quantification has indeed shown that there are about 1,000 times more necrotic cells (13,600 myocytes in the left ventricle and 9,000 in the right one at 24 month) than apoptotic cells (874 cells in the left ventricle at 24 month). The combiantion of the two processes was found in 1,150 cells at 3 month and in 14,5500 cells at 24 month (41). Since the completion of the apoptotic process may require only few hours, the window for detection of fragmented DNA using the TUNEL method may be very short, suggesting that the finding of only a low percentage of apoptotic cell death at a given point in time may actually reflect an important number of cells undergoing apoptosis. Apoptosis (which was evaluated both by the terminal deoxynucleotidyl transferase assay and DNA laddering) during aging is localised into the left ventricle suggesting that it is initiated by mechanical factors.

The observation of increased apoptotic cardiocyte death has not been confirmed in humans. In a recent abstract (42), the percentage of myocyte cell death by apoptosis in 27 autopsy samples from patients who died of extra-cardiac disease has been determined using the TUNEL method. Several myocardial regions were examined including the anterior, lateral and posterior regions of the left ventricle, the septum and the right ventricle, and an average of 76,609 myocyte nuclei was examined from each heart. The percentage of cardiomyocyte death ranged from 0% to 0.04% with no correlation between age and the apoptotic index (Figure 1).

However, the percentage of apoptotic cardiomyocytes was found to be 3-fold higher in men than in women (unpublished data). In this study, increased apoptotic myocyte death was found in 2 subjects who died after prolonged anoxia. This underscores the necessity of making a strict and careful selection of subjects before attributing any change in the rate of apoptotic myocyte death to aging per se. Further studies are needed to confirm these findings and to examine the relative importance of apoptosis versus necrosis during the aging process.

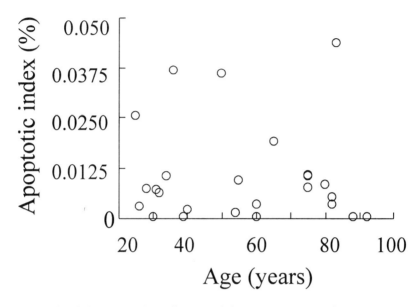

Figure 1 The relation between the cardiac apoptotic index (%) and the age of the subject at the time of death.

PATHOGENESIS OF THE SENESCENT HEART

Senescent versus pressure-overload heart

As explained previously, careful clinical investigations have demonstrated that the senescent heart has normal myocardial performances at rest and during exercise because it uses several compensatory mechanisms to maintain a normal output. Experimental investigations have indeed confirmed these findings and have shown several modifications both at the molecular, cellular and multicellular (papillary muscle) levels in the aging rat heart, which are very similar to those observed during experimental pressure-overload, while in vivo studies showed essentially normal myocardial functions (2).

Fibrosis is also a common feature found both during overload and in senescence. Nevertheless, although fibrosis is a constant finding in the aging heart, there are several examples of mechanically overloaded hearts in which the collagen concentration remains normal, and it has recently been suggested that fibrosis in these particular conditions is under hormonal control (43). Arrhythmias and a loss in heart rate variability are a common feature between the two conditions both in humans and in animals, nevertheless the types of arrhythmias, their frequency and prognostic value are extremely different. The β adrenergic/muscarinic receptor ratio remains unchanged during cardiac hypertrophy, while the same ratio is increased during senescence in the rat heart due to a much more pronounced decrease in muscarinic compared to β-adrenergic receptor density (44).

Finally, although increased cell death is a common feature between the two conditions in animals, it remains to be shown whether increased cell death also occurs during normal senecence in humans. Also, the relative contribution of necrosis versus apoptosis deserves further investigation.

Changes in the senescent heart are multifactorial

Several alterations, but not all, observed in the heart of elderly results from the general process of adaptation of any muscle to a mechanical overload. In the case of senescence, mechanical overload results from an increased characteristic impedance and stiffness of the aorta and a dilatation of all the major arteries which are a major finding in the senescent vessels. In other words, the senescent heart is firstly an overloaded heart and reflects the vascular effects of aging.

Nevertheless, there are several changes occuring in the aged myocardium which cannot be explained by a simple mechanical overload, including the myocyte loss, the pronounced fibrosis and its clinical consequences (permanent, or nearly permanent, arrhythmias), and the several changes that occur in the right ventricle. The origins of these modifications can be related to the endocrine modifications linked to aging or to the general process of senescence. Aging does not seem, for the moment, to affect cardiomyocyte apoptosis in humans.

SUMMARY

During aging, clinical studies have revealed a modest left ventricular hypertrophy in response to an increased cardiac afterload resulting from an aged-related arterial dilatation and a loss of vascular compliance. The decreased ventricular compliance induced by fibrosis, leads to a reduced efficiency of early ventricular diastolic filling. However, no decrease in left ventricular end-diastolic volume is observed because the atrial contribution is increased. During exercise, the cardiac output is maintained in the elderly, since an increase in stroke volume compensates for the decline in maximal heart rate. Permanent arrhythmias are present in the senescent human heart. The senescent heart is able to hypertrophy in response to overload and to adapt to the new requirements. Similar alterations are observed both in the senescent heart and in the overloaded heart, in clinical as well as in experimental studies, however differences do exist especially in terms of fibrosis and arrhythmias.

Experimental studies have revealed various cellular changes with aging: In the rat ventricle, the expression of a myosin heavy chain is replaced by that of the isogene β which leads to a decreased myosin ATPase activity. In consequence, the contraction is slower and more economical as shown by calculating the Hill's equation. The Ca^{2+} ATPase of the sarcoplasmic reticulum and Na^+/Ca^{2+} exchange activity which are the two principal determinants of relaxation are decreased which probably explains the reduced velocity of relaxation observed in isolated rat papillary muscle. Cell loss is an important determinant of the senescent myocardial function, and is compensated for by hypertrophy of the remaining myocytes with associated fibrosis. Investigations are needed to examine the relative role of necrosis, apoptosis (and proliferation) in the occurrence of myocyte loss with aging and to examine the potential determinants of these processes. The few studies available for the moment suggest that normal aging may not be associated with increased cardiocyte apoptosis.

References

1. Brock DW, Guralnik JM, Brody JA. Demography and epidemiology of aging in the United States. In Handbook of the biology of aging Chap 1 Schneider EL, Rowe JW eds Academic Press, San Diego, 1990, p 3.
2. Lakatta E. Cardiovascular regulatory mechanisms in advanced age. Physiol Rev 1993;73:413.
3. Folkow B, Svanborg A. Physiology of cardiovacular aging. Physiol Rev1993;73:725.
4. Assayag P, Besse S, Delcayre C, Hardouin S, Carré F, Moalic JM, Swynghedauw B. Biological and molecular characteristics of the senescent heart, in Recent Advances in Aging Science, Beregi, E, Gergely, I A, and Rajczi, K, eds Monduzzi Editore, Bologna,1993, 341.
5. Besse S, Delcayre C, Chevalier B, Hardouin S, Heymes C, Bourgeois F, Moalic JM, Swynghedauw B. Is the senescent heart overloaded and already failing? A review. Cardiovasc Drugs Ther 8, 581, 1994.
6. Celermajer DS. Noninvasive detection of atherosclerosis. N Engl J Med 1998;339:2014-5.
7. Swynghedauw B. Biological mechanisms of myocardial remodeling. Physiol Rev 1999;in press.
8. Linzbach AJ, and Akuamoa-Boateng E. Die Altersveränderungen des menschlichen Herzens-I-Das Herzgewicht im Alter. Klin Wschr 1973;51:156.
9. Yin FCP, Spurgeon HA, Weisfeldt ML, Lakatta EG. Mechanical properties of myocardium from hypertrophied rat hearts A comparison between hypertrophy induced by senescence and by aortic banding. Circ Res 1980;46:292.
10. Besse S, Assayag P, Delcayre C, Carré F, Cheav SL, Lecarpentier Y, Swynghedauw B. Normal and hypertrophied senescent rat heart Mechanical and molecular characteristics. Am J Physiol 1993;265:H183.
11. Hasenfuss G, Holubarsch C, Hermann H-P, Astheimer K, Pieske B, Just H. Influence of the force-frequency relationship on the haemodynamic and left ventricular function in patients with non-failing hearts and in patients with dilated cardiomyopathy. Eur Heart J 1994;15:164-70.
12. Guarnieri T, Filbaum CR, Zitnik G, Roth G, Lakatta EG.Contractile and biochemical correlates of b-adrenergic stimulation of the aged heart. Am J Physiol 1980;239:H501-08.
13. Orchard CH, Lakatta EG. Intracellular calcium transients and developed tension in heart muscle. J Gen Physiol 1985;86: 637-51.
14. Assayag P, Carré F, Chevalier B, Delcayre C, Mansier P, Swynghedauw B. Compensated cardiac hypertrophy Arrhythmogenecity and the new myocardial phenotype. Part 1: Fibrosis. Cardiovasc Res 1997;34:439-44.
15. Swynghedauw B, Chevalier B, Charlemagne D, Mansier P, Carré F. Compensated cardiac hypertrophy Arrhythmogenicity and the new myocardial phenotype. Part 2: The cellular adaptational process. Cardiovasc Res 1997;35:6-12.
16. de la Bastie D, Levitsky D, Rappaport L, Mercadier JJ, Marotte F, Wisnewsky C, Brokovich V, Schwartz K, Lompre AM. Function of the sarcoplasmic reticulum and expression of its Ca^{2+}ATPase gene in pressure overload-induced cardiac hypertrophy in the rat. Circ Res 1990;66:554.
17. Maciel LMZ, Polikas R, Rohrer D, Popovich BK, Dillmann WH. Age-induced decreases in the messenger RNA coding for the sarcoplasmic reticulum Ca^{2+} ATPase of the rat heart. Circ Res 1990;67:230.
18. Froehlich JP, Lakatta EG, Beard E, Spurgeon HA, Weisfeld ML, Gerstenblith G. Studies of sarcoplasmic reticulum function and contraction duration in young and aged rat myocardium. J Mol Cell Cardiol 1978;10:427.
19. Wei JY, Spurgeon HA, and Lakatta EG. Excitation-contraction in rat myocardium: alterations with adult aging. Am J Physiol 1984;246:H784.

20. Heyliger CE, Prakash AR, McNeill JH. Alterations in membrane Na^+-Ca^{2+} exchange in the aging myocardium. Age 1988;11:1.

21. Besse S, Trouvé P, Assayag P, Swynghedauw B, Charlemagne, D. Expression of the a catalytic subunit messenger RNAs of the Na-K ATPase in the normal and hypertensive senescent rat heart. In Proc GRRC 94 Crozatier B, and Seguin, J, Eds, Montpellier 7-8 Avril 1994 (Abstract).

22. Orchard CH, Lakatta EG. Intracellular calcium transients and developed tension in rat heart muscle. J Gen Physiol 1985;86:637.

23. Rumberger E, Timermann J. Age changes of the force-frequency relationship and the duration of action potential of isolated papillary muscles of guinea pig. Eur J Appl Physiol 1976;35:277.

24. Swynghedauw B. Cardiac hypertrophy and failure. INSERM-J Libbey, Paris-London, 1990.

25. Haller BG, Zust H, Shaw S, Gnadinger MP, Uehlinger DE, Weidmann P. Effects of posture and aging on circulating atrial natriuretic peptide levels in man. Hypertension 1987;5:551.

26. Heymes C, Swynghedauw B, Chevalier B. Activation of angiotensinogen and angiotensin converting enzyme gene expression in the left ventricle of senescent rats. Circulation 1994;90:1328-33.

27. Heymes C, Silvestre J-S, Llorens-Cortes C, Chevalier B, Marotte F, Levy BI, Swynghedauw B, Samuel J-L. Cardiac senescence is associated with enhanced expression of angiotensin II receptors subtypes. Endocrinology 1999;in press.

28. Tummala PE, Dananberg J, Grekin RJ. Alterations on the secretion of arial natriuretic factor in atria from aged rats. Hypertension 1992;20:85.

29. Chevalier B, Mansier P, Teiger E, Callens-El Amrani F, Swynghedauw B. Alterations in b adrenergic and muscarinic receptors in aged rat heart Effects of chronic administration of propranolol and atropine. Mech Ageing Dev1991;60:215.

30. Hardouin S, Bourgeois F, Besse S, Machida CA, Swynghedauw B, Moalic JM. Decreased accumulation of b1 adrenergic receptors, Gas and total myosin heavy chain messenger RNAs in the left ventricle of senescent rat heart. Mech Ageing Develop 1993;71:169.

31. Baker SP, Marchand S, O'Neil E, Nelson CA, Posne P. Age-related changes in cardiac muscarinic receptors: decreased ability of the receptors to form a high affinity agonist binding state. J Gerontol 1985;40:141.

32. Narayanan N, Derby JA. Alterations in properties of b1-adrenergic receptors of myocardial membranes in aging: impairments in agonist-receptors interactions and guanidine nucleotide regulation accompany diminished catecholamine-responsiveness of adenylate cyclase. Mech Ageing Dev 1982;19:127.

33. Besse S, Robert V, Assayag P, Delcayre C, Swynghedauw B. Non-synchronous changes in myocardial collagen mRNA and protein during aging Effect of DOCA-salt hypertension. Am J Physiol 1999;in press.

34. Lompré AM, Schwartz K, d'Albis A, Lacombe G, Thiem NV, Swynghedauw B. Myosin isozymes redistribution in chronic heart overloading. Nature 1979;282:105-7.

35. Anversa P, Palackal T, Sonnenblick EH, Olivetti G, Meggs LG, Capasso JM. Myocyte cell loss and myocyte cellular hyperplasia in the hypertrophied aging rat heart. Circ Res 1990;67:871.

36. Eghbali M, Eghbali M, Robinson TF, Seifter S, Blumenfeld OO. Collagen accumulation in heart ventricles as a function of growth and aging. Cardiovasc Res 1980;23:723.

37. Tomanek RJ, Taunton CA, Liskop KS. Relationship between age, chronic exercise, and connective tissue of the heart. J Gerontol 1972;27:33.

38. Robert R, Besse S, Sabri A, Silvestre J-S, Assayag P, Thiem NV, Swynghedauw B, Delcayre C. Differential regulation of matrix metalloproteinases associated with aging and hypertension in the rat heart. Lab Invest 1997;76:729-38.

39. Mann DL, Spinale FG. Activation of matrix metalloproteinases in the failing human heart: breaking the tie that binds. Circulation 1998;98:1699-702.

40. Olivetti G, Giordano G, Corradi D, Melissari M, Lagrasta C, Gambert SR, Anversa P. Gender differences and aging : effects on the human heart. J Am Coll Cardiol 1995;26:1068-79.

41. Kajstura J, Cheng W, Sarangarajan R, Li P, Li B, Nitahara JA, Chapnick S, Reiss K, Olivetti G, Anversa P. Necrotic and apoptotic myocyte cell death in the aging heart of Fischer 344 rats. Am J Physiol 1996;271: H1215-28.

42. Mallat Z, Costagliola R, Fornes P, Belmin J, Lecomte D, Tedgui A. No evidence for increased cardiomyocyte apoptosis with aging in humans. Circulation 1998;I-75.Abstract.

43. Weber KT. Wound healing in cardiovascular disease. Armonk, NY: Futura Publishing Cy, 1995.

44. Carré F, Lessard Y, Coumel P, Ollivier L, Besse S, Lecarpentier Y, Swynghedauw B. Spontaneous arrhythmias in various models of cardiac hypertrophy and senescence of rats. A Holter monitoring study. Cardiovasc Res 1992;26:698.

III.2.4
Apoptosis during cardiac surgery

Hermann Aebert, M.D., Joachim P. Schmitt, M.D.,
and Heribert Schunkert, M.D.
Universität Regensburg, Regensburg, Germany

INTRODUCTION

Open heart surgery involves substantial stress for cardiac myocytes and thus the risk of cellular damage. Particularly, open heart surgery implies cardiac arrest for a quiet and bloodless surgical field. The physiological blood flow via the coronary arteries is interrupted by cross-clamping of the ascending aorta and the heart is perfused temporarily with some type of cardioplegic solution. These solutions contain non-physiologic ion concentrations to arrest electromechanic coupling. Together with hypothermia, cardioplegia results in reduction of the energy requirements of the heart by up to 97% (1, 2). Nevertheless, a distinct depression of cardiac contractility is observed early in the postoperative period (3). The extent of this depression is directly related to patient survival (4). The reasons for the delayed recovery of the heart are poorly understood but cellular trauma or potentially apoptosis may be involved (5). Given this background information, a better understanding and further improvements of cardioplegic strategies are certainly needed.

The composition of nowadays cardioplegic solutions varies considerably between different centers (6). This diversity is explained by the lack of good determinants of cellular protection in the clinical setting. Particularly, patients are characterized by a multitude of different factors like age, concomitant diseases, anesthesia, drugs, previous myocardial damage, and surgical technique that all may influence postsurgical hemodynamics, serum levels of heart specific enzymes and clinical outcome. Moreover, at the time of chest closure, i.e. 30 - 60 minutes after the start of reperfusion following cardioplegia, the heart is no longer accessible for tissue sampling such that many biochemical and histological parameters may not yet show any alterations.

Therefore, we looked for other parameters to evaluate the effect of cardioplegic solutions on the hearts of patients during cardiac surgery. A prerequisite was that changes of these parameters occur early after termination of cardiac arrest and would therefore be available in the clinical setting. Immediate early genes seemed promising in these respects.

IMMEDIATE EARLY GENES

Heat shock proteins are a family of proteins supporting cellular homeostasis. In the heart they are induced experimentally by different forms of stress including hyperthermia, wall stress, and ischemia (7, 8). This induction is accompanied by a better tolerance against ischemia (9, 10, 11). The protective effects of heat shock proteins were impressively demonstrated in hearts of mice expressing a human hsp 70 transgene in the heart that conferred a high resistance against ischemia when compared to normal controls (12). In cells, heat shock proteins function as chaperones and mediators of protein translocation between different cell compartments. Recently, an antiapoptotic action (13, 14) of hsp 70 was discovered.

We observed a significantly increased expression of inducible hsp 70 on the mRNA and protein level after cardioplegic arrest and reperfusion in isolated rat hearts and in hearts of patients undergoing open heart surgery (5, 15). With different cardioplegic solutions expression of hsp 70 was increased about 2-fold compared to precardioplegia controls. During the limited time period of about 2 hours after administration of cardioplegia, when hearts of patients where accessible to cardiac biopsy, a positive correlation between hsp 70 protein levels as determined by western blots and the time of cardioplegic arrest and reperfusion was observed (unpublished data).

Protein and mRNA levels of several protooncogenes where found to be increased after cardioplegic arrest and reperfusion (5, 15) . Specifically, c-fos and c-jun which have been linked to apoptosis (16, 17, 18) showed a 2- to 5-fold increase compared to precardioplegia controls. Like for hsp 70, the induction of protooncogenes showed a positive correlation with the time periods of cardioplegic arrest and reperfusion. However, in contrast to hsp 70 induction, which was similar with different cardioplegic solutions, significant differences were observed for protooncogene induction with different cardioplegic solutions in the hearts of patients undergoing open heart surgery (5).

Immunohistochemical studies with monoclonal antibodies directed against inducible hsp 70 and protooncogenes demonstrated positive staining in cardiac myocytes and endothelial cells following cardioplegic arrest and reperfusion. No staining was observed in other cell types of the heart.

Taken together, these findings indicated an induction of several immediate early genes after cardioplegic arrest and reperfusion in cardiac myocytes and endothelial cells. These cell types are known as prime targets for injury following cardioplegic arrest and reperfusion. Since a role of the induced immediate early genes in apoptosis had been demonstrated, we examined additional biopsies of human hearts for evidence of apoptosis.

TUNEL TECHNIQUE

Biopsies of human hearts taken after cardioplegic arrest (mean time 62 min) and reperfusion (mean time 38 min) showed positive staining for *in situ* nick end labeling of DNA fragments in an average of 1% of cardiac myocytes (5) .

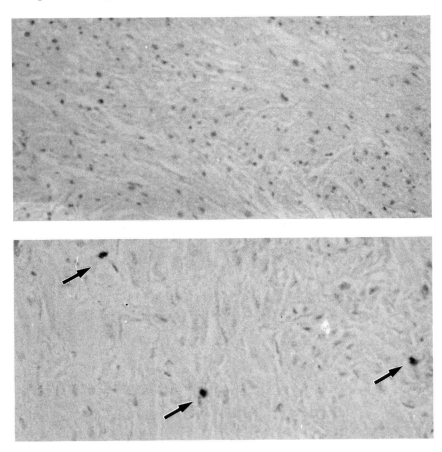

Figure 1 In situ nick-end labeling of DNA fragments in tissue sections of human heart biopsies of the same patient removed before (upper panel) and after cardioplegic arrest and reperfusion (lower panel). Positive staining in cardiomyocytes is only observed after cardioplegia and reperfusion (arrows).

However, quantification of positive cells appeared difficult for several reasons. Labeled cells were found most prominently in the subendocardial layers and the thickness of the atrial wall varied in the biopsy specimens. In addition, distinctive differences in the relative number of labeled cells occurred even in patients receiving the same cardioplegic solution. Positive staining was also observed in some endothelial cells. However, virtually no positive staining for in *situ nick* end labeling was detected in biopsies removed before cardioplegic arrest and reperfusion. There are several limitations of the TUNEL technique (19) and we consecutively tried to confirm our findings with other methods.

ELECTRON MICROSCOPY

No morphological changes typical for late stages of apoptosis like nuclear fragmentation or membrane budding (20, 21) were observed in human biopsies taken after cardioplegic arrest and reperfusion. However, some myocytes exhibited beginning condensation and margination of nuclear chromatin typical for early stages of apoptosis. In contrast to the nucleus and other organelles, the mitochondria of these myocytes displayed severe damage (unpublished data). These mitochondria were massively swollen with rarefied christae. Ruptures of mitochondrial membranes clearly indicated irreversible apoptotic changes. Interestingly, some mitochondria in the affected myocytes showed intermediate forms between normal and massive swelling, indicating the dynamic process occurring during early apoptotic stages (Figure 4). After transmission of a death inducing signal to some mitochondria, membrane changes are propagated in a feedforward amplification loop by release of cytochrome c and other cell death promoting substances. Myocytes with these mitochondrial changes were surrounded by completely normal cells. There were no signs of pericellular inflammation, edema, or invasion of leukocytes. All these morphological changes argue much in favor of apoptosis and against necrosis.

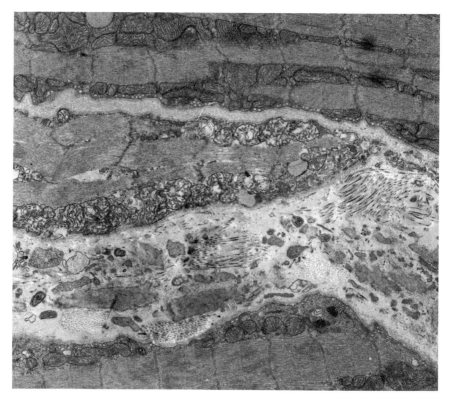

Figure 2 Electron microsopy of a human heart biopsy taken after cardioplegia and reperfusion. Two normal cardiomyocytes (top and bottom) are framing a myocyte with severely swollen mitochondria in the centre adjacent to connective tissue.

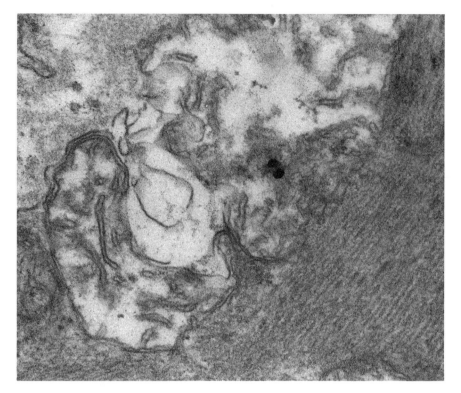

Figure 3   Higher magnification displays ruptures of mitochondrial membranes.

RELEASE OF CYTOCHROME C

Cytochrome c is an enzyme localized between the inner and outer mitochondrial membrane. By rupture of the outer mitochondrial membrane cytochrome c and other death promoting substances are released to the cytosol (22, 23, 24). Using differential centrifugation and western blot analyses with monoclonal antibodies we examined the cytosol fraction of human heart biopsies. After cardioplegic arrest and reperfusion we observed a 3.4 ± 0.4 fold increase ($p < 0.0001$) of cytosolic cytochrome c when compared to biopsies taken from the same patients before cardioplegic arrest (unpublished data).

Some cytochrome c was also detected in precardioplegia controls. Electron microscopy of the mitochondrial fraction showed some completely destroyed mitochondria in these samples, which we attributed to physical disruption during the process of tissue homogenization and centrifugation (unpublished data).

Analysis of citrate synthase in the cytosol fraction substantiated this assumption. This enzyme is localized exclusively within the inner mitochondrial membrane (25). In all cytosolic preparations including controls citrate synthase activity was observed supporting mitochondrial damage during tissue preparation. Since cardiomyocytes are exceedingly rich in mitochondria, we speculate that this high concentration may account for a little citrate synthase activity in the cytosolic fraction due to membrane damage during processing. It seems noteworthy that after cardioplegic arrest and reperfusion citrate synthase activity was increased 2.0 ± 0.3 fold ($p < 0.005$) compared to precardioplegia controls (unpublished data). We do not know whether this is due to i) affection of also the inner mitochondrial membrane during the process of apoptosis, ii) the transition of apoptosis to necrosis, iii) a small percentage of cells that undergo necrosis independently of apoptosis, or iv) an *ex vivo* artifact since mitochondria with apoptotic changes of the outer membrane may be more prone to disruption of the inner membrane during tissue processing. No matter what the reason may be, we assumed that the ratio of cytochrome c to citrate synthase might reflect the actual amount of damage to outer mitochondrial membranes inflicted by cardioplegia and reperfusion rather than cytosolic cytochrome c levels alone. Calculation of the quotients for all samples revealed 1.7 ± 0.2 fold ($p < 0.05$) higher cytochrome c / citrate synthase ratios after cardioplegia and reperfusion when compared to precardioplegia controls (unpublished data). It is noteworthy that we also found a significant positive correlation between these ratios and the time of cardioplegic arrest and reperfusion. This was not the case for the isolated values of cytochrome c and citrate synthase.

Together with our morphological findings, these data support the idea of a dynamic process within the limited time period for biopsy removal during the surgical setting and the model of a feed forward loop of mitochondrial membrane damage (Figure 4).

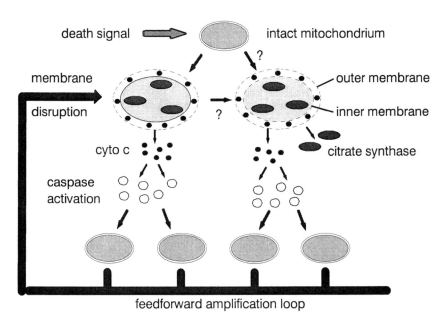

Figure 4 Simplified model of early stages of apoptosis due to mitochondrial changes. This model incorporates our findings on mitochondrial changes in different stages and increasing cytochrome c release during reperfusion after cardioplegic arrest as well as previously published models (see text).

CLINICAL SIGNIFICANCE OF APOPTOSIS DURING OPEN HEART SURGERY

In situ nick end labeling has been a mainstay for detection and quantification of apoptosis in many studies. However, there are several reports calling its specificity in question (19, 26). We found quantification particularly difficult since marked cells were concentrated in the subendocardium and the thickness of the atrial wall varied considerably in different biopsy specimens. Bare counting of labeled cells and comparing them to unmarked myocytes did not seem very reliable. We think that biochemical measurements using the ratio of cytochrome c and citrate synthase may offer a new way for quantification. This is supported by the positive correlation between this ratio and the time of cardioplegic arrest and reperfusion. However, this needs to be reexamined in further studies and different settings.

The data on cytochrome c release and electron microscopy provide strong evidence on the occurrence of apoptosis in hearts of patients undergoing open heart surgery. Temporal depression of myocardial function following cardioplegic arrest and reperfusion is a well known phenomenon (3). It is of major clinical significance since postoperative survival of patients is directly related to the degree of myocardial depression early after surgery (4). The cause of this depression is unknown. Depletion of cellular ATP stores, edema, disturbance of enzyme and membrane function as a consequence of cardioplegic arrest have been alleged in the past (27, 28). Cell death was denied as a possible cause since this depression occurred even with normal serum levels of heart specific enzymes like creatinine-kinase. In apoptosis, cellular contents are not spilled to the intercellular space, in fact, coordinated elimination of dead cells without such spillage is one of the key features of programmed cell death.

Clinical outcome is good in the majority of patients after open heart surgery. Probably the apoptotic loss of myocytes is compensated long term by alleviation of underlying cardiac pathology, e.g. ischemia in coronary artery disease by bypass grafting, and by the remaining cells, e.g. by hypertrophy. However, in the early time frame after surgery, the loss of disseminated myocytes throughout the myocardium may have profound implications for the cellular network. Myocyte slippage, in particular, may be substantially affected with greater implications on cardiac function than assumed on the basis of the relatively low percentage of apoptotic myocytes (29). Moreover, patients with extensive preoperative damage to the myocardium like in severely reduced ejection fraction after previous myocardial infarction exhibit a drastic increase of postoperative morbidity and mortality (30). We speculate that in these patients the ability of the remaining myocytes to compensate for the apoptotic loss is reduced to an even greater extent. A further possibility is a reduced threshold to undergo apoptosis of cardiomyocytes of failing hearts due to chronic changes. Only further studies will be able to clarify these issues.

There is no doubt that cardioplegic arrest is an unphysiological condition for the heart. This is not only evident in patients with severe preoperative myocardial damage but also in hearts that undergo prolonged cardioplegic arrest like in cardiac transplantation (31). A highly significant correlation exists between the cardioplegic time of transplanted hearts and one year survival of transplant recipients. Our data on induction of early immediate genes and apoptosis of cardiomyocytes following cardioplegic arrest and reperfusion may be helpful in better evaluating and comparing as well as in newly designing cardioplegic strategies in the future. Several experimental and *post mortem* studies included in this book and published elsewhere illustrate the importance of apoptosis in cardiac biology and pathology. Further efforts to clarify the role and mechanisms of apoptosis in the setting of cardiac surgery are extremely important because this holds the promise for interference with frequent postsurgical problems. In particular, a better understanding of apoptotic cell death and, based on this information, improved techniques for cardiac preservation during open heart surgery may ultimately lead to improved clinical results, especially in patients with preexisting heart failure, and thus, high risk for perioperative morbidity and mortality.

References

1. Buckberg DG. Myocardial protection: an overview. *Semin Thorac Cardiovasc Surg.* 1993;5:98-106.
2. Bretschneider HJ, Gebhard MM, Preusse CJ. „Cardioplegia. Principles and problems." In *Physiology and pathophysiology of the heart,* N. Sperrlohn, ed. Boston: M. Nijhoff Publishers, 1984;605-616.
3. Breisblatt WM, Stein KL, Wolfe CJ, Follansbee WP, Capozzi J, Armitage JM, Hardesty RL. Acute myocardial dysfunction and recovery: a common occurence after coronary bypass surgery. *J Am Coll Cardiol.* 1990;15:1261-1269.
4. Kirklin JW and Barrat-Boyes BG. „Myocardial management during cardiac surgery with cardiopulmonary bypass." In *Cardiac Surgery,* 2nd edn., JW Kirklin and BG Barrat-Boyes, eds. New York, London, Tokyo: Churchill Livingston, 1993;133-165.
5. Aebert H, Cornelius T, Birnbaum DE, Siegel AV, Riegger GA, Schunkert H. Induction of immediate early genes and programmed cell death following cardioplegic arrest in human hearts. *Eur J Cardio-thorac Surg.* 1997;12:261-267.
6. Demmy TL, Haggerty SP, Boley TM, Curtis JJ. Lack of cardioplegia uniformity in clinical myocardial preservation. *Ann.-Thorac-Surg.* 1994;57:648-51.
7. Izumo S, Nadal-Ginard B, Mahdavi V. Protooncogene induction and reprogramming of cardiac gene expression produced by pressure overload. *Proc Natl Acad Sci U S A.* 1988;85:339-343.
8. Currie RW, Tanguay RM, Kingma JG Jr. Heat-shock response and limitation of tissue necrosis during occlusion/reperfusion in rabbit hearts. *Circulation.* 1993;87:963-971.
9. Amrani M, Corbett J, Boateng SY, Dunn MJ, Yacoub MH. Kinetics of induction and protective effect of heat-shock proteins after cardioplegic arrest. *Ann Thorac Surg.* 1996;61:1407-1412.
10. Currie RW, Karmazyn M, Kloc M, Mailer K. Heat-shock response is associated with enhanced postischemic ventricular recovery. *Circ Res.* 1988;63:543-549.
11. Hutter MM, Sievers RE, Barbosa V, Wolfe CL. Heat shock protein induction in rat hearts. A direct correlation between the amount of heat shock protein induced and the degree of myocardial protection. *Circulation* 1994;89:355-360.
12. Plumier JC, Ross BM, Currie RW. Transgenic mice expressing the human heat shock protein 70 have improved post-ischemic myocardial recovery. *J Clin Invest.* 1995;95:1854-1860.
13. Kwak HJ, Jun CD, Pae HO, Yoo JC, Park YC, Choi BM, Na YG, Park RK, Chung HT, Chung HY, Park WY, Seo JS. The role of inducible 70-kDa heat shock protein in cell cycle control, differentiation, and apoptotic cell death of the human myeloid leukemic HL-60 cells. *Cell Immunol.* 1998;187:1-12.
14. Buzzard KA, Giaccia AJ, Killender M, Anderson RL. Heat shock protein 72 modulates pathways of stress-induced apoptosis. *J Biol Chem.* 1998;273:17147-17153.
15. Aebert H, Cornelius T, Ehr T, Holmer SR, Birnbaum DE, Riegger GA, Schunkert H. Expression of immediate early genes after cardioplegic arrest and reperfusion. *Ann Thorac Surg.* 1997;63:1669-1675.

16. Preston GA, Lyon TT, Yin Y, Lang JE, Solomon G, Annab L, Srinivasan DG, Alcorta DA, Barrett JC. Induction of apoptosis by c-Fos protein. *Mol Cell Biol.* 1996;16:211-218.
17. Smyne RJ, Vendrell M, Hayward M, Baker SJ, Miao GG, Schilling K, Robertson ML, Curran T, Morgan JI. Continous c-fos expression preceeds programmed cell death in vivo. *Nature* 1993;363:166-169.
18. Steller H. Mechanisms and genes of cellular suicide. *Science* 1995;267:1445-1449.
19. Grasl-Kraupp B, Ruttkay-Nedecky B, Koudelka H, Bukowska K, Bursch W, Schulte-Hermann R. In situ detection of fragmented DNA (TUNEL assay) fails to discriminate among apoptosis, necrosis, and autolytic cell death: a cautionary note. *Hepatology* 1995;21:1465-1468.
20. Majno G, and Joris I. Apoptosis, oncosis, and necrosis. An overview of cell death. *Am J Pathol* 1995;146:3-15.
21. Martin SJ and Green DR. Protease activation during apoptosis: death by a thousand cuts? *Cell* 1995;82:349-352.
22. Yang J, Liu X, Bhalla K, Kim CN, Ibrado AM, Cai J, Peng TI, Jones DP, Wang X. Prevention of apoptosis by Bcl-2: release of cytochrome c from mitochondria blocked. *Science* 1997;275:1129-1132.
23. Vander Heiden MG, Chandel NS, Williamson EK, Schumacker PT, Thompson CB. Bcl-xl regulates the membrane potential and volume homeostasis of mitochondria. *Cell* 1997;91:627-637.
24. Green DR and Reed JC. Mitochondria and Apoptosis. *Science* 1998;281:1309-1312.
25. Robinson Jr. JB, Brent LG, Sumegi B, Srere PA. In *Mitochondria, a practical approach*, VM Darley-Usmar, D Rickwood, MT Wilson, eds. Oxford, Washington DC: IRL Press, 1987;160, 161.
26. Freude B, Masters TN, Kostin S, Robicsek F, Schaper J. Cardiomyocyte apoptosis in acute and chronic conditions. *Basic Res Cardiol.* 1998;93:85-89.
27. Birdi I, Angelini GD, Bryan AJ. Biochemical markers of myocardial injury during cardiac operations. *Ann Thorac Surg.* 1997;63:879-884.
28. Prasad K, Kalra J, Bharadwaj B, Chaudhary AK. Increased oxygen free radical activity in patients on cardiopulmonary bypass undergoing aortocoronary bypass surgery. *Am Heart J.* 1992;123:37-45.
29. Cheng W, Li B, Kajstura J, Li P, Wolin MS, Sonnenblick EH, Hintze TH, Olivetti G, Anversa P. Stretch-induced programmed myocyte cell death. *J Clin Invest.* 1995;96:2247-2259.
30. Milano CA, White WD, Smith LR, Jones RH, Lowe JE, Smith PK, Van-Trigt P. Coronary artery bypass in patients with severely depressed ventricular function. *Ann Thorac Surg.* 1993;56:487-493.
31. Hosenpud, J.D., Bennet, L.E., Keck, B.M., Fiol, B., Novick, R.J. The Registry of the International Society for Heart and Lung Transplantation: fourteenth official report-1997. *J Heart Lung Transplant.* 1997;16:691-712.

PART FOUR:
Therapeutical options

IV.1
New opportunities for heart disease therapeutics

Giora Z. Feuerstein, M.D.
DuPont Pharmaceuticals Corporation
Wilmington, DE, USA

INTRODUCTION

Apoptosis was first introduced into biology in a seminal paper by a group of pathologists studying cell population regulation (1). In this paper, the authors described a form of cell death marked by its singularity, a unique morphology and resolution without apparent "traces" (e.g., inflammation) in the tissue of origin. These features of cell death were contrasted to various forms of cell death by necrosis, due to noxious stimuli leading to cell membrane disruption, swelling, disintegration, cell-content leakage and local inflammation. Featuring prominently in the apoptotic process are the "apoptotic bodies" (fragments of dense DNA surrounded by an apparently intact plasma membrane), DNA condensation and fragmentation (the latter noted as "ladder" when separated on DNA-gel electrophoresis). The apoptosis phenotype has been later on associated with "programmed cell death" (PCD) described first in the nematode, C. elegance, where genetically specified deletions of cells during development followed a highly timed activation of specific genes (ced-3/4) (2). It is now quite common to use apoptosis and PCD interchangeably; in this review, apoptosis represents the cellular phenotype resulting from activation of genomic programs that lead to DNA damage and cell death. The objectives of this review are: a. to highlight the key evidence on apoptosis in human cardiac myocytes; b. review the key stimuli and signal transduction pathways identified in cardiac myocytes; c. discuss the significance of apoptosis in cardiac function and disease; d. suggest potential novel therapeutic strategies for cardiac diseases based on modulation of selected molecular targets in cardiomyocyte apoptosis.

APOPTOSIS IN CARDIAC DISEASE - THE EVIDENCE

Reports on cardiomyocyte apoptosis in human cardiac disease were only recently published (3,4). Using the key markers: 1. DNA "ladder" and 2. Markers of doublestranded DNA damage by TUNEL (Terminal deoxy-Uridine-Nick-End-Labeling) histochemistry, apoptosis of cardiomyocytes and non-myocytes were identified in the following cardiac diseases: 1. Ischemic and idiopathic dilated cardiomyopathy, associated with clinical heart failure; 2. Acute myocardial infarction; 3. Congenital arrhythmogenic dysplasias; 4. Myocarditis; 5. Arrhythmias. The incidence of cardiac myocyte apoptosis in these conditions varies considerably with estimates of 0.1 % to 30%, depending on the disease specimen, methodology, and area of sampling. However, the rate of cardiac cell deletion (myocytes and non-myocytes) by apoptosis is difficult to assess in vivo especially in the human situation; however, in vitro, the resolution of the apoptotic process from initiation to complete engulfment is quite rapid: hours or few days and, therefore, even a low prevalence, e.g., 0.1 %, recycled over years, may lead to substantial depletion of cardiac cells. At the present time, the contribution of cardiac myocyte apoptosis to initiation and progression of the above-cited heart diseases cannot be accurately estimated.

STIMULI THAT ELICIT CARDIOMYOCYTE APOPTOSIS

Significant research has been launched over the past 5 years to identify stimuli that elicit cardiomyocyte apoptosis and to decipher their signal transduction pathways (5). It is important to note that much of the information is derived from 1. in vitro studies; 2. Nonhuman (and often non-adult) cardiomyocytes; 3. Highly controlled (artificial) conditions.

Circumstantial evidence supports the existence of many of these stimuli also in human cardiac disease, including: 1. Stress conditions such as ischemia (especially when followed by reperfusion) and oxygen radicals (H_2O_2, O_2^-, OH^-). The capacity of oxygen radicals to elicit cardiomyocytes apoptosis has been demonstrated in both cell cultures and isolated cardiac perfusion studies (6,7). In the former condition, deprivation of growth factors, energy sources (glucose), and endogenous antioxidants are usually present; 2. Cytokines, such as TNFα have been shown to produce cardiomyocyte apoptosis in culture. Cytokines may figure prominently, especially in the advanced heart failure where very high levels of circulating TNFα (and other cytokines) are present. Endogenous synthesis of TNFα in the heart (where its receptors are present) may be equally important; 3. Nitric oxide (NO) produced primarily by the Type II iNOS (inducible nitric oxide synthase) elicits cardiomyocyte apoptosis possibly in association with peroxinitrite iNOS ($ONOO^-$) production. Activation of iNOS in heart failure has been established; 4. Neurohormonal factors such as angiotensin II (ATII) acting via the AT-receptors have been shown to produce cardiomyocyte apoptosis (8). Elevated circulating levels of ATII, correlating to disease stage, and in situ cardiac ATII production, (possibly by a non-ACE pathway) may play an important role in this respect. It remains to be shown whether drugs that effectively block ATII production (ACE inhibitors) or action (ATII-receptor antagonists) reduce cardiac apoptosis while improving heart failure condition; 5. Mechanical stress has been shown to elicit apoptosis in cardiac muscle preparation in vitro. This physical form of stress is likely to exist in situations of cardiac remodeling leading to dilated cardiomyopathy and sphericity where increase in wall tension/stress is fundamental to the heart failure condition.

Taken together, diverse stimuli are capable to produce apoptosis in cardiac myocytes, many of which co-exist in advanced heart failure. It is difficult at this time to dissect out the most important contributing factors in chronic human cardiac diseases where multiple humoral and local pro-apoptotic stimuli exist.

SIGNALING PATHWAYS OF APOPTOSIS IN CARDIAC MYOCYTES

A complex network of biochemical pathways transduces signals of diverse apoptotic stimuli in cardiac myocytes. Five possible pro-apoptotic signaling pathways in cardiac myocytes have emerged which may provide opportunities for specific interventions.

These signal transduction pathways were largely derived from in vitro and mostly neonatal cardiomyocytes. Discrete stimuli may activate multiple signal transduction pathways and "cross talk" between various pathways are likely to be the common situation. Activation of apoptotic pathways may be 'intercepted' and aborted by anti-apoptotic regulatory mechanisms, thus, checkpoints that provide 'rescue' opportunities may be important in determining execution of the apoptotic. programs.

The five major signaling pathways that have been suggested to convey apoptotic stimuli in cardiac myocytes are:

I.   Redox-regulated systems such as NFκB and SAPKs.
II.   Fas/TNFα family of cytokine receptors operating via unique "death domains" that are linked to several signaling pathways.
III. Caspases, a family of cystein proteases operating in a cascade that is activated either by receptor-originating signals or mitochondria-associated cytochrome C
      The diversity and mode of activation and operation of the caspases cascade has been recently reviewed in great detail (5,9,10).
IV.   G-protein coupled receptors that mediate stimuli induced by ligands/agonists to 7 transmembrane receptors; one such system is the angiotensin II and its receptor signaling system Gαi, but novel GPCR pathways associated with Gαq have also been described (11).
V.   Phospholipase-C type biochemical reactions that lead to sphingomyelinase activation and generation of sphingolipids like ceramide (12).

The scope of this brief review may not accommodate detailed deliberations of each of the discrete signaling events enumerated above, for which the reader is encouraged to resort to recent reviews (5). More important though, are emerging principles that can be summarized as follows: a. single pro-apoptotic stimuli may lead to activation of single or multiple pathways of apoptosis; b. the final common pathway of apoptotic signaling pathways involves breakdown of numerous nuclear proteins of cytoarchitectural function, transcription modulation and cell cycle regulation; c. 'checkpoints' that regulate the apoptotic process are present in cardiomyocytes as it is also the case for other cells; in this respect, the Bc1-2 family of proteins and the Bax associated proteins may modulate both cell membrane or mitochondria-activated apoptosis (13).

THE SIGNIFICANCE OF CARDIAC CELL APOPTOSIS IN THE EVOLUTION OF HEART DISEASES

The emerging evidence in recent literature on cardiac apoptosis strongly suggests that this form of cell death indeed exists in the human heart at various disease conditions. Although the evidence derived from human specimens is largely based on histology/phenotype observation, cell based systems provide strong support for the existence of pro-apoptotic pathways in cardiomyocytes. However, a key question that remains unanswered is whether cardiac cell apoptosis has a significant role in any of the cardiac diseases where apoptosis is found. While this question cannot be decisively answered at this time, some suggestions as for possible mechanisms whereby apoptosis contributes to heart disease can be offered: 1. Loss of cardiomyocytes leads to loss of "cardiac mass" and hence -"diminished pump power". This possibility although plausible, is difficult to assess as the rate and incidence of the apoptotic cycle in the heart has not been assessed. However, Adams et al (11) have shown that robust apoptosis induced by Gαq overexpression in transgenic mice results in severe heart failure with markedly dilated chambers and perinatal death, indicating that robust apoptosis exercised over a brief period may, on its own (without ischemia or growth factor deprivation) result in fulminant heart failure. Furthermore, in cardiac selective "knock out" mice where gp130 gene is deleted, heart failure develops following pressure overload by apoptosis without ischemic or inflammatory component (14). While "quantity" cannot be dismissed as a possible mechanism, other possible factors might be: a. loss of cardiomyocytes may result in electrical conduction inhomogeneity that may lead to arrhythmias; b. apoptosis may lead to "cardiac remodeling", due to 're-alignment' of 'neighboring' cardiomyocytes. This latter mechanism is unique to the heart, where function is extremely dependent on optimal geometrical and structural alignment. Thus, apoptosis, even if limited in scope, may result in widespread mechanical and electrical disturbances.

NOVEL THERAPEUTIC OPPORTUNITIES FOR HEART DISEASES BASED ON ANTI-APOPTOTIC AGENTS

The potential for development of cardioprotective agents that are mechanistically based on modulation of apoptosis is rapidly emerging. Diverse opportunities may be exploitable, emanating both from enhancing anti-apoptotic capacities within cardiac myocytes such as the bcl-2 system or inhibition of key pro-apoptotic stimuli and/or their signal transduction pathways. The former option, enhancing anti-apoptotic pathways may turn to be a difficult task as the discrete regulatory pathways of the anti-apoptotic genes have not been clarified as yet. However, some interesting "proof of concept" studies have been recently reported. Experiments conducted in bcl-2 transgenic (TG) mice provided prove of concept that enhanced expression of anti-apoptotic pathways may provide protection from ischemic injury (15). In the latter study, bcl-2 TG mice were exposed to transient cerebral ischemia and neuronal death followed over extended periods; the bcl-2 TG mice demonstrated significant protection against ischemia induced neuronal loss. While such studies have not yet been reported in experimental models of cardiac ischemia (or heart failure), an in vitro model of cardiomyocyte apoptosis evoked by p53 overexpression has been studied with co-transfection with bcl-2 (13). In this model of cardiac myocyte apoptosis, bcl-2 provided strong anti-apoptotic action and prevented cell death. This data suggest that there is a potential of developing pharmacological strategies aimed at enhancing the expression and/or action of bcl-2 in view of arresting cardiac cell apoptosis. However, specific strategies that enable this objective have not yet been reported. Alternatively, it may be more plausible to expect that agents acting at critical 'checkpoints' downstream of the key "final common pathway(s)" elements leading to apoptosis may prove a superior strategy to prevent apoptosis. Several anti-apoptotic agents that may provide cardioprotection due to anti-apoptotic mechanism, have been reported: a. p38/MAPK inhibitors; b. caspase inhibitors; c. β-adrenergic receptor blockers; d. antioxidant/SAPK inhibitors; e. growth factors. These agents will be discussed below in more detail.

p38/MAPK INHIBITORS

Recent studies have demostrated that c-Jun N-terminal kinase (JNKs)/stress-activated protein kinase (SAPKs) and p38/MAPK are activated by a variety of cellular stresses that lead to apoptosis. In particular, myocardial ischemia and reperfusion (17) was shown to activate p38/MAPK in vivo. In order to establish whether activation of p38/MAPK plays a role in myocardial cell apoptosis and infarction, we have used a potent and selective inhibitor of p38/MAPK, SB203580 (16) in a rabbit heart (Langendorff preparation) model of ischemia and reperfusion.(17) In this model, ischemia alone caused a moderate increase in p38/MAPK (3.5 fold over baseline) while reperfusion after ischemia further increased p38/MAPK by 6.3 fold. Activation of p38/MAPK is a rapid (minutes) event that precedes cellular and organ lesions. Administration of SB203580 before the ischemic insult resulted in dose-dependent inhibition of p38/MAPK and markedly diminished the consequences of the ischemia/reperfusion injury, including apoptosis (>50%), creatinine kinase loss (34%) and infarct size (>50%). Confirmation of inhibition of apoptosis was done by both TUNEL and DNA-"ladder" criteria. Most importantly, the p38/MAPK inhibitor accelerated the recovery of coronary flow, cardiac contractility and left ventricular pressure. It is also of interest to note that the agent, SB203580, did not inhibit SAPK, another kinase activated by stress/ischemia, indicating the specific role of p38/MAPK in myocardial injury associated with ischemia and reperfusion. These data, while preliminary, should encourage more detailed work in many other models of cardiac injury, including heart failure. If such studies are consistently positive, clinical investigations will be warranted pending on the safety and tolerability of the p38/MAPK inhibitors.

CASPASE INHIBITORS

Activation of caspases in cardiac tissue in response to a variety of stimuli has been demonstrated in vitro and in vivo (6,16). However, only limited information is available on the capacity of agents that modulate caspase actions to modify cardiac injury induced by chemical or pathological stress situations. Yaoita et al. (6) have recently reported that a non-selective caspase inhibitor, Z-Val-Ala-Asp (OMe)-CH2F (ZVAD-fmk) was effective in reducing myocardial injury in rats induced by transient (30 min) coronary ligation and reperfusion over 24 hrs. In this in vivo model, ZVAD reduced the number of apoptotic cardiac cells and also blocked DNA-"laddering" along with reduction in infarct size. However, while the attenuation of apoptosis was most notable, the reduction in infarct size was slight. Similar data were also reported by Yue et al. (18) using staurosporine to induce apoptosis in cultured rat neonatal cardiomyocytes. These studies, while preliminary, suggest the involvement of some caspases in cardiac cell death by diverse stimuli. Key issues that need to be resolved are: 1. which specific caspase(s) are critical in cardiac cell apoptosis? 2. what are the discrete stimuli that lead to activation of these caspase(s) in human cardiac disease? 3. which specific caspase(s) needs to be inhibited to salvage the myocardial cells? Since ZVAD is a non-selective caspase inhibitor, including caspase-I (the Interleukin- 1 converting enzyme) data generated with this inhibitor do not allow the identification of a specific caspase at this time.

β-ADRENERGIC RECEPTOR BLOCKERS

Beta-adrenergic receptor (BAR) blockers are proven drugs for cardioprotection in a variety of heart diseases including myocardial infarction and heart failure. While the primary mechanism of cardioprotection by BAR blockers is believed to be reduction in cardiac work, new information derived from studies with the multiple-action BAR blocker, carvedilol (19,20,21) and the non-selective BAR blocker propranolol indicate that these agents may prevent apoptosis of cardiac myocytes subjected to ischemia and reperfusion injury. In a rabbit model of in vivo ischemia (30 minutes) and reperfusion (I/RP, 4 hours), robust apoptosis has been demonstrated by TUNEL and "DNA ladder" markers. Administration of carvedilol (a multiple action BAR blocker, α_1-AR blocker and antioxidant, immediately before reperfusion, reduced the number of apoptotic myocytes by 77% (Figure 1).

Protective Effect of Carvedilol Against Ischemia/Reperfusion Induced Apoptosis in Rabbit Cardiomyocytes

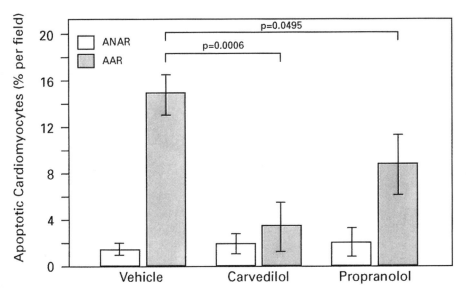

Figure 1 Protective effect of carvedilol and propranolol from ischemia/reperfusion induced cardiac myocyte apoptosis in the rabbit.
AAR = area at risk; ANAR = area not at risk; Aptotic cells were counted on TUNEL positive cardiac myocytes.

Propranolol, the non-selective beta-blocker, administered at equipotent doses as carvedilol, also provided significant protection against I/RP induced apoptosis, although to a lesser extent (39%). In this model, I/RP, resulted in robust activation of stress-activated protein kinase (SAPK) in the ischemic myocardium only; this increase of SAPK was significantly diminished by carvedilol (53%) yet no consistent effect on SAPK activation was found in propranolol treated rabbits (Figure 2). Furthermore, expression of Fas in the ischemic myocardiurn was also significantly reduced by carvedilol (7). The antioxidant properties of carvedilol might have contributed to the anti-apoptotic and cardiac protection of carvedilol since propranolol, an equipotent BAR blocker, that lacks anti-oxidant actions, displayed less anti-apoptotic capacity.

Effect of Carvedilol on Ischemia/Reperfusion-Induced SAPK/JNK Activation in Heart

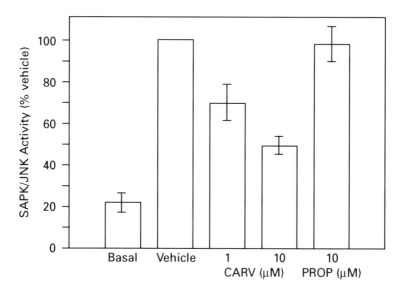

Figure 2 Effect of carvedilol or propranolol on ischemia/reperfusion induced SAPK activation. CARV = carvedilol; PROP = propranolol; SAPK = stress activated protein kinase.

CONCLUSION

Apoptosis is now recognized as a fundamental process in cell biology that is critical for tissue/organ development, physiologic adaptation and disease. The heart is no exception to other organs - apoptosis plays a role in cardiac development, maturation and diverse disease conditions. At this time, the evidence on the existence of apoptosis in human cardiac disease is largely based on histologic markers of cell morphology (light and EM) and histochemistry ("LADDER" and TUNEL). The discrete stimuli and the molecular mechanisms that initiate and propagate apoptosis in human heart disease are largely unknown. In vitro studies in experimental models (largely cultured animal myocytes) suggest multiple stimuli that activate highly diverse signal pathways. The pathways of apoptosis display redundancies, regulatory "checkpoints" and possibly convergence into a final common pathway where a "point of no return" completes the process. It is quite clear that numerous proteins within the nucleus are degraded leading to fatal aberrations in DNA structure, integrity and function ultimately compromising cell viability. The scope and function of nuclear protein degradation in apoptotic cardiomyocytes is largely unknown.

Three possible consequences of cardiac myocytes apoptosis are envisioned: 1. Compromise in cardiac contractility due to loss of myocytes; 2. Conduction disturbances leading to arrhythmias; 3. Cardiac remodeling due to disruption or geometrical alignment of cardiac myocytes. The precise role of any of these processes needs to be investigated. Finally, the significance of cardiac myocyte apoptosis must also be viewed in the perspective of the pharmaceutical opportunity. If indeed cardiomyocyte apoptosis plays an important role in initiation and progression of cardiac diseases, drugs that effectively and specifically inhibit apoptosis might be useful therapeutic agents for diverse cardiac diseases. Opportunities may emerge from either enhancing anti-apoptotic mechanisms (e.g., up-regulation of bcl-2) or inhibition of key targets in the pro-apoptotic pathways. In conclusion, the recognition of apoptosis as a discrete, genomically mediated cell death in the myocardium, has opened new conceptual paradigms in heart disease research. Most importantly, the understanding, on a molecular basis, of the key executioners of apoptosis in cardiac myocytes may provide new opportunities for development of novel cardioprotective agents.

SUMMARY

Apoptosis is a form of cell death that involves discrete genetic and molecular programs, de novo protein expression and a unique cellular phenotype. Evidence for the existence of apoptosis in the human heart has been reported in various cardiac diseases, including ischemic and non-ischemic heart failure, myocardial infarction and arrhythmias. Among the most potent stimuli that elicit cardiomyocyte apoptosis are: oxygen radicals (including NO), cytokines (FAS/TNF α-receptor-signaling), stress or mitogen activated protein kinases (SAPK/MAPK), sphingolipids metabolites (ceramide), G-protein coupled receptor (GPCR) signaling (Gαi, Gαq), the caspase cascade of proteases and NFkB activation. Apoptosis of cardiac myocytes may contribute to progressive pump-failure, arrhythmias and cardiac remodeling. The recognition of numerous molecular targets associated with cardiomyocyte apoptosis may provide novel therapeutic strategies for diverse cardiac ailments, as recently suggested by pharmacologic studies in experimental animals.

References

1. Kerr JFR, Wyllie AH, Currie AR. Apoptosis: A basic biological phenomenon with wide ranging implications in tissue kinetics. *Br J Cancer* 1972; 26: 239-257.
2. Yuan, J, Shaham S, Ledoux S, Ellis HM, Horvitz HR. The C. elegans cell death gene ced-3 encodes a protein similar to mammalian interleukin-1β-converting enzyme. Cell 1993; 75: 641-652.
3. Anversa P, Leri A, Behrami CA, Guerra S, Kajstura J. Myocyte death and growth in failing heart. Lab Invest 1998; 78: 767-786.
4. Narula J, Haider N, Virmani R, DiSalvo TG, Kolodgie FD, Hajar RJ, Schmidt U, Semigran MJ, Dec GW, Khaw BA. Apoptosis in myocytes in end-stage heart failure. New Engl J Med 1996; 335: 1182-1189.
5. Haunstetter A, Izumo S. Apoptosis. Basic mechanisms and implications for cardiovascular disease. Circ *Res* 1998; 82: 1111-1129.

6. Yaoita H, Ogawa K, MaeLare K, Maruyama Y. Attenuation of ischemia/repercussion injury in rats by a caspase inhibitor. Circulation 1998; 97: 276-281.
7. Yue T-L, Wang X-K, Romanic Am, Liu G-L, Louden C, Gu J-L, Kumai S, Poste G, Ruffolo RR Jr., Feuerstein GZ. Possible involvement of stress-activated protein kinase signaling pathway and Fas receptor expression in prevention of ischemia/reperfusion- induced cardiomyocyte apoptosis by carvedilol. Circ Res 1998; 82: 166-174.
8. Fortuno MA, Ravassa S, Etayo JC, Diez J. Overexpression of Bax protein and enhanced apoptosis in the left ventricle of spontaneously hypertensive rats. Effects of AT₁ blockade with losartan. Hypertension 1998; 32:280-286.
9. Salvesen GS, Dixit VM. Caspases: intracellular signaling by proteolysis. Cell 1997: 91: 443-446.
10. Black SC, Huang JQ, Rezaiefar P, Rodinovic S, Eberhardt A, Nicholson DW, Rodger IW. Co-Localization of the cystein protease caspase-3 with apoptotic myocytes after in vivo myocardial ischemia and reperfusion in rats. J Mol Cell Cardiol 1998; 30: 733-742.
11. Adams JW, Sokata Y, Davis MG, Sah V, Wang Y, Liggett SB, Chien KR, Brown JH, Dom GW. Enhanced Galphaq signaling: a common pathway mediates cardiac hypertrophy and apopotic heart failure. Proc Natl Acad Sci 1998; 95: 10140-10145.
12. Hofmann K, Dixit VM. Ceramide in apoptosis-does it really matter? Trends in Biochem Science. 1998; 374-377.
13. Kirshenbaum LA, Moissac D. The bcl-2 gene product prevents programmed cell death of ventricular myocytes. Circulation 1997; 96: 1580-1585
14. Hirota H, Chen J, Betz UAK, Rajewsky K, Gu Y, Ross J, Muller W, Chien KA. Loss of a 8PB30 cardiac muscle cell survival pathway is a critical event in the onset of heart failure during biomedrinical stress. Cell 97: 189-198 1999
15. Kitogawa K, Matsumoto M, Tsujimoto Y, Ohtsuki T, Kuwabara K, Matsushita K, Yang G, Tanabe H, Martinou J-C, Hori M, Yanagibara T. Amelioration of hippocampal neuronal damage after global ischemia by neuronal over expression of bcl-2 in transgenic mice. Stroke 29; 2616-2621, 1998.
16. Lee JC, Laydon JT, McDonnell PC, Gallagher TF, Kumar S, Green D, Blumenthal MJ, Heys JR, Landvatter SW, Strickler SM, McLaughlin MM, Siemens IR, Fisher SM, Livi GP, White JR, Adams JL, Young PR. A protein kinase involved in the regulation of inflammatory cytokine biosynthesis. Nature 1994; 372: 739-746.
17. Ma X-L, Kumar S, Gao F, Louden C, Lopez BL, Christopher TA, Wang C, Lee JC, Feuerstein G, Yue T-L. Inhibition of p38 mitogen activated protein kinase decreases cardiomyocyte apoptosis and improves cardiac function after myocardial ischemia and reperfusion. Circulation 99; 1685-1691, 1999.
18. Yue T-L, Wang C, Romanic AM, Kikly K, Keller P, DeWolf WE, Hart TK, Thomas HC, Storer B, Gu J-L, Wang XK, Feuerstein G. Staurosporine-induced apoptosis in cardiomyocytes: a potential role of caspase 3. J. Mol Cell Cardiol 30; 495-507 1998.
19. Feuerstein GZ, Shusterman NH, Ruffolo RR Jr. Carvedilol Update IV: prevention of oxidative stress and cardiac remodeling in heart failure progression. Drug of today 1997; 33: 453-473.
20. Packer M, Colucci WS, Sackner-Bernstein J, Liang C-S, Goldscher DA, Freeman I, Kukin ML, Kinhal V, Udelson JE, Klapholz M, Gottlieb SS, Pearle D, Cody RJ, Gregory JJ, Kantrowitz NE, LeJemtel TH, Young ST, Lukas MA, Shusterman NH. Double blind, placebo-controlled study of the effects of carvedilol in patients with moderate to severe heart failure. The PRECISE trial. Circulation 1996; 94: 2793-2799.
21. Australia/New Zealand Heart Failure Collaborative Group. Randomized, placebo controlled trial of carvedilol in patients with congestive heart failure due to ischemic heart disease. Lancet 1997; 349: 375-380..
22. Wang L, Ma W, Markovich R, Chen J-W, Wang PH. Regulation of cardiomyocyte apoptotic signaling by Insulin-like growth Factor 1. Circ Res 1998; 83: 516-522.
23. Okubo Y, Blakesley VA, Stannard B, Gutkind S, LeRoith D. Insulin-like growth factor-I inhibits the stress- activated protein kinase - Jun N-terminal kinase. J Biol Chem 1998; 273: 25961-25966.

IV.2
Beta blocker therapy and prevention of apoptosis

Andreas V. Sigel, M.D., and Heribert Schunkert M.D.

Universität Regensburg, Regensburg, Germany

INTRODUCTION

Chronic congestive heart failure, initiated by ischemic or hypertensive damage of the myocardium, can continue to worsen over months or years, despite the absence of clinically apparent acute events. Electron microscopic studies using myocardial specimen obtained from failing human hearts (1) and hearts of dogs with experimental heart failure (2) have clearly established the existence of cardiomyocyte apoptosis. Thus, it has been hypothesized that progressive cell loss by myocyte apoptosis may accelerate the natural course of congestive heart failure. Activation of neurohormonal mechanisms including the beta adrenergic system has been suggested to induce myocyte apoptosis and, thus, to promote the course of heart failure.

With beta-blocker therapy evolving to a new cornerstone in treating chronic congestive heart failure, the choice of drugs raises important theoretical and practical questions. In this respect, it is essential to (1.) document the underlying mechanisms responsible for their profound cardioprotection on a molecular basis, (2.) to investigate whether all beta-blockers are equally effective, (3.) to define the role of potential cardioprotective mechanisms beyond beta-blockade and (4.) to document whether this cardioprotection may be due to inhibition of apoptosis.

Most importantly, the precise mechanism of cardioprotection deserves further attention. Drugs that could address this question are the second-generation compounds metoprolol or bisoprolol and the third-generation compound carvedilol. While metoprolol and bisoprolol are β_1-selective, carvedilol is a hybrid drug involving nonselective β-antagonism, α-blockade and antioxidant effects (3,4). *Experimental* data suggest that carvedilol may show superior cardioprotection due to its additional pharmacological properties (5,6). However, a prospective *clinical* comparison of carvedilol and metoprolol showed parallel beneficial effects over 6 months in the treatment of congestive heart failure, with no relevant between-group differences (7), suggesting that the beta-blockade by itself is the key for cardioprotection.

Accordingly, evaluating more precisely the effect of different beta-blockers on programmed cell death in patients or experimental models of myocardial infarction or congestive heart failure may document the mechanism of cardioprotective effects.

SYMPATHETIC STIMULATION OF APOPTOSIS

A variety of pathophysiological processes are activated in patients with congestive heart failure, and some of these events have been implicated in the progress of the disease (8,9).

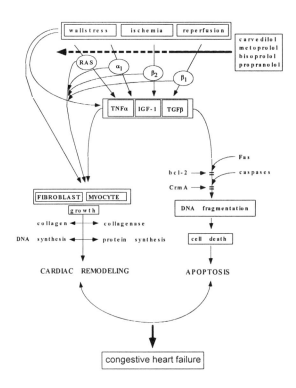

Figure 1 Possible crosstalk between the sympathetic nervous system, the renin angiotensin system (RAS), cardiac remodeling and apoptosis leading to congestive heart failure. Beta-blockers share an inhibition of the β_1 receptor, some of the agents, e.g. carvedilol, also block the β_2 and α_1 receptors. The renin angiotensin system is indirectly downregulated since renin secretion is under control of the β_1 receptor.

The most important mechanisms to be activated in congestive heart failure involve neurohumoral systems, including the renin-angiotensin system and the sympathetic nervous system (10,11). Increased sympathetic nervous system activity in patients with heart failure may help to support cardiovascular function in the short term. However, increased sympathetic nervous system activity, particularly, if prolonged, may exert deleterious effects on cardiovascular structure and function. These events stimulate various growth factors, such as TNF-α, IGF-1 or TGF-β, leading to pathophysiological myocardial remodeling (figure 1).

Furthermore, stimulation of the beta-adrenergic pathway has been shown to stimulate apoptosis of cardiac myocytes (12). Moreover, neurohormonal cross talk involves the β-adrenergic system also in the regulation of atrial natriuretic peptides and the renin angiotensin system. Specifically, chronic β-adrenergic stimulation blocks ANP and BNP (27), whereas renin release is augmented (28). These interactions may further stress the heart and create a pro-apoptotic condition. Thus, increased sympathetic nervous activity, acting via the beta-adrenergic receptors, may play an important role in the progression of myocardial failure by acting directly on myocytes and on other cells in the heart (table 1). This interaction may regulate fundamental biological properties such as growth, the composition of the cardiac extracellular matrix and programmed cell death.

Table 1   Distribution of beta-adrenoceptors over heart and kidney, and the effect of receptor stimulation and blockade. Blockade leads to decreased oxygen consumption and inhibition of the renin-angiotensin system, thus, reducing events that may trigger apoptosis in the heart.

Organ	Receptor	β-adrenergic Stimulation:	β-adrenergic Blockade:
Heart	$\beta_1 > \beta_2$	Tachycardia increased AV conduction increased contractility = *increased oxygen consumption*	Bradycardia decreased AV conduction decreased contractility = *decreased oxygen consumption*
		DNA synthesis RNA synthesis Protein synthesis = *remodeling of cardiac cells and the cardiac extracellular matrix*	Inhibition of DNA synthesis Inhibition of RNA synthesis Inhibition of protein synthesis = *inhibition of pathological remodeling*
		ANP, BNP suppression	ANP, BNP stimulation
Kidney	β_1	Renin release = *activation of the renin-angiotensin system*	Inhibition of renin release = *inhibition of the renin-angiotensin system*
Blood vessels	β_2	*Vasodilation*	*Vasoconstriction*

Therefore, the hypothesis is presented that beta-adrenergic antagonism may inhibit or reverse pathological remodeling and apoptosis, and, thus, may improve nyocardial structure and function leading to prolonged patient survival (13,14).

BETA-BLOCKER THERAPY AND PREVENTION OF APOPTOSIS

Experimental studies

Accumulating evidence suggests that beta-blocker therapy can inhibit programmed cell death during acute ischemia and, thus, reduce infarct size in several experimental settings (table 2). However, at present, most of the studies on beta-blocker therapy and apoptosis used the hybrid drug carvedilol, which involves nonselective $\beta_{1/2}$- and α-antagonisms as well as antioxidative properties. In four animal models of acute myocardial infarction in three different species, carvedilol has shown that it is efficious in salvaging acutely ischemic myocardium (15). In addition, the results suggest that carvedilol prevents myocardial ischemia / reperfusion-induced apoptosis possibly by downregulation of the SAPK signaling pathway, and by inhibition of Fas receptor expression (16).

Table 2   Experimental studies on beta-blocker therapy and cardioprotection / apoptosis.

Sepcies		Model	Drug	Reference
In vivo	*Dog*	ischemia / reperfusion myocardial infarction	c p c p	15 15
	Pig	ischemia / reperfusion	c p	15
	Rabbit	ischemia / reperfusion	c p	16
	Rat	ischemia / reperfusion	c	15
Ex vivo	*Rat*	ischemia / reperfusion	c	17
In vitro	***Rat***	hypoxia / reoxygenation	c p	18

C: carvedilol, **P** : propranolol.

To further investigate different effects of carvedilol, antioxidants and other beta-blockers on myocardial injury, we used an in-vitro cell culture model of hypoxia and reoxygenation-induced programmed cell death (18). Carvedilol and its antioxidative metabolite BM ˙91.0228 partially inhibited LDH and CK leakage (figure 2) and completely inhibited morphological features of apoptosis as well as DNA laddering (figure 3). Furthermore, both drugs prevented the induction of Fas receptor protein, cytochrome c release and caspase 3 activation in cardiac myocytes.

These features could not be seen in propranolol or vehicle treated cardiac myocytes. In addition, propranolol neither prevented LDH leakage into the medium nor DNA fragmentation.

These data suggest that additional pharmacological properties, such as antioxidative capacity may inhibit apoptosis and, thus, may enhance cardioprotection. However, at present, this hypothesis could not be confirmed by large prospective clinical trials. In addtion, other beta-blockers with well known clinical cardioprotection, haven't been investigated.

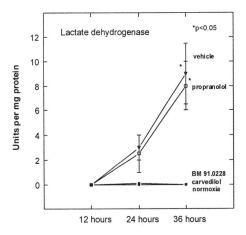

Figure 2 Differential effects of carvedilol, propranolol and BM 91.0228 on LDH leakage into the medium in cultured neonatal rat cardiac myocytes. Carvedilol and BM 91.0228 prevented myocardial injury following hypoxia (0-24 hours) and hypoxia (0-24 hours) and reoxygenation (24-36 hours).

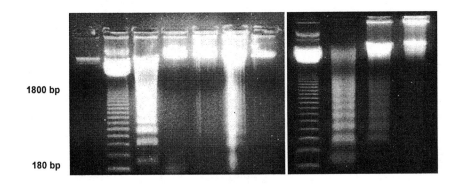

Figure 3 Effect of hypoxia and reoxygenation on apoptosis in cardiac myocytes using DNA laddering. *lane 1*: high molecular weight DNA control, *lane 2*: 123 ladder, *lane 3*: thymus cell DNA positive apoptosis control, *lane 4*: normoxic myocyte DNA, *lane 5*: myocyte DNA after 36 of hypoxia, *lane 6*: apoptotic myocyte DNA after 24h of hypoxia followed by 12 hours of reoxygenation, *lane 7*: carvedilol pre reoxygenation, *lane 8*: 123 ladder, *lane 9*: reoxygenated myocytes, *lane 10*: propranolol pre reoxygenation, *lane 11*: BM 91.0228 pre reoxygenation.
Significant DNA fragmentation only occurs in reoxygenated cardiac myocytes in vehicle- and propranolol-treated myocytes. Carvedilol and BM 91.0228 prevented DNA fragmentation.

Clinical studies

Since the first report in 1975 (26) demonstrated that heart failure can be improved by long term treatment with a beta-blocker multiple studies documented the beneficial effects of beta-blocker therapy (table 3). At present, there is no doubt that reduction of sympathetic nervous system activity may lead to decreased morbidity and mortality in chronic congestive heart failure patients. However, the current clinical data are not sufficient to show any anti-apoptotic effect of beta-blockers. Only one clinical study investigated the effect of thiobarbituric acid-reactive substances (TBARS), indirect markers of free radical activity (7). The data demonstrated that beta-blocker therapy significantly reduced TBAR production, thus, possibly indicating inhibition of apoptotic processes. Thus far, no clinical studies compared various beta-blockers in their efficacy to suppress myocyte apoptosis. Accordingly, there is no recommendation to either use selective or non-selective beta-blockers, with or without additional antioxidative properties. Finally, multiple large clinical trials have addressed the question whether the superior in-vitro cardioprotection of carvedilol can be confirmed in the in-vivo situation (table 3). However, no clinical study showed that the cardioprotection of carvedilol is significantly superior to other beta-blockers.

Table 3 Clinical hallmark studies on beta-blocker therapy and mortality/apoptosis.

Abbreviation	Title	Apoptosis as Endpoint	Reference
BEST	Beta-Blocker Evaluation Survival Trial	-	19
CIBIS I/II	Cardiac Insufficiency Bisoprolol Study	-	17, 20
COMET	Carvedilol Or Metopolol Evaluation Trial	-	21
COPERNICUS	Carvedilol Prospective rRandomized Cumulative Survival Trilal	-	22
MDC	Metoprolol in Dilated Cardiomyopathy Trial	-	14
MERIT-HF	Metoprolol Randomized Intervention Trial in Congestive Heart Failure	-	23
MOCHA	Multicenter Oral Carvedilol Heart Failure Assessment	-	24
PRECISE	Prospective Randomized Evaluation of Carvedilol on Symptoms and Exercise	-	25
	Prospective Comparison of Metropolol and Carvedilol	(+)	7

Thus, the promising in-vitro data on beta-blockers with additional anti-oxidative properties are currently not supported by large clinical trials. In fact, both β_1-selective and $\beta_{1/2}$ and α-blocking beta-blockers appear to be highly beneficial in the treatment of congestive heart failure. However, given the important role of oxygen free radical production in the induction of apoptosis may raise the question whether treatment with beta-blockers having antioxidative properties may be effective during or shortly after an ischemic event and/or reoxygenation. Representing the major stimulus of oxygen free radical production, reperfusion should be protected by antioxidative compounds, thus eliminating oxidative stress-induced apoptosis.

Future studies may be of interest that specifically evaluate the ability of hybrid compounds in this setting.

SUMMARY

Multiple in-vitro studies implying models of hypoxia and reoxygenation could clearly show the cardioprotective effect of various beta-blockers. The significant cardioprotection may, at least in part, be due to inhibition of programmed cell death. In addition, beta-blockers with additional antioxidative properties showed superior cardioprotection in experimental settings. This effect may be due to the importance of oxygen free radical formation during reoxygenation.

However, while beta-blockers may be highly efficacious in the treatment of patients with myocardial infarction or congestive heart failure the role of antiapoptotic mechanisms could not yet be demonstrated. Specifically, a large number of randomised studies demonstrated that patients with congestive heart failure of various causes show improvement of cardiac function and functional class when administered long-term beta-blocker therapy. However, at present, only one study could link cardioprotection to apoptotic processes.

Therefore, clinical studies should address the question, whether beta-blocker therapy can inhibit programmed cell death. In addition, they should document more precisely the underlying mechanisms which are responsible for the well known cardioprotective effect. Despite these open questions, beta-blocker therapy constitutes a major advantage in the treatment of congestive heart failure.

References

1. Olivetti G, Abbi R, Quaini F, Kajstura J, Cheng W, Nitahara JA, Quaini E, Loreto C, Beltrami CA, Krajewski S, Reed JC, Anversa P. Apoptosis in the failing human heart. N Engl J Med 1997; 336: 1131-1141.
2. Sabbah HN, Sharov VG. Apoptosis in heart failure. Prog Cardiovasc Dis 1998; 40: 549-562.
3. Feuerstein G, Yue TL, Ma X, Ruffolo RR. Novel mechanism in the treatment of heart failure: inhibition of oxygen radicals and apoptosis by carvedilol. Prog Cardiovasc Dis 1998; 48 (Suppl 1): 17-24.
4. Ruffolol RR, Feuerstein GZ. Carvedilol: preclinical profile and mechanisms of action in preventing the progression of congestive heart failure. Eur Heart J 1998; 19 (Suppl B): 19-24.
5. Ruffolo RR, Feuerstein GZ, Ohlstein EH. Recent observations with beta-adrenoceptor blockade. Beneficial effects in hypertension and heart failure. Am J Hypertension 1998; 11: 9-14.
6. Feuerstein GZ, Bril A, Ruffolo RR. Protective effects of carvedilol in the myocardium. Am J Cardiol 1997; 80: 41L-45L.
7. Kukin MK, Kalman J, Charney RH, Levey DK, Buchholz-Varley C, Ocampo ON, Eng C. Prospective, randomized comparison of effect of long-term treatment with metropolol or carvedilol on symptoms, exercise, ejection fraction, and oxidative stress in heart failure. Circulation 1999; 99: 2645-2651.
8. Katz AM. Cardiomyopathy of overload: a major determinant of prognosis in congestive heart failure. N Engl J Med 1990; 322: 100-109.
9. Jennings GL, Esler MD. Circulatory regulation at rest and exercise and the functional assessment of patients with congestive heart failure. Circulation 1990; 81 (Suppl II): 5-11.
10. Hasking GJ, Esler MD, Jennings GL. Norepinephrine spillover to plasma in patients with congestive heart failure. Evidence of increased overall and cardiorenal sympathetic nervous activity. Circulation 1986; 73: 615-625.

11. Rose CP, Burgess JH, Cousineau D. Tracer norepinephrine kinetics in coronary circulation of patients with heart failure secondary to chronic pressure and volume overload. J Clin Invest 1985; 76: 1740-1751.

12. Communal C, Singh K, Pimentel DR, Colucci WS. Norepinephrine stimulates apoptosis in adult rat ventricular myocytes by activation of the beta-adrenergic pathway. Circulation 1998; 98: 1329-1334.

13. Swedberg K, Hjalmarson A, Waagstein F, Wallentin I. Beneficial effects of long-term beta-blockade in congestive cardiomyopathy. Br Heart J 1980; 44: 117-133.

14. Waagstein F, Bristow MR, Swedberg K, Camerini F, Fowler MB, Silver MA, Gilbert EM, Johnson MR, Goss FG, Hjalmarson A, for the metropolol in dilated cardiomyopathy (MDC) trial study group: beneficial effects of metropolol in idiopathic dilated cardiomyopathy. Lancet 1993; 342: 1441-1446.

15. Ruffolo RR, Bril A, Feuerstein GZ. Cardioprotective potential of carvedilol. Cardiology 1993; 82 (Suppl 3): 24-28.

16. Yue TL, Ma XL, Wang X, Romanic AM, Liu GL, Louden C, Gu JL, Kumar S, Poste G, Ruffolo RR Jr, Feuerstein GZ. Possible involvement of stress-activated protein kinase signaling pathway and Fas receptor expression in prevention of ischemia/reperfusion-induced cardiomyocyte apoptosis by carvedilol. Circ Res 1998; 82: 166-174.

17. CIBIS-II investigators and committees. The cardiac insufficiency bisoprolol study II (CIBIS II): a randomised trial. Lancet 1999; 353:9-13.

18. Sigel AV, Romanic AM, Peng CF, Schunkert H, Feuerstein G, Riegger GAJ and Yue TL. Hypoxia and reoxygenation related injuries in cardiac myocytes are enhanced by programmed cell death: Differential protective effects of beta-adrenergic receptor blockers. Circulation 1998; 19: 742A.

19. Design of the beta-blocker evaluation survival trial (BEST). The BEST steering committee. Am J Cardiol 1995: 1220-1223.

20. CIBIS investigators and Committees: A randomized trial of β-blockade in heart failure. The cardiac insufficiency bisoprolol study (CIBIS). Circulation 1994; 1765-1773.

21. Gilbert EM, Abraham WT, Olsen S, Hattler B, White M, Mealy P, Larrabee P, Bristow MR. Comparative hemodynamic, left ventricular functional, and antiadrenergic effects of chronic treatment with metoprolol versus carvedilol in the failing heart. Circulation 1996; 94: 2817-2825.

22. Australian-New Zealand Heart Failure Research Colloborative Group: Randomised, placebo-controlled trial of carvedilol in patients with congestive heart failure due to ischaemic heart disease. Lancet 1997; 349: 375-380.

23. Rationale, design, and organization of the metoprolol CR/XL randomized intervention trial in heart failure (MERIT-HF). The international steering committee. Am J Cardiol 1997; 80: 54J-58J.

24. Bristow MR, Gilbert EM, Abraham WT, Adams KF, Fowler MB, Hershberger RE, Kubo SH, Narahara KA, Ingersoll H, Krueger S, Young S, Shudterman N, for the MOCHA investigators: Carvedilol produces dose-related improvements in left ventricular function and survival in subjects with chronic heart failure. Circulation 1996; 94: 2807-2816.

26. Waagstein F, Hjalmarson A, Varnauskas E, Wallentin I. Effect of chronic beta-adrenergic receptor blockade in congestive cardiomyopathy. Br Heart J 1975; 37: 1022-1036.

27. Luchner A, Burnett JC, Jougasaki M, Hense HW, Riegger GA, Schunkert H. Augmentation of the cardiac natriuretic peptides by beta-receptor antagonism: evidence from a population-based study. J Am Coll Cardiol 1998; 32: 1839-1844.

28. Holmer SR, Hense HW, Danser AH, Mayer B, Riegger GA, Schunkert H. Beta adrenergic blockers lower renin in patients treated with ACE inhibitors and diuretics. Heart 1998; 80: 45-48.

IV.3
Apoptosis in cardiac myocytes – Role of the renin-angiotensin-system

Daniela Grimm, M.D., Gilbert Schönfelder, M.D.,
and Martin Paul, M.D.

Freie Universität Berlin, Berlin, Germany

INTRODUCTION

Apoptosis is considered as a form of physiological cell death, characterized by chromatin condensation, cytoplasmatic blebbing and DNA fragmentation. It plays a key role during development, homeostasis, and several diseases including cardiovascular disorders. Apoptosis occurs through the activation of a cell-intrinsic suicide program. The activation of the cell suicide program is regulated by many different signals that originate from both the intracellular and extracellular milieu (1). Experimental evidence suggests that exaggerated apoptosis may account for the loss of cardiomyocytes in heart failure. Furthermore, several factors intrinsic and extrinsic to the cardiomyocytes have been suggested as potential candidates to trigger apoptosis.

Regulation of apoptosis involves a variety of cytokines, genes and growth factors that have been found to be expressed in the myocardium and in interstitial cells. In general, they can be classified into four categories. These include (1.) genes that primarily suppress apoptosis, such as some members of the Bcl-2 family, (2.) growth factors and cytokines, that initiate or prevent programmed cell death, such as myc, TNFα, TGFß, or IGF-1. (3.) genes that act as effectors of apoptosis, such as the ICE family of genes, and (4.) intermediate genes such as Fas and Fas ligand. There is also evidence that apoptosis is accompanied by oxidative stress (2). It has also been shown that the protooncogen Bcl-2 promotes cell survival by inhibiting adapters needed for the activation of the caspases that dismantle the cell. Bcl-2 family members are essential for maintenance of major organ structures. The proapoptotic gene caspase CED-3 which encodes a cysteine protease received much attention (3). Recent studies have demonstrated that cardiac myocyte apoptosis also occurs in the hypertrophied heart, after acute myocardial infarction and in the aging heart, conditions frequently associated with the development of heart failure. Available data support the existence of myocyte apoptosis in the failing heart. The role of the vasoconstrictor and growth modulator Angiotensin II (ANG II) in this process has gained wide attention. If ANG II and the renin angiotensin system (RAS) are triggers of myocyte apoptosis in the heart, blockers of the RAS such as angiotensin converting enzyme (ACE) inhibitors and ANG II receptor antagonists could provide therapeutic tools in preventing or reducing apoptosis in cardiac disorders such as left ventricular hypertrophy and heart failure. In addition, the development of novel therapeutic modalities aimed to prevent and retard the process of progressive ventricular dysfunction and the transition towards end-stage heart failure by interference with apoptotic mechanisms will be a major focus of research.

APOPTOSIS AND MYOCARDIAL INFARCTION

Normally, apoptosis is not detected in left ventricular myocardium. In general, myocyte death in myocardial infarction is attributed to necrosis, but recently myocardial apoptosis has been observed in human acute myocardial infarction. Apoptosis is the early and predominant form of cell death in infarcted human myocardium. It occurs mainly in cardiac myocytes, and is shown to be limited to hypoxic regions during acute infarction. The existence of a p53-independent pathway that mediates myocyte apoptosis during myocardial infarction was demonstrated by Bialik (4). Apoptosis not only occurs in acute myocardial infarction but it is also accelerated in the reperfused myocardium. Therapies directed at early rescue of apoptotic cardiomyocytes may, therefore, prove very valuable (5).

The ratio of Bcl-2 protein, an inhibitor of apoptosis, to Bax protein, an inducer of programmed cell death, determines survival or death after an apoptotic stimulus. It has been shown that Bcl-2 protein is induced in salvaged myocytes at the acute stage of anterior myocardial infarction but Bax protein is overexpressed at a later stage. The changes in the expression of these genes were present at day 1 and 7 after coronary artery occlusion. The expression of Bcl-2 and the overexpression of Bax plays an important pathophysiological role in the protection or acceleration of the apoptosis of human myocytes after ischemia and /or reperfusion (6). Mechanical load produced by myocardial infarction and ventricular failure may affect the regulation of Bcl-2 and Bax in viable cardiomyocytes triggering programmed cell death and the remodeling of the ventricular wall (7). Recently Chen et al. (8) investigated apoptosis in hypoperfused myocardium of pigs with severe coronary stenosis. Using in situ end-labeling and deoxyribonucleic acid laddering, apoptosis was detected in focal fibrotic areas and also in areas without fibrosis or patchy infarction. Programmed cell death was found not only in 24-h hypoperfused myocardium, but also in 4-week hypoperfused myocardium. The severity of myocyte apoptosis correlated significantly with regional blood flow reduction.

These results demonstrated that there is ongoing cardiomyocyte death through myocyte apoptosis in hypoperfused hibernating myocardium.

Anversa and coworkers (9) investigated quantitatively the contribution of apoptotic and necrotic myocyte cell death in the rat model of myocardial infarction. Myocyte necrosis was absent in the viable myocardium after infarction. Myocyte cell death by apoptosis involved 2.8 million cells at 2 hours after coronary artery occlusion and necrosis only 90.000 cells. Apoptosis of the cardiomyocytes continued to represent the major form of cell death, affecting 6.6 million cells at 4.5 hours, whereas necrosis peaked at 1 day, including 1.1 million cells. DNA ladders were found at 2-3h, 4.5h, 1 day and 2 days after infarction. Finally the expression of Bcl-2 and Fas in myocytes increased 18-fold and 131-fold, respectively. Myocyte apoptosis was also present in the surviving portion of the wall adjacent to and remote from the ischemic area.

In general, apoptosis seems to be the major form of myocardial damage following myocardial infarction, whereas necrotic cell death follows apoptosis and contributes to the progressive cell loss over time after myocardial infarction. The enhanced expression of Fas may activate apoptosis in spite of the increase in Bcl-2, which tends to preserve cell survival (10).

Some authors have attempted to determine whether acute left ventricular failure associated with myocardial infarction leads to architectural changes in the spared nonischemic portion of the ventricular wall. Side-to-side slippage of myocytes in the myocardium occurs in association with ventricular dilatation after a large MI and contributes to the occurrence of decompensated eccentric hypertrophy (11). The persistence of elevated myocardial and cellular loads sustained the progression of heart failure.

APOPTOSIS AND LEFT VENTRICULAR HYPERTROPHY – ROLE OF ANG II

Hypertrophy has been recognized to be a compensatory response to chronic pressure overload. However, it appears that after a certain time of compensation, left ventricular dysfunction and the process of deterioration will become evident. Myocyte hypertrophy, myocyte loss, fibrosis and remodeling of the extracellular matrix proteins are well recognized in end-stage left ventricular hypertrophy (12,13). In contrast to passive necrosis involving groups of cells where mitochondrial dilatation, loss of metabolic integrity, nuclear flocculation, cell swelling and lysis occur in response to injury, apoptosis is an active process which is under genetic control and tends to involve single cells which undergo cytoplasmatic and nuclear condensation. Chronic hypertrophy or increased workload has been shown to result in apoptosis and to contribute to myocardial dysfunction and heart failure (14). Left ventricular failure imposes an elevated diastolic load on myocytes, resulting in stretching of sarcomeres (15) and the stimulation of multiple second messenger systems which have been linked to the initiation of myocyte reactive hypertrophy in the heart (16-21).

Cheng and coworkers showed that stretching is coupled with oxidant stress, expression of Fas, programmed cell death, architectural rearrangement of myocytes, and impairment in force development of the myocardium (22).

ANG II has been shown to activate programmed myocyte cell death *in vitro*. Ligand binding of ANG II-AT_1 receptors initiated programmed myocyte cell death via an elevation in cytosolic calcium and the stimulation of calcium-dependent endogenous endonuclease. The latter produced DNA fragmentation followed by nuclear fragmentation, cellular shrinkage, and the formation of apoptotic bodies.

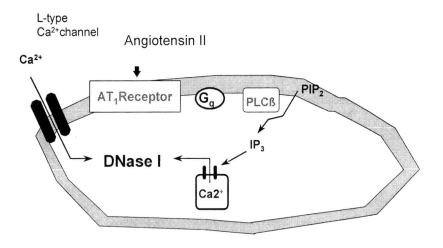

Figure 1 Activation of DNase I by ANG II via the AT1 receptor.

The effect of ANG II on myocyte apoptosis was inhibited by the selective AT_1 receptor blocker losartan, whereas an AT_2 receptor antagonist had no influence on myocyte cell death (23).

Sarcomere stretching, applied in vitro to mimic cardiac decompensation in vivo, is coupled with the cellular release of ANG II. Importantly, diastolic stretch in vitro and in vivo is associated with myocyte apoptosis. The latter encountered in the postinfarcted heart, is characterized by an increase in Bax and a decrease in Bcl-2 in myocytes, suggesting that the apoptotic process may involve the tumor suppressor protein p53 (25,26). p53 is a transcriptional regulator of the Bcl-2 and Bax genes, and the induction of p53 may downregulate Bcl-2 and upregulate Bax in the cells. However changes in the relative proportion of Bcl-2 and Bax are not sufficient to trigger programmed cell death (27). The ability of p53 to induce programmed cell death may involve the transmission of a death signal that may be modulated by the p53-dependent genes Bax and Bcl-2. Pierzchalski and coworkers (28) showed that p53 enhances the myocyte renin-angiotensin system and decreases the Bcl-2-Bax ratio in the cells, triggering apoptosis. The induction of p53 is proposed as a proximate event in the initiation of the suicide program in the decompensated heart.

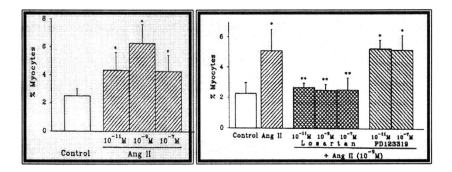

Figure 2 ANG II mediates apoptosis in cardiac myocytes via the AT1 receptor. <u>Left panel</u>: Induction of apoptosis in neonatal ventricular myocytes. The percentages of apoptotic myocytes in control cultures (open bar) and cultures treated with various concentrations of ANG II (hatched bars) are shown. <u>Right panel</u>: Effects of different concentrations of the AT1 blocker, losartan (cross-hatched bars) and the AT2 receptor antagonist, PD 123319 (hatched bars) on apoptosis in neonatal ventricular myocytes. Shown are percentages of apoptotic cells compared to negative control and ANG II stimulated cells (23).

Recently, it has been demonstrated that myocyte apoptosis increased after stretching. p53 binding to the promoter regions of angiotensinogen and the AT1 receptor was demonstrated, in parallel to an increase in Bax expression. In addition specific binding sites for P53 were identified on the promoters.

p53 Consensus Binding Sequences

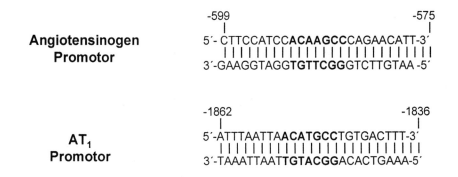

Figure 3 Consensus binding sites for p53 (bold letters) on the angiotensinogen and AT1 promoter sequences (28).

Expression of angiotensinogen increased and Bcl-2 decreased in stretched myocytes whereas ANG II concentration was elevated. The AT1 blocker, losartan, in contrast, abolished apoptosis in stretched myocytes. These data demonstrate that stretch-mediated release of ANG II is coupled with apoptosis and the activation of p53 which may be responsible for the prolonged upregulation of the local renin-angiotensin system and the increased susceptibility of myocytes to undergo apoptosis (29).

Strech-mediated Myocyte Apoptosis

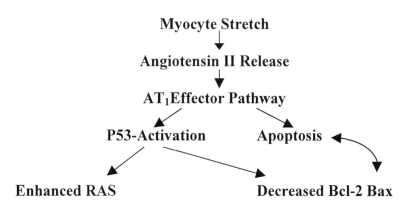

Figure 4 Mediation of apoptosis after myocyte stretching via the AT1 effector pathway.

It has been suggested by these studies that cell viability after an apoptotic stimulus may depend on the ratio of the level of Bcl-2 to that of Bax. A high level of Bcl-2 relative to Bax promotes survival, whereas an excess of Bax relative to Bcl-2 promotes cell death. (30). *In vivo*, increased apoptosis has been demonstrated in the hypertrophied left ventricle of young, adult and aged SHR (31-33).

Cardiac apoptosis in adult SHR could result from an exaggerated local production of ANG II (32). This hypothesis was supported by the findings that ANG II induces apoptosis of adult rat ventricular cells in vitro through a mechanism triggered by the interaction of the peptide with AT_1 receptors (23,24). These in vitro findings were supported with the in vivo investigations of Fortuno (34). Compared with Wistar-Kyoto (WKY) rats, untreated spontaneously hypertensive rats (SHR) exhibited increased apoptosis, increased Bax, and similar Bcl-2. The Bcl-2/Bax ratio was lower in untreated SHR than in WKY. Chronic administration of losartan was associated with the normalization of apoptosis, Bax expression, and the Bcl-2-Bax-ratio in treated SHR. Chronic blockade of AT_1 receptors prevents Bax overexpression and normalizes apoptosis in the left ventricle of SHR independently of its hemodynamic effect. This finding suggests that the interaction of angiotensin II with the AT_1 receptor may participate in the stimulation of Bax protein, which in turn renders cells from the left ventricle of SHR more susceptible apoptosis.

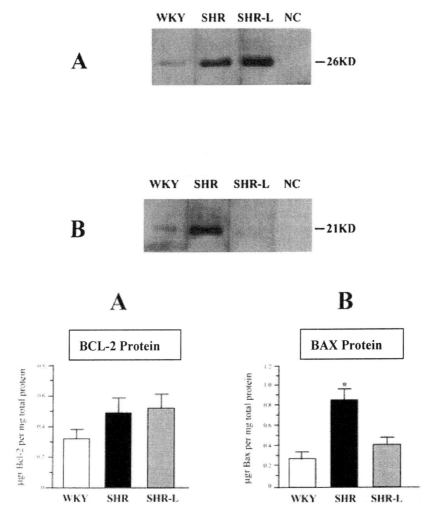

Figure 5 Influence of AT1-blockade on apoptosis in left ventricular hypertrophy. Spontaneously hypertensive rats (SHR) which develop left ventricular hypertrophy, were treated with the AT1-blocker losartan (SHR-L) and compared to Wistar Kyoto control rats (WKY). Upper panel: Western blot data of cardiac Bvl-2 (A) and Bax (B) protein levels. NC: negative control. Lower panel: Western blot analysis of Bcl-2 (A) and Bax (B) proteins from the left ventricles in each experimental group. Each bar represents an n of 9-10 animals. Shown is mean and SEM of the Bcl or bax/total protein ratio. The asterisk represents a statistical significant difference of $p < 0.01$ compared to WKY and $p < 0.05$ compared to SHR-L (34).

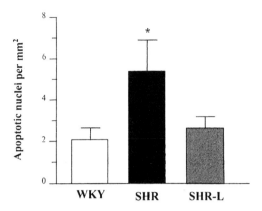

Figure 6 Values for apoptotic density measured in the ventricles of each experimental group of the experiment shown in figure 5. Bars represent the means and SEMs of 9-10 animals. The asterisk represents a statistical significance of p<0.01 compared with the WKY and the SHR-L groups (34).

APOPTOSIS IN THE FAILING HUMAN HEART – ROLE OF ANG II

It is well known that a variety of pathologic processes are activated in patients with congestive heart failure. The most important processes to be activated in heart failure are the neurohormonal systems, including the renin-angiotensin system, the sympathetic nervous system, and the endothelin system. In addition to the neurohormonal systems, the formation of reactive oxygen free radicals is increased in patients with heart failure and may be responsible for the loss of cardiomyocytes being an important factor in the development of heart failure of both ischemic or nonischemic origin. Morphological and biochemical features of cardiomyocyte apoptosis were detected in left ventricular myocardium of dogs with chronic heart failure (35). Treatment with enalapril attenuated cardiomyocyte apoptosis in dogs with moderate heart failure (36). Attenuation of cardiomyocyte apoptosis may be one mechanism by which ACE inhibitors preserve global LV function in heart failure.

In addition to treatment with ACE inhibitors, application of carvedilol, a potent antioxidant and non-selective beta-blocker with vasodilatative properties was applied in heart failure therapy. It has been shown to be effective in the management of heart failure (37). Recent results suggest that carvedilol prevents myocardial ischemia/reperfusion-induced apoptosis in cardiomyocytes by downregulation of Fas receptor expression and stress-activated protein kinase signaling pathway (38).

It has been shown that programmed cell death of cardiomyocytes occurred in the decompensated human heart in spite of enhanced expression of Bcl-2. Bcl-2 was 1.8-fold increased in patients with heart failure as compared to control persons (39). Bcl-2 overexpression, therefore, may contribute to the progression of cardiac dysfunction.

324

CONCLUSIONS AND OUTLOOK

A large body of data concerning programmed cell death in the myocardium has accumulated over the last 5 years. It has been shown that complex mechanisms are involved in this process such as P53 dependent and independent pathways, cytokine-induced pathways (TNF, Fas) and others. It has also become clear that ANG II and the RAS play a central role in myocyte apoptosis in cardiac disorders such as heart failure and left ventricular hypertrophy.

Since loss of cardiomyocytes through programmed cell death has been shown to be an important contributor to the progression of heart failure, and since factors that trigger cardiac apoptosis could be identified, the development of novel therapeutic strategies aimed at preventing or slowing heart failure will be mandatory. It has also helped us to better understand current therapeutic options. The prevention or inhibition of apoptotic mechanisms in heart disease by inhibitors of the RAS could explain, at least in part, the beneficial effects of these substances under these conditions. This knowledge may also be helpful in the development of new drugs that prevent progressive loss of cardiac myocytes.

References

1. Steller H. Mechanisms and genes of cellular suicide. *Science.* 1995;267:1335-1449.
2. Buttke TM, Sandstrom PA. Oxidative stress as a mediator of apoptosis. *Immunol Today.* 1994;15:7-10.
3. Adams JM, Cory S. The Bcl-2 protein family: Arbiters of cell survival. *Science.* 1998;281:1322-1326.
4. Bialik S, Geenen DL, Sasson IE, Cheng R, Horner JW, Evans SM, Lord EM, Koch CJ, Kitsis RN. Myocyte apoptosis during acute myocardial infarction in the mouse localizes to hypoxic regions but occurs independently of p53. *J Clin Invest.* 1997;100:1991-1999.
5. Veinot JP, Gattinger DA, Fliss H. Early apoptosis in human myocardial infarcts. *Human Pathol.* 1997;28:485-492.
6. Misao J, Hayakawa Y, Ohno M, Kato S, Fujiwara T, Fujiwara H. Expression of bcl-2 protein, an inhibitor of apoptosis, and Bax, an accelerator of apoptosis, in ventricular myocytes of human hearts with myocardial infarction. *Circulation.* 1996;94:1506-1512.
7. Cheng W, Kajstura J, Nitahara JA, Li B, Reiss K, Liu Y, Clark WA, Krajewski S, Reed JC, Olivetti G, Anversa P. Programmed myocyte cell death affects the viable myocardium after infarction in rats. *Exp Cell Res.* 1996;226:316-327.
8. Chen C, Ma I, Linfert DR, Lai T, Fallon JT, Gillam LD, Waters DD, Tsongalis GJ. Myocardial cell death and apoptosis in hibernating myocardium. *J Am Coll Cardiol.* 1997; 30:1407-1412.
9. Anversa P, Cheng W, Liu Y, Leri A, Redaelli G, Kajstura J. Apoptosis and myocardial infarction. *Basic Res Cardiol.* 1998;93:Suppl3:8-12.
10. Kajsura J, Cheng W, Reiss K, Clark WA, Sonnenblick EH, Krajewski S, Reed JC, Olivetti G, Anversa P. Apoptotic and necrotic myocyte cell deaths are independent contributing variables of infarct size in rats. *Lab Invest.* 1996;74:86-107.
11. Olivetti G, Capasso JM, Sonnenblick EH, Anversa P. Side-to-side slippage of myocytes in ventricular wall remodeling acutely after myocardial infarction in rats. *Circ Res .*1990;67:23-34.
12. Grimm D, Kromer EP, Böcker W, Bruckschlegel G, Holmer SR, Riegger GAJ, Schunkert H. Regulation of extracellular matrix proteins in pressure-overload cardiac hypertrophy: effects of angiotensin-converting enzyme inhibition. *J Hypertens.* 1998;1345-1355.
13. Weber KT, Brilla CG. Pathological hypertrophy and cardiac interstitium. Fibrosis and renin-angiotensin-aldosterone system. *Circulation.* 1991;83:1849-1865.
14. Bing OHL. Hypothesis: apoptosis may be a mechanism for the transition to heart failure with chronic pressure overload. *J Mol Cell Cardiol.* 1994; 26:943-948.

15. Ross J, Sonnenblick EH, Taylor HM, Covell JW. Diastolic geometry and sarcomeric lengths in the chronically dilated left ventricle. *Circ Res.* 1971; 28:49-61.
16. Vitali-Mazza L, Anversa P, Tedeschi F, Mastandrea R, Mavilla V, Visioli O. Ultrastructural basis of acute left ventricular failure from severe acute aortic stenosis in the rabbit. *J Mol Cell Cardiol.* 1972; 4:661-671.
17. Komuro I., Kaida T, Shibazaki Y, Kurabayashi M, Katoh Y, Hoh E, Takaku F, Yazaki Y. Stretching cardiac myocytes stimulates protooncogene expression. *J Biol Chem.* 1990; 265: 3595-3598.
18. Schneider MD, Roberts R, Parker TG. Modulation of cardiac genes by mechanical stress. The oncogene signaling hypothesis. *Mol Biol Med.* 1991; 8: 167-183.
19. Sadoshima J, Jahn L, Takashashi T, Kulik TJ, Izumo S. Molecular characterization of the stretch-induced adaptation of cultured cardiac cells. An in vitro model of load-induced cardiac hypertrophy. *J. Biol. Chem.* 1992;267:10551-10660.
20. Sadoshima J, Takahashi T, Jahn L, Izumo S. Roles of mechano-sensitive ion channels, cytoskeleton, and contractile activity in stretch-induced immediate-early gene expression and hypertrophy of cardiac myocytes. *Proc Natl Acad Sc. USA.* 1992;89: 9905-9909.
21. Sadoshima J, Izumo S. Mechanical stretch rapidly activates multiple signal transduction pathways in cardiac myocytes: potential involvement of an autocrine/paracrine mechanism. *EMBO.* (Eur. Mol. Biol. Organ.). 1993;2:1681-1692.
22. Cheng W, Li B, Kajstura J, Li P, Wolin MS, Sonnenblick EH, Hintze TH, Olivetti G, Anversa P. Stretch-induced programmed myocyte cell death. *J Clin Invest.* 1995;96:2247-2259.
23. Cigola E, Kaijstura J, Li B, Meggs LG, Anversa P. Angiotensin II activates programmed cell death in vitro. *Exp Cell Res.* 1997;231:363-371.
24. Kajstura J, Cigola E, Malhotra A, Li P, Cheng W, Meggs LG, Anversa P. Angiotensin II induces apoptosis of adult ventricular myocytes in vitro. *J Mol Cell Cardiol.* 1997;29:859-870.
25. Miyashita T, Reed J. Tumor suppressor p53 is a direct transcriptional activator of the human Bax gene. *Cell.* 1995; 80: 293-299.
26. Miyashita T, Harigai M, Hanada M, Reed JC. Identification of a p53-dependent negative response element in the Bcl-2 gene. *Cancer Res.* 1994;54: 3131-3135.
27. Veis DJ, Sorenson CM, Shutter JR, Korsmeyer SJ. Bcl-2 deficient mice demonstrated fulminant lymphoid apoptosis, polycystic kidneys and hypopigmented hair. *Cell.* 1993;75:229-240.
28. Pierzchalski P, Reiss K, Cheng W, Cirielli C, Kajstura J, Nitahara JA, Rizk M, Capogrossi MC, Anversa P. p53 induces myocyte apoptosis via the activation of the renin-angiotensin system. *Exp. Cell Res.* 1997;234: 57-65.
29. Leri A, Claudio PP, Li Q, Wang X, Reiss K, Wang S, Malhotra A, Kajstura J, Anversa P. Stretch-mediated release of Angiotensin II induces myocyte apoptosis by activating p53 that enhances the local renin-angiotensin system and decreases the Bcl-2-to Bax protein ratio in the cell. *J Clin Invest.* 1998;101:1326-1342.
30. Oltvai ZN, Korsmeyer SJ. Checkpoints of dueling dimers foil death wishes. *Cell.* 1994; 79:189-192.
31. Hamet P, Richard L, Dam TV, Teiger E, Orlov SN, Gaboury L, Gossard F, Tremblay J. apoptosis in target organs in hypertension. *Hypertension.* 1995;26:642-648.
32. Diez J, Panizo A, Hernandez M, Vega F, Sola I, Fortuno MA, Pardo J. Cardiomyocyte apoptosis and cardiac angiotensin-converting enzyme in spontaneously hypertensive rats. *Hypertension.* 1997;30:1029-1034.
33. Li Z, Bing OHL, Long X, Robinson KG, Lakatta EG. Increased cardiomyocye apoptosis during the transition to heart failure in the spontaneously hypertensive rat. *Am J Physiol.* 1997;272:H2313-H2319.
34. Fortuno MA, Ravassa S, Etayo JC, Diez J. Overexpression of Bax protein and enhanced apoptosis in the left ventricle of spontaneously hypertensive rats. Effects of AT_1 blockade with losartan. *Hypertension.* 1998;32:280-286.
35. Sharov VG, Sabbah HN, Shimoyama H, Goussev AV, Lesch M, Goldstein S. Evidence of cardiocyte apoptosis in myocardium of dogs with chronic heart failure. *Am J Pathol.* 1996;148:141-149.
36. Goussev A, Sharov VG, Shimoyama H, Tanimura M, Lesch M, Goldstein S, Sabbah HN. Effects of ACE inhibition on cardiomyocyte apoptosis in dogs with heart failure. *Am J Physiol.* 1998;275:H626-631.

37. Ruffolo RR Jr. Feuerstein GZ. Neurohormonal activation, oxygen free radicals, and apoptosis in the pathogenesis of congestive heart failure. *J Cardiovasc Pharmacol* 1998;32 Suppl 1:S22-30.
38. Yue TL, Ma XL, Wang X, Romanic AM, Liu GL, Louden C, Gu JL, Kumar S, Poste G, Ruffolo RR Jr. Feuerstein GZ. Possible involvement of stress-activated protein kinase signaling pathway and Fas receptor expression in prevention of ischemia/reperfusion-induced cardiomyocyte apoptosis by carvedilol. *Circ Res.* 1998;82:166-174.
39. Olivetti G, Abbi R, Quaini F, Kajstura J Cheng W, Nitahara JA, Quaini E, Di Loreto C, Beltrami CA, Krajewski S, Reed JC, Anversa P. Apoptosis in the failing heart. *N Engl J Med.* 1997;336:1131-1141.

IV.4
Estrogens and the prevention of cardiac apoptosis

Christian Grohé, M.D., Rainer Meyer, Ph.D., and Hans Vetter, M.D.
Universität Bonn, Bonn, Germany

INTRODUCTION

A large array of cardiac diseases such as hypertensive heart disease and cardiac remodeling after myocardial infarction display significant gender-based differences (1, 2, 3). In this context it has been shown that during the process of aging cardiac number and diameter vary significantly between men and women. While cardiac myocytes of male patients tend to develop hypertrophy and polyploidy, cardiac myocytes of female patients remain consistent over time in terms of size and number of nuclei (4). The underlying mechanisms of this process remain to be elucidated. However, it is remarkable that the incidence of cardiac disease in female gender reveals a significant increase after the onset of menopause (5). Therefore it has been hypothesized that the decline of ovarian sex hormones after the onset of menopause, in particular estrogens, play an important role in the pathogenesis of cardiac disease in women. The role of estrogen in the pathogenesis of this process is currently under investigation (6-11). The influence of estrogen on the development of cardiac diseases can be divided in systemic and direct effects on the cardiovascular system. Systemic effects include the influence of sex hormones on lipid and insulin metabolism (12, 13). Furthermore, it has become evident that estrogens display a variety of genomic and non-genomic effects on cardiovascular tissues that may modulate the respective phenotype of these tissues. Two different estrogen receptors have been identified so far, estrogen receptor α and estrogen receptor β. These two subtypes differ in ligand binding as well as in DNA binding properties (14-18). These differences offer a variety of potential interactions of the respective estrogen receptor and its specific estrogenic ligand depending on the tissue specific distribution of the receptors. Estrogen receptors have been characterized in vascular smooth muscle cells as well as in cardiac myocytes and cardiac fibroblasts (19-20). These cardiac estrogen receptors act as transcription factors on a variety of cardiac genes involved in the pathogenesis of heart disease such as connexin 43, the endothelial as well as the inducible form of nitric oxide synthases (10, 20-22). The induction of these genes may help to protect female individuals to develop congestive heart failure before menopause. In addition rapid, so called non-genomic effects of estrogen on cardiac myocytes have been described, which may contribute to the cardioprotective effect of estrogen (21-25).

New observations suggest that programmed cell death (apoptosis) may play a major role in cellular mechanisms involved in heart failure. In particular, the regulatory pathways that lead to apoptosis are currently under investigation in patients with cardiac remodeling and hypertensive heart disease (26-28). However, little is known about the role of estrogen in this context. While the circulating estrogen level in premenopausal women obviously exerts a cardioprotective effect, the decrease in endogenous estrogen metabolites is associated with an increase in cardiovascular disease in postmenopausal women. Therefore it seems to be critical to understand if estrogen replacement therapy in postmenopausal subjects leads to a modulation of apoptotic pathways in the myocardium. To further elucidate the potential effect of estrogen on apoptosis in cardiac disease, we investigated if estrogen replacement alters expression of proteins involved in the regulatory cascade leading to apoptosis in a model of hypertensive heart disease. We chose to investigate spontaneously hypertensive rats (SHR) as it is established that these animals display a sexual dimorphic pattern of blood pressure regulation and contain the classical features of elevated blood pressure and consecutive left ventricular hypertrophy (29).

Female spontaneously hypertensive rats were ovariectomized or sham-operated 14 weeks after birth (Harlan Winkelmann, Borchen, Germany). In a subset of experiments ovariectomized rats were substituted with estrogen by subcutaneous implantation of 17β-estradiol (E2) slow release pellets (Innovative Research of America, Sarasota, FL, USA). Tissue samples were harvested ten weeks post surgery.

In a first step we determined if the antiapoptotic protein bcl2 p29 protein is expressed in cardiac myocytes. bcl 2 has been shown to be regulated by cytokines such as interleukin-1β, tumor necrosis factor α and interferon γ in rat neonatal ventricular cardiomyocytes (30). We studied the expression of bcl2 in isolated neonatal and adult cardiac myocytes (Wistar-Kyoto strain) in the absence and presence of E2. Previously we demonstrated the expression of bcl 2 in isolated neonatal and adult cardiac myocytes (data not shown). We then studied the expression pattern of bcl2 in lysates obtained from SHR female rats, but failed to demonstrate the presence of this protein in left ventricular tissue (Figure 1).

S   O   O+E   St

29kD -

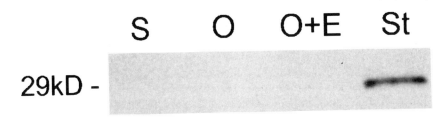

Figure 1 Cardiac expression of bcl2 p29 protein. The protein was detectable at the expected size of 29 kD only in control lysates from isolated adult cardiac myocytes (Wistar-Kyoto strain) treated with the apoptosis inducing agent staurosporine (St) in representative immunoblots. In sham-operated female rats (S), ovarectomized (O) and in protein lysates of ovarectomized rats which had been substituted with estrogen (O+E) the respective protein could not be detected. One of three similar studies is shown.

Control experiments using lysates from isolated adult cardiac myocytes from female Wistar-Kyoto rats treated with staurosporine (apoptosis inducing agent) clearly demonstrated the presence of the protein in adult cardiac myocytes (Figure 1). Our findings complement the observations from Fortuno et al. (26), who showed that the expression of bcl2 in the myocardium of male SHR rats is regulated by an AT_1 receptor antagonist. Furthermore, it is likely that other members of the bcl2 family such as bcl_{xl} are expressed and play an important role in apoptotic pathways in the myocardium (30). In a next step we investigated the expression pattern of the protein bax which counteracts the function of bcl2 and is designated as an proapoptotic protein (28, 31). Interstingly, the expression of bax in left ventricular tissue of female SHR rats was altered by estrogen. In intact females, the expression of the protein was low. In ovariectomized animals, however, the protein expression increased significantly in the left ventricle. Estrogen treatment of ovariectomized animals inhibited the upregulation of bax (Figure 2).

S   O   O+E

21kD -

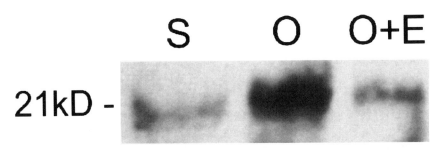

Figure 2 Cardiac expression of bax protein. In representative immunoblots the protein was detectable at the expected size of 21 kD. In sham-operated female rats (S), only a very weak signal could be detected. The amount of protein increased after ovariectomy (O). In protein lysates of ovariectomized rats which had been substituted with estrogen (O+E) the expression was significantly lower than in the myocardium of ovariectomized animals. One of three similar studies is shown.

These data suggest that the proapoptotic protein bax is upregulated in the myocardium of ovariectomized animals and that estrogen treatment can reverse this effect as samples from animals, which were estrogen-supplemented after ovariectomy, had a significantly lower level of bax expression compared to ovariectomized animals. As bcl2 and bax are critical proteins in the onset of the regulatory cascade leading to apoptosis, an additional set of proteins are involved in this cascade further downstream. An important member of the apoptotic pathway is the family of aspartate-specific cysteinyl proteases (caspases). This family has been identified as critical mediators of apoptosis in Caenorhabditis elegans and mammals (32). One important member of this family is caspase 3 also designated CPP32, apopain, YAMA (32). The caspases cleave different substrates. Gelsolin has been characterized as a potential target and then in turns leads to disruption of actin filaments which lead to nuclear fragmentation and cellular degradation. To further investigate the apoptotic cascade in the myocardium of female SHR rats we analysed the expression of caspase 3 in lysates obtained from the animals mentioned above. We were able to demonstrate that the expression of caspase 3 in intact (sham) animals was low. In ovariectomized animals the protein level increased significantly, demonstrating an upregulation of caspase 3 in the myocardium. Finally, estrogen treatment of ovariectomized animals inhibited the upregulation of the protein clearly demonstrating that the regulation of this protein in the myocardium of female SHR rats is estrogen-dependent (Figure 3).

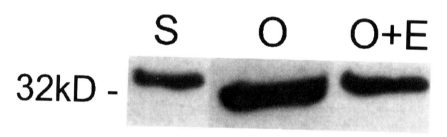

Figure 3 Cardiac expression of caspase 3 protein. In representative immunoblots the protein was detectable at the expected size of 32 kD. In sham-operated female rats (S), only a very weak signal could be detected. The amount of protein increased after ovariectomy (O). In protein lysates of ovariectomized rats which had been substituted with estrogen (O+E) the expression was significantly lower than in the myocardium of ovariectomized animals observed. One of three similar studies is shown.

We therefore were able to show that estrogen affects the expression of another member of the cascade leading to apoptosis. The functional implications of these findings have to be addressed in forthcoming studies since the activity rather than the expression level of these proteins determines the disposition to undergo apoptosis. In particular the influence of estrogen on the cleavage of caspases such as caspase 3 or caspase 9 has to be demonstrated.

Finally, we examined the expression of p53 in the myocardium of the chosen animal model. The data presented here show that the expression level of p53 is high in cardiac tissue obtained from all three groups studied. However significant differences in protein expression were not detectable between the three groups studied (Figure 4).

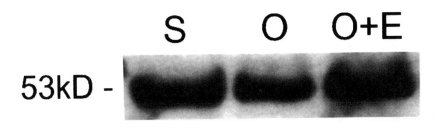

Figure 4 Cardiac expression of p53 protein. In representative immunoblots the protein was detectable at the expected size of 53 kD. In sham-operated female rats (S), expression of the respective protein could be detected at a high level. The amount of protein did not increase after ovariectomy (O). In protein lysates of ovariectomized rats which had been substituted with estrogen (O+E) the expresion level was not significantly different. One of three similar studies is shown.

The role of estrogen in the regulation of apoptosis is currently under investigation. In classical estrogenic target tissues such as human mammary gland tumour cell lines (MCF 7), estrogen increases the intracellular p26bcl-2 to p21 bax ratio and therefore modulates the apoptotic pathway in these cells (33). Estrogen withdrawal does not only lead to apoptosis of osteocytes as studied by DNA nick translation (34). In addition, estrogen withdrawal causes a reduced expression of endothelial and neuronal isoforms of the nitric oxide synthase and increased apoptosis in the rat vagina (35). In cardiovascular tissues such as endothelial cells, treatment with E2 inhibits tumor factor-alpha induced apoptosis as studied by the expression pattern of interleukin-1β converting enzyme (ICE). The protective effect of E2 in this cell model was abrogated by the use of an estrogen receptor antagonist (36). These antiapoptotic properties of E2 may be mediated by increased endothelial cell interaction with the substratum and increased tyrosine phosphorylation of pp125 focal adhesion kinase (37). These observations demonstrate that estrogen has a modulatory effect on the onset of apoptosis in the respective target tissue. However, little is known about the effect of estrogen on apoptosis in the myocardium. There is a growing body of evidence, that apoptosis plays a major role in regulation of processes of the myocardium such as heart development, cardiac remodeling following myocardial ischemia or cardiac hypertrophy (28). We here show that the observed gender based differences may be partially due to the effect of estrogen on the apoptotic pathway in the myocardium. Estrogen withdrawal leads to the activation of critical propapoptotic proteins involved in the regulatory cascade leading to programmed cell death in our animal model. This effect can be prevented by estrogen supplementation in postmenopausal subjects.

Estrogen replacement therapy in primary and secondary prevention of cardiovascular disease is well established, however the route of administration as well as the composition of the respective drug regimen (estrogen alone or in combination with progesterone) remains controversial. In addition, estrogen replacement therapy has been attributed with an increased risk of thromboembolic complications. The design of selective estrogen receptor modulators (SERMS) during the last decade may be helpful in the light of the debate if the classical estrogen replacement therapy may also have detrimental effects (12,13). SERMS may potentially exert cardioprotective effects but avoid the complications such as thromboembolism. In summary, we have shown that estrogen modulates apoptotic pathways in the myocardium. Estrogen replacement after ovariectomy leads to an inhibition of propapoptotic proteins such as bax or caspase 3. The regulatory pathways leading to apoptosis in the myocardium, however, consist of a large array of complex regulatory processes. In this context it is interesting to observe that also nitric oxide has an impact on apoptosis in the myocardium (39). Previously we have shown that estrogen regulates the expression of the endothelial and inducible nitric oxide synthase (40) in the myocardium. Therefore it is tempting to speculate how the interaction between NO release and estrogen modulates the apoptotic pathway in cardiac myocytes (Figure 5). Further studies, however, are required to characterize the impact of apoptosis on heart failure and how estrogen may influence this process.

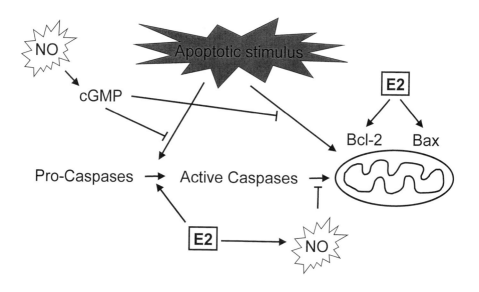

modified after [39]

Figure 5 Apoptosis and the interaction of NO and estrogen.
The pathways leading to apoptosis involve mitochondrial proteins such as Bcl-2 and Bax. These proteins interact with a family of proenzymes designated as pro-caspases. Apoptotic stimuli activate these proenzymes which in turn modulate the activity of downstream apoptotic effector proteins. NO as well as estrogen (E2) may interact with these processes. Estrogen modulates the expression of NO synthases as well as caspase 3 and bax. These regulatory pathways may play an important role in the onset of apoptosis in the myocardium.

ACKNOWLEDGEMENTS

This work was supported by a grant from the Deutsche Forschungsgemeinschaft (ME 1502/1-1, GR 729/8-1). The authors would like to thank Kerstin Löbbert, Simone Nüdling, Stefan Kahlert, and Martin van Eickels for their expertise and contribution to this work.

References

1. Dahlberg ST. Gender difference in the risk factors for sudden cardiac death. Cardiology 1990; 77: suppl 2: 31–40.
2. Marcus R, Krause L, Weder AB, Dominguez-Mejia AN, Schork D, Julius S. Sex-specific determinants of increased left ventricular mass in the Tecumseh blood pressure study. Circulation 1994; 90: 928–936.
3. Gardin, JM, Wagenknecht LE, Anton-Culver H, Flack J, Gidding S, Jurosaki T, Wong ND, Manolio TA. Relationship of cardiovascular risk factors to echocardiographic left ventricular mass in healthy young black and white adult men and women. Circulation 1995; 92: 380–387.
4. Olivetti G, Giordano G, Corradi D, Melissari M, Lagrasta C, Gambert SR, Anversa P. Gender differences and aging: effects on the human heart: J Am Coll Cardiol 1995; 26: 1068-1079.
5. Kannel WB, Hjortland MC, McNamara PM, Gordon T. Menopause and the risk of cardiovascular disease: The Framingham Study. Ann Intern Med 1976; 85: 447-452.
6. Node K, Kitakaze M, Kosaka H, Minamino T, Sato H, Kuzuya T, Hori M. Roles of NO and Ca^{2+}-activated K^+ channels in coronary vasodilation induced by 17β-estradiol in ischemic heart failure. FASEB J 1997; 11: 793-799.
7. Caulin-Glaser T, Garcia-Gardena G, Sarrel P, Sessa WC, Bender JR. 17β-estradiol regulation of human endothelial cell basal nitric oxide release, independent of cytosolic calcium Ca^{2+} mobilization. Circ Res 1997; 81: 885-892.
8. Rubanyi GM, Freay AD, Kauser K, Sukovich D, Burton G, Lubahn DB, Couse JF, Curtis SW, Korach KS. Vascular estrogen receptors and endothelium-derived nitric oxide production in the mouse aorta. Gender differences and effect of estrogen receptor gene disruption. J Clin Invest 1997; 99: 2429-2437.
9. MacRitchie AM, Jun SS, Chen Z, German Z, Yuhanna IS, Sherman TS, Shaul PW. Estrogen upregulates endothelial nitric oxide synthase gene expression in fetal pulmonary artery endothelium. Circ Res 1997; 81: 355-362.
10. Grohé C, Kahlert S, Löbbert K, Karas RH, Stimpel M, Vetter H, Neyses L. Cardiac myocytes and cardiac fibroblasts contain functional estrogen receptors. FEBS-Letters 1997; 416: 107–112.
11. Grohé C, Kahlert S, Löbbert K, van Eickels M, Stimpel M, Vetter H, Neyses L. Effects of moexiprilat on estrogen-stimulated cardiac fibroblast growth. Br J Pharm 1997; 121: 1350–1354.
12. Blum A, Cannon RO. Effects of oestrogens and selective oestrogen receptor modulators on serum lipoproteins and vascular function. Curr Opin Lipidol 1998; 9: 575–586.
13. Gustaffson JA. Therapeutic potential of selective estrogen receptor modulators. Curr Opin Chem Biol 1998; 2: 508-511.
14. Walter P, Green S, Green G, Krust A, Bornert JM, Jeltsch JM, Staub A, Jensen E, Scrace G, Waterfield M, Chambon P. Cloning of the human estrogen receptor cDNA. Proc Natl Acad Sci USA 1985; 82: 7889-7893.
15. Kuiper GGJM, Enmark E, Pelto-Huikko M, Nilsson S,Gustafsson JA. Cloning of a novel estrogen receptor expressed in rat prostrate and ovary. Proc Natl Acad Sci 1996; 93: 5925–5930.
16. Paech K, Webb P, Kuiper GGJM, Nilsson S, Gustaffson JA, Kushner PJ, Scanlan TS. Differential ligand activation of estrogen receptors ERα and ERβ at AP 1 sites. Science 1997; 277: 1508–1510.
17. Kuiper GGJM., Carlsson B, Grandien K, Enmark E, Häggblad J, Nilsson S, Gustafsson JA. Comparison of the ligand binding specifity and transcript tissue distribution of estrogen receptors α and β. Endocrinology 1997; 188: 863-870.
18. Cowley SM, Hoare S, Mosselman S, Parker MG. Estrogen receptors α and β form heterodimers on DNA. J Biol Chem 1997; 32: 19858-19862.

19. Grohé, C, Kahlert S, Löbbert K, Vetter H. Expression of oestrogen receptor a and b: role of local oestrogen synthesis. J Endocrinol 1998; 156: R1-R7.
20. Karas RH, Patterson BL, Mendelsohn ME. Human vascular smooth muscle cells contain functional estrogen receptors. Circulation 1994; 89: 1943-1950.
21. Meyer R, Linz KW, Surges R, Meinardus S, Vees J, Hoffmann A, Windholz O, Grohé C. Rapid modulation of L-type calcium current by acutely applied oestrogens in isolated cardiac myocytes from human, guinea pig, and rat. Experimental Physiology 1998; 83: 305-321.
22. Grohé C, Kahlert S, Nüdling S, Vetter H, Meyer R. Oestrogen activates the MAPK and JNK signal transduction pathway in rat cardiac myocytes. J Physiol (abstract) 1997; 11: 821.
23. Migliaccio A, Di Domenico M, Castoria G, deFalco A, Bontempo P, Nola, E, Auricchio F. Tyrosine kinase/p21ras/MAP-kinase pathway activation by estradiol-receptor complex in MCF-7 cells. EMBO J 1996; 15: 1292-1300.
24. Jiang C, Poole-Wilson PA, Sarrel PM., Mochizuki S, Collins P, Mcleod KT. Effect of 17β-oestradiol on concentration, Ca^{2+} current and intracellular free Ca^{2+} in guinea-pig isolated cardiac myocytes. Brit J Pharm 1992; 106: 739-745.
25. Morley P, Whitfield JF, Vanderhyden BC, Tsang BK, Schwartz JL. A new, nongenomic estrogen action: the rapid release of intracellular calcium. Endocrinology 1992; 131: 1305–1312
26. Fortuno MA, Ravassa S, Etayo JC, Diez J: Overexpression of bax protein and enhanced apoptosis in the left ventricle of spontaneously hypertensive rats: effects of AT1 blockade with losartan. Hypertension 1998; 32: 280-286.
27. Diez J, Fortuno MA, Ravassa S: Apoptosis in hypertensive heart diease. Curr Opin Cardiol 1998; 13: 317-325.
28. Brömme HJ, Holtz J: Apoptosis in the heart: when and why? Mol Cell Biochem 1996; 163/164: 261-275.
29. Bachmann J, Wagner J, Haufe C, Wystrychowski A, Ciechanowicz A, Ganten D: Modulation of blood pressure and the renin-angiotensin system in transgenic and spontaeously hypertensive rats after ovariectomy. J Hypertens 1993; 11, (suppl 5): 226-227.
30. Ing DJ, Zang J. Dzau VJ, Webster KA, Bishopric NH: Modulation of cytokine-induced cardiac myocyte apoptosis by nitric oxide, bak, and bcl x. Circ Res 1999; 84: 21-33.
31. Hetts SW: To die or not to die. JAMA 1998; 279: 300-307.
32. Kothaka S, Azuma T, Reinhard C, Klippel A, Tang J, Chu K, McGarry TJ, Kirschner MW, Koths K, Kwiatkowski DJ, Williams LT: Caspase-3-generated fragment of gelsolin: effector of morphological change in apoptosis. Science 1997; 278: 294-298.
33. Huang Y, Ray S, Reed JC, Ibrado AM, Tang C, Nawabi A, Bhalla K: Estrogen increases intracellular p26bcl-2 to p21bax ratios and inhibits taxol-induced apoptosis of human breast cancer MCF-7 cells. Breast Cancer Res Treat 1997; 42: 73-81.
34. Tomkinson A, Reeve J, Shaw RW, Noble BS: The death of osteocytes via apoptosis accompanies estrogen withdrawal in human bone. J Clin Endocrinol Metab 1997; 82: 3128-3135.
35. Berman JR, McCarthy MM, Kyprianou N: Effect of estrogen withdrawal on nitric oxide synthase expression and apoptosis in the rat vagina. Urology 1998; 51: 650-656.
36. Spyridopulos I, Sullivan AB, Kearney M, Isner JM, Losordo DW: Estrogen-receptor-mediated inhibition of human endothelial cell apoptosis. Estradiol as a survival factor. Circulation 1997; 95: 1505-1514.
37. Alvarez Rj, Gips SJ, Moldovan N, Wilhide CC, Milliken EE, Hruban RH, Silverman HS, Dang CV, Goldschmidt-Clermont PJ: 17-beta estradiol inhibits apoptosis of endothelial cells. Biochem Biophys Res Commun 1997; 237: 372-381.
38. Simoncini T, De Caterina R, Genazzani AR: Selective estrogen receptor modulators: different actions on vascular cell adhesion molecule-1 (VCAM-1) expression in human endothelial cells. J Clin Endocrinol Metab 1999; 84: 815-818.
39. Kim YM, Bombeck CA, Billiar TR: Nitric oxide as a bifunctional regulator of apoptosis. Circ Res. 1999;84:253-256.
40. Nuedling S, Kahlert S, Loebbert K, Doevendans P, Meyer R, Vetter H, Grohé C: 17β-Estradiol stimulates expression of endothelial and inducible NO synthase in rat myocardium in-vitro and in-vivo. Cardiovasc Res 1999, in press.

IV.5
Open questions on apoptosis in cardiac biology

Heribert Schunkert, M.D.
Universität Regensburg, Regensburg, Germany

INTRODUCTION

As summarized in this volume, most if not all cardiac cell types entertain the complex machinery of programmed cell death. Specifically, histochemical and molecular studies document beyond any doubt that cardiac myocytes, endothelial as well as vascular smooth muscle cells may undergo apoptosis. Moreover, death receptors, pro- and antiapoptotic factors as well as enzymatic cascades that -if activated- result in digestion of critical cellular structures have been localized to these cells. The stimuli that force cardiac cells into programmed death are also well characterized and include ischemia and/or reoxygenation, pressure overload or extensive stretching, or, finally, excessive stimulation with neurohormones or free radicals, just to name a few. While we are just at the beginning to understand these phenomena, a series of new questions emerges that asks for the appropriate integration of apoptosis in the pathophysiology of cardiac disease.

CHECKPOINTS OF APOPTOSIS

From a teleological point of view, apoptosis of a postmitotic and largely irreplacable cardiac myocyte should to be restricted to an extreme derangement of the cell. Especially, a well coordinated dissembling of a myocyte appears to be the preferable alternative only when irreversible loss of function, necrosis, or malignant transformation confer an even larger threat for the multicellular organism. Thus, under physiological circumstances apoptosis of cardiac myocytes needs to be prevented and, if falsely initiated, reversed. In this respect, further research is required to define the stringent checkpoints that have to be passed before programmed cell death is being executed in cardiac cells.

Indeed, these hurdles need to be high enough so that physiological concentrations of pro-apoptotic factors such as tumor necrosis factor alpha or fas-ligand are being ignored by cardiac cells. It may be interesting in this respect that fas-ligand concentrations display a gender-related difference with significantly higher circulating levels found in men (1). In parallel, middle-aged men are known to have an accelerated myocyte loss (2) and a prevalence of heart failure that is three times higher than that in women (3). Thus, one may raise the question as to whether leaks at the checkpoints of apoptosis may occur and achieve -over time- functional relevance.

POINT-OF-NO-RETURN

Another pertinent question asks for the point-of-no-return. Specifically, given that some activation of death receptors or some damage of mitochondrial membranes with cytochrome c leakage may affect cardiac cells constantly, the cascades of apoptosis may be activated locally within an otherwise healthy cell. Can such small bursts of pro-apoptotic signaling be extinguished? Probably, yes. However, it appears to be important to clearly define the extent and the quality of damage that can be reversed before a cell is definitively dead as well as the healing mechanisms that are involved. Moreover, we need to learn what sort of damage can be repaired without subsequent functional deficits!

KEY PLAYERS

Another difficulty is to define the key players in apoptosis, its abrogation, and cellular repair. In particular, there is ample redundancy of both pro- and anti-apoptotic pathways in each cell. Even within a given pathway, it appears that critical signaling steps can be handled by alternative members of large protein families. For example, Bcl-2, Bcl-X short and long form, Bax, Bad, Bak, Mcl-1 etc. are all members of the Bcl-2 family. Moreover, in a model of myocardial infarction the disruption of the p53 gene (4) or the overexpression of the insulin-like growth factor-1 (IGF-1) gene (5) had no affect on the extend of myocyte death in the ischemic region. By contrast, IGF-1 overexpression inhibited apoptosis and necrosis in the overloaded but nonischemic myocardium (5). Thus, quantitative alterations of individual players may be sufficient to ameliorate apoptotic cell death depending on the degree of pro-apoptotic stimulation.

DIFFERENT SUSCEPTIBILITIES

With the exception of myocardium that is ischemic during acute infarction, apoptosis affects only a minority of cells. Thus, in general, the critical checkpoints of apoptosis as well as the healing mechanisms that are activated after incomplete apoptotic signaling appear to be fairly strong in cardiac myocytes. However, other cell types such as cardiac fibroblasts are even more resistant against pro-apoptotic stimuli. Specifically, under co-culture condition, prolonged ischemia and subsequent reperfusion leave cardiac fibroblasts virtually untouched while the vast majority of cardiac myocytes undergoes apoptosis (6). *In vivo*, e.g. during myocardial infarction, this quality of fibroblasts may be of enormous benefit as they can fill in for necrotic or apoptotic myocytes to form a scar that resists the continuous wall stress of the beating heart. On the other hand, this phenomenon raises the obvious question on how cardiac fibroblasts can escape apoptosis.

Not only fibroblasts can resist to apoptosis. Also, non-beating cardiac myocytes appear to be largely insensitive to pro-apoptotic conditions (7). At least under cell culture conditions, proper beating of the cells appears to be important to study pro-apoptotic signaling in cardiac myocytes (7). The *in vivo* analogy of this phenomenon may be hibernation which, therefore, may be a well suited mechanism for cardiac myocytes to escape apoptotic cell death. However, this speculation needs to be proven and the mechanisms that protect non-beating myocytes from apoptosis need to be defined.

NECROSIS VERSUS APOPTOSIS

Depending on the pathophysiological context, apoptosis may occur as a separate entity affecting only a small minority of cells (e.g. chronic heart failure). However, apoptosis may also occur in parallel with necrosis (e.g. border zone of a myocardial infarction), or as a predecessor of necrosis (e.g. ischemic zone of a myocardial infarction, reperfusion injury). Obviously, the mechanisms threatening a cell are quite different under these circumstances and, consequently, the intracellular mechanisms causing apoptosis may be different as well.

The close physical or temporal neighborhood of apoptosis and necrosis may also ask for a clear distinction of the two modes of cell death. Particularly, how can apoptotic myocytes that are rich in large structural proteins be removed from a tissue that in itself is highly organized and specialized? Can this procedure be achieved entirely without spillage of intracellular contents and subsequent inflammation? Which cells clear the remainder of an apoptotic myocyte and how long does it take? Obviously, timing becomes a critical issue. Most importantly, during acute myocardial infarction 85% of the ischemic cells display features of apoptosis initially while at later time points most of these cells will undergo necrosis (8). Under these circumstances it is unclear whether apoptosis helps the heart to maintain its structural integrity or whether wide spread apoptosis only increases the extent of cell loss. Moreover, prevention of apoptosis may not be beneficial necessarily when it only affects the point in time at which necrosis takes place. Thus, it appears important to define the acute and chronic functional implications of apoptosis and necrosis especially when both take place simultaneously.

MARKER FOR FAILING ORGAN PRESERVATION

The rapid and distinctive detectability of morphological and biochemical criteria of apoptosis may be highly suitable for the assessment of therapeutical strategies that aim for tissue preservation and protection. For example, donor hearts that undergo prolonged transportation before transplantation or hearts that are arrested for bypass or valve surgery may undergo an apoptotic loss of cardiac myoctes. Positive TUNEL labeling, electron microscopical evidence of mitochrondrial damage and nuclear condensation, or translocation of cytochrome c all become detectable within minutes during such procedures (9,10). Thereby, these markers of apoptosis may signal tissue damage long before traditional markers of necrosis, e.g. creatine kinase or troponin T release, become evident. Moreover, the signs of apoptosis may be more specific for tissue trauma. Thus, signs of apoptosis may be instrumental for the assessment of cardioplegic strategies, that are currently rather non-standardized, in part, due to a lack of good endpoints for comparison.

FUNCTIONAL CONSEQUENCES

Finally, the functional implications of apoptosis need to be defined for each pathophysiological context in which programmed cell death occurs. The first step in this respect requires a consistent estimate on the quantitative contribution of apoptosis to cell loss in each model. With respect to chronic heart failure the percentage of apoptotic cells has been reported to range from 0.02% to 35% (8,11,12). No matter what the precise number will be, myocyte cell loss appears to occur in various forms of cardiac myopathies, particularly, at the transition to heart failure. Even moderate losses of cardiac myocytes, scattered throughout the myocardium, may affect cardiac performance profoundly. In fact, diffuse myocyte loss may have greater impact, on the basis of the number of affected cells, than regional myocyte loss during myocardial infarction (13). Moreover, the structural organization of the heart may be severely altered if side-to-side slippage of myocytes occurs throughout the myocardium on the basis of diffuse myocyte apoptosis (14). Ultimately, ventricular dilatation, the hall mark of end stage heart failure, may be the consequence.

The final task, after the phenomenon of apoptosis is well integrated in the pathophysiology of heart failure, will be to clarify whether its abrogation will be of therapeutical value. Initial studies are very much in favor of this notion. Particularly, inhibition of the renin angiotensin system has been shown to diminish apoptosis and, in parallel, improve cardiac function of spontaneously hypertensive rats (15). Likewise, caspase inhibition in an ischemia/reperfusion model has improved cardiac function in the rat (16). However, the direct link between prevention of apoptosis and long-term cardiac outcome needs further intensive investigation before this tool will enter the clinical arena. This applies specially to acute myocardial infarction in which apoptosis and necrosis are closely linked to each other. Nevertheless, it is easily foreseeable that the improved recognition of apoptosis in cardiac biology will ultimately have enormous impact on the treatment of patients with heart failure and myocardial infarction.

References

1. Sigel AV, Hense HW, Laberer S, Riegger GAJ, Schunkert H. Estrogen prevents Fas-ligand production. Evidence for a apoptosis-protective effect from a population based study. *J Am Coll Cardiol* 1999;33 (Suppl A);206A.
2. Olivetti G, Giordano G, Corradi D, Melissari M, Lagrasta C, Gambert SR, Anversa P. Gender differences and aging: effects on the human heart. *J Am Coll Cardiol* 1995;26:1068-79.
3. Schunkert H, Broeckel U, Hense HW, Keil U, Riegger GAJ. Left ventricular systolic dysfunction in the population. *Lancet* 1998;351:372.
4. Bialik S, Geenen DL, Sasson IE, Cheng R, Horner JW, Evans SM, Lord EM, Koch CJ, Kitsis RN Myocyte apoptosis during acute myocardial infarction in the mouse localizes to hypoxic but occurs independently of p53. *J Clin Invest* 1997;100:1363-72.
5. Li Q, Li B, Wang X, Leri A, Jana KP, Liu Y, Kajstura J, Baserga R, Anversa P. Overexpression of insulin-like growth factor-1 in mice protects from myocyte death after infarction, attenuating ventricular dilation, wall stress, and cardiac hypertrophy. *J Clin Invest* 1997;100:1991-9.
6. Lakatta EG, Long X, Crow M. Differential suceptibility of cardiac myocyteand fibroblasts to hypoxia and p53 mediated apoptosis. In: Schunkert H, Riegger G (Eds). Apoptosis in cardiac biology. Kluwer Academic Publishers, Boston 1999 (in press).
7. Sigel AV. Apoptosis in myocardial infarction. In: Schunkert H, Riegger G (Eds). Apoptosis in cardiac biology. Kluwer Academic Publishers, Boston 1999 (in press).
8. Kajstura J, Cheng W, Reiss K, Clark WA, Sonnenblick EH, Krajewski S, Reed JC, Olivetti G, Anversa P. Apoptotic and necrotic myocyte cell deaths are independent contributing variables of infarct size in rats. *Lab Invest* 1996 Jan;74(1):86-107.
9. Aebert H, Cornelius T, Ehr T, Sigel AV, Birnbaum DE, Schunkert H. Induction of early immediate genes and programmed cell death following cardioplegic arrest in human hearts. *Eur J Cardiothorac Surg* 1997;12:261-267.
10. Aebert H, Schunkert H. Apoptosis during cardiac surgery. In: Schunkert H, Riegger G (Eds). Apoptosis in cardiac biology. Kluwer Academic Publishers, Boston 1999 (in press).
11. Narula J, Haider N, Virmani R, DiSalvo TG, Kolodgie FD, Hajjar RJ, Schmidt U, Semigran MJ, Dec GW, Khaw BA. Apoptosis in myocytes in end-stage heart failure. *N Engl J Med* 1996;335:1182-9.
12. Saraste A, Voipio-Pulkki LM, Parvinen M, Pulkki K. Apoptosis in the heart. *N Engl J Med* 1997;336:1025-6.
13. Anversa P, Zhang X, Li P, Capasso JM. Chronic coronary artery constriction leads to moderate myocyte loss and left ventricular dysfunction and failure in rats. *J Clin Invest* 1992;89:618-29.
14. Anversa P, Leri A, Beltrami CA, Guerra S, Kajstura J. Myocyte death and growth in the failing heart. *Lab Invest* 1998;78:767-86.
15. Diez J, Panizo A, Hernandez M, Vega F, Sola I, Fortuno MA, Pardo J Cardiomyocyte apoptosis and cardiac angiotensin-converting enzyme in spontaneously hypertensive rats. *Hypertension* 1997;30:1029-34.
16. Yaoita H, Ogawa K, Maehara K, Maruyama Y. Attenuation of ischemia/reperfusion injury in rats by a caspase inhibitor. *Circulation* 1998;97:276-81.

Index

D

E